MEDICAL

APARTHEID

**The Dark History of Medical
Experimentation on Black Americans
from Colonial Times to the Present**

HARRIET A. WASHINGTON

ANCHOR BOOKS

A Division of Random House, Inc.

New York

FIRST ANCHOR BOOKS (BROADWAY BOOKS) EDITION, 2008

LIBRARY OF CONGRESS CATALOGING-IN-PUBLICATION DATA
Washington, Harriet A.
Medical apartheid : the dark history of medical experimentation on black
Americans from colonial times to the present /
by Harriet A. Washington.
p. cm.
1. Human experimentation in medicine—United States—
History. 2. African Americans—Medical care—History. I. Title.

R853.H8W37 2006
174.2'8—dc22
2005051873

Anchor ISBN: 978-0-7679-1547-2

www.anchorbooks.com

PRINTED IN THE UNITED STATES OF AMERICA
10 9

For Ron DeBose, my husband,

with undying love and gratitude

When I began working at the institute, I recalled my adolescent dream of becoming a medical research worker. Daily I saw young . . . [white] boys and girls receiving instruction in chemistry and medicine that the average black boy or girl could never receive. When I was alone, I wandered and poked my fingers into strange chemicals, watched intricate machines trace red and black lines upon ruled paper. At times I paused and stared at the walls of the rooms, at the floors, at the wide desks at which the white doctors sat; and I realized—with a feeling that I could never quite get used to—that I was looking at the world of another race.

—RICHARD WRIGHT, 1944

The wrongs which we seek to condemn and punish have been so calculated, so malignant and so devastating that civilization cannot tolerate their being ignored because it cannot survive their being repeated.

—CHIEF U.S. PROSECUTOR ROBERT JACKSON, OPENING STATEMENT, NUREMBERG DOCTORS' TRIAL, DECEMBER 9, 1946

CONTENTS

PART 3   Race, Technology, and Medicine

INTRODUCTION

The American Janus of Medicine and Race

Science without conscience is the soul's perdition.
—FRANÇOIS RABELAIS, PANTAGRUEL

On a sylvan stretch of New York's patrician upper Fifth Avenue, just across from the New York Academy of Medicine, a colossus in marble, august inscriptions, and a bas-relief caduceus grace a memorial bordering Central Park. These laurels venerate the surgeon James Marion Sims, M.D., as a selfless benefactor of women. Nor is this the only statuary erected in honor of Dr. Sims. Marble monuments to his skill, benevolence, and humanity guard his native South Carolina's statehouse, its medical school, the Alabama capitol grounds, and a French hospital. In the mid-nineteenth century, Dr. Sims dedicated his career to the care and cure of women's disorders and opened the nation's first hospital for women in New York City. He attended French royalty, his Grecian visage inspired oil portraits, and in 1875, he was elected president of the American Medical Association. Hospitals still bear his name, including a West African hospital that utilizes the eponymous gynecological instruments that he first invented for surgeries upon black female slaves in the 1840s.

But this benevolent image vies with the detached Marion Sims portrayed in Robert Thom's *J. Marion Sims: Gynecologic Surgeon,* an oil representation of an experimental surgery upon his powerless slave Betsey. Sims stands aloof, arms folded, one hand holding a metroscope (the forerunner of the speculum) as he regards the kneeling woman in a coolly evaluative medical gaze. His tie and morning coat contrast with her simple servants' dress, head rag, and bare feet.

The painting, commissioned and distributed by the Parke-Davis pharmaceutical house more than a century after the surgeries as one of its A History of Medicine in Pictures series, takes telling liberties with the historical facts. Thom portrays Betsey as a fully clothed, calm slave woman who kneels complacently on a small table, hand modestly raised to her breast, before a trio of white male physicians. Two other slave women peer around a sheet, apparently hung for modesty's sake, in a childlike display of curiosity. This innocuous tableau could hardly differ more from the gruesome reality in which each surgical scene was a violent struggle between the slaves and physicians and each woman's body was a bloodied battleground. Each naked, unanesthetized slave woman had to be forcibly restrained by the other physicians through her shrieks of agony as Sims determinedly sliced, then sutured her genitalia. The other doctors, who could, fled when they could bear the horrific scenes no longer. It then fell to the women to restrain one another.

I wanted to reproduce Thom's painting on the cover of this book, or at least in the text, but when I asked permission of its copyright holder, Pfizer Inc., the company insisted on reviewing the entire manuscript of this book before making a decision. As an independent scholar I could not acquiesce to this, and I used another cover image. When I renewed my request to use the image within the text, Pfizer agreed to base its decision upon reading this chapter and an outline of the book.

The Pfizer executives apparently were uncomfortable with what they read, because they refused to grant permission to reproduce this telling image or even respond to my query after I supplied the requested chapter and outline. This act of censorship exemplifies the barriers some choose to erect in order to veil the history of unconscionable medical research with blacks.

Betsey's voice has been silenced by history, but as one reads Sims's biographers and his own memoirs, a haughty, self-absorbed researcher emerges, a man who bought black women slaves and addicted them to morphine in order to perform dozens of exquisitely painful, distressingly intimate vaginal surgeries. Not until he had experimented with his surgeries on Betsey and her fellow slaves for years did Sims essay to cure white women.

Was Sims a savior or a sadist? It depends, I suppose, on the color of the women you ask. Marion Sims epitomizes the two faces—one benign, one malevolent—of American medical research.

"Of all the forms of inequality, injustice in health is the most shocking and the most inhumane." In 1965, Martin Luther King, Jr., spoke these words in Montgomery, Alabama, at the end of the Selma to Montgomery march that had been attended by the black and white physicians of the Medical Committee for Human Rights. King had invited the doctors not only to give medical succor to injured marchers but also to witness the abuse suffered at the hands of segregationists. With these almost unnoticed words, King ushered in a new era in civil rights, because as Delegate to Congress Donna Christian-Christensen, M.D., chair of the Congressional Black Caucus Health Braintrust, has declared, "Health disparities are the civil rights issue of the 21st century." Thus Dr. King's alarm over racial health injustice was prescient, and were he alive today, his concern would be redoubled. Mounting evidence of the racial health divide confronts us everywhere we look, from doubled black infant death rates to African American life expectancies that fall years behind whites'. Infant mortality of African Americans is twice that of whites, and black babies born in more racially segregated cities have higher rates of mortality. The life expectancy of African Americans is as much as six years less than that of whites.

Old measures of health not only have failed to improve significantly but have stayed the same: some have even worsened. Mainstream newspapers and magazines often report disease in an ethnocentric manner that shrouds its true cost among African Americans. For example, despite the heavy emphasis on genetic ailments among blacks, fewer than 0.5 percent of black deaths—that's less than one death in two hundred—can be attributed to hereditary disorders such as sickle-cell anemia. A closer look at the troubling numbers reveals that blacks are dying not of exotic, incurable, poorly understood illnesses nor of genetic diseases that target only them, but rather from common ailments that are more often prevented and treated among whites than among blacks.

Three times as many African Americans were diagnosed with diabetes in 1993 as in 1963. This rate is nearly twice that of white Americans and is sorely underestimated: The real black diabetes rate is probably double that of whites. As with most chronic diseases, African Americans suffer more complications, including limb loss, blindness, kidney disease, and terminal heart disease. Cancer, the nation's second greatest killer, is diagnosed later in blacks and carries off proportionately more African Americans than whites. African Americans suffer the nation's highest rate of cancer and cancer deaths.

The distortion of African American death rates is illustrated by the common dismissal of black women's breast-cancer risks as "lower than white women's." This characterization implies that black women are at low risk from breast cancer, but their risk is only *slightly* lower, because the estimated lifetime risk of developing breast cancer is ten per one hundred for white women born in 1980, and seven per one hundred for black women born that year. Moreover, this lower risk of developing breast cancer is overshadowed by blacks' much higher risk of dying from it: Eighty-six percent of white women with breast cancer are alive five years later; only 71 percent of black women survive that long. A black woman is 2.2 times as likely as a white woman to die of breast cancer. Black women have been undergoing mammograms at the same rate as white women but are more likely to receive poorer-quality screening, which may not detect a cancer in time for a cure. A black woman is also more likely to develop her cancer before age forty, too early for recommended mammograms to catch it, and black women are diagnosed at a more advanced stage than either Hispanic or white breast-cancer patients. Black breast-cancer patients have a worse overall prognosis, and a worse prognosis at each stage. Black men have the nation's highest rates of developing and of dying from prostate and lung cancers.

Despite its image as a disease that affects middle-aged white men, heart disease claims 50 percent more African Americans than whites and African Americans die from heart attacks at a higher rate than whites. African Americans are more likely to develop serious liver ailments such as hepatitis C, the chief cause of liver transplants. They are also more likely to die from liver disease, not because of any inherent racial susceptibility, but because blacks are less likely to receive aggressive treatment with drugs such as interferon or lifesaving liver transplants.

Even the legion of newest illnesses—emerging disease such as HIV/AIDS and hepatitis C—kills blacks at much higher rates than whites. AIDS, the scourge of our time, has become a disease of people of color here and abroad: Forty-nine percent of HIV-infected Americans are African Americans and 86 percent of children with AIDS are African American or Hispanic. Blacks are ten times as likely to develop AIDS as whites.

Mental ailments are destroying blacks, as well: Black women suffer the highest rates of stress and major depression in the nation and suicide rates soared *200 percent* among young black men within just twenty years.

These are dire statistics, born of complex interactions among unhealthy environments, social pressures and limitations, lifestyle factors, and limited access to health care, including very limited access to cutting-edge *therapeutic* medical research that is meant to help treat or cure a patient with a disorder. But this dearth of therapeutic research is accompanied by a plethora of nontherapeutic research with African Americans, which is meant to investigate medical issues for the benefit of future patients or of medical knowledge.

And this brings us to the subject of this book, which documents a peculiar type of injustice in health: the troubled history of medical experimentation with African Americans—and the resulting behavioral fallout that causes researchers and African Americans to view each other through jaundiced eyes. In his 1909 preface to *The Doctor's Dilemma,* George Bernard Shaw scathingly observed, "The tragedy of illness at present is that it delivers you helplessly into the hands of a profession which you deeply mistrust." He could have been speaking for contemporary African Americans, because studies and surveys repeatedly confirm that no other group as deeply mistrusts the American medical system, especially medical research.

The problem is growing. As the *Wall Street Journal* observed several years back, "It hasn't been a good time for scientists who experiment on people—or the people they experiment on." This is a masterpiece of understatement, especially if you consider the recent history of medical research with African Americans.

The Office for Protection from Research Risks (OPRR) has been busily investigating abuses at more than sixty research centers, including experimentation-related deaths at premier universities, from Columbia to California. Another important subset of human subject abuse has been scientific fraud, wherein scientists from the University of South Carolina to MIT have also been found to have lied through falsified data or fictitious research agendas, often in the service of research that abused black Americans. Within recent years, the OPRR has also suspended research at such revered universities as Alabama, Pennsylvania, Duke, Yale, and even Johns Hopkins.

Many studies enrolled only or principally African Americans, although some included a smattering of Hispanics. Some research studies specifically excluded white subjects according to the terms of their official protocols, the federally required plans that detail how research studies are conducted. However, in other human medical experiments, the recruitment of blacks and the poor is a tacit feature of the study because they recruit subjects from heavily black inner-city areas that tend to surround American teaching hospitals. American university research centers have historically been located in inner-city areas, and accordingly, a disproportionate number of these abuses have involved experiments with African Americans.

These subjects were given experimental vaccines known to have unacceptably high lethality, were enrolled in experiments without their consent or knowledge, were subjected to surreptitious surgical and medical procedures while unconscious, injected with toxic substances, deliberately monitored rather than treated for deadly ailments, excluded from lifesaving treatments, or secretly farmed for sera or tissues that were used to perfect technologies such as infectious-disease tests. A few African American medical institutions have suffered their own run-ins with federal oversight agencies concerned about how they treated their own research subjects.

But the considerable concern raised by governmental oversight agencies has been dwarfed by the periodic hue and cry raised in the popular press. The news media seize upon and decry new experimental abuses with regularity. Moreover, it is newspapers, not research oversight organizations, that have been instrumental in unveiling and ending egregious abuses, from the Tuskegee Syphilis Study in the 1970s to the 1996 jailing of poor black mothers who were unwitting research subjects in South Carolina, to the 1998 infusion of poor black New York City boys with the cardiotoxic drug fenfluramine.

However, newspapers and magazines have given such abuses episodic rather than analytic treatment, expending their outrage, then falling silent until the next wave of research deaths, missing consent forms, or unwitting subjects steals headlines. Subjects are often identified not as black but, using coded references, as "the urban poor," "socioeconomically disadvantaged," or "inner-city residents." This episodic approach treats the exploitation of black experimental subjects as isolated events, so that even while the repeated reports buttress widespread distrust of medical research, these stories fail to discern the stubborn and illuminating *patterns* characterizing the medical abuse of African Americans.

In fact, the news media often fail to perceive unethical experimentation, even as they write about it. Scientists promulgate novel drugs and technologies, such as Norplant use among adolescents and psychosurgery for rioters, as new therapies that are necessarily extreme remedies. But despite the "treatments" ' untried nature and the vulnerability of their subjects, the news media often swallow such euphemistic labels as "breakthrough" and "new therapy" whole.

Research is an utterly essential and desirable component of treatment, but its subjects must be aware that they are participating, must be informed, must consent, and must be allowed to weigh the possible risks and benefits. As this book will show, these conditions are only haphazardly met, or not at all, when the subjects are African Americans.

A Historical Vacuum

The experimental exploitation of African Americans is not an issue of the last decade or even the past few decades. Dangerous, involuntary, and nontherapeutic experimentation upon African Americans has been practiced widely and documented extensively at least since the eighteenth century.

Attempts to understand the distrust this history generates are confused and distorted because few know its facts beyond a few oft-cited experimental outrages, notably the Tuskegee Syphilis Study. History of medicine courses, medical museums, and even much medical scholarship leave one unaware of the long tragic history of medical research with African Americans.

There *are* fine books that address more general issues in the history of African Americans in medicine. These include *The History of the Negro in Medicine,* by Herbert M. Morais; *Making a Place for Ourselves,* by Vanessa Northington Gamble, M.D.; and the sweepingly ambitious *An American Health Dilemma,* by Drs. Linda Clayton and Michael Byrd.

Other works deal with discrete instances of African American experimental exploitation, such as James Jones's *Bad Blood* and Susan M. Reverby's *Tuskegee's Truths. The Plutonium Files,* by Eileen Welsome, meticulously details government radiation experiments in a gripping exposé; *Bones in the Basement,* by Robert Blakely and Judith Harrington, documents the archaeological evidence that revealed how the Medical College of Georgia used stolen African American bodies for physician training; Allen Hornblum's *Acres of Skin* chronicles experimentation in Philadelphia's Holmesburg prison complex; and *The Treatment,* by Martha Stephens, does the same with Cincinnati's radiation experiments. Most of the abuses detailed in these books targeted African Americans. *Killing the Black Body,* by Dorothy Roberts, includes research in its examination of the reproductive constraints on African American women in a historical context; and Sharla M. Fett's *Working Cures* and Todd L. Savitt's *Medicine and Slavery* are seminal histories of antebellum medicine that discuss research issues, but not exclusively.

A few scholars have devoted books to research with blacks abroad, such as Clarence Lusane's fine *Hitler's Black Victims,* Wolfgang U. Eckart's *Medizin und Kolonialimperialismus,* on medical colonialism in Germany's African holdings, and Jan-Bart Gewald's *Herero Heroes,* on the German medical abuse of Namibia's Herero people.

But none of the works listed above attempts anything like a comprehensive history of the racial research wars. There have been no inclusive treatments of African American medical research, and only a few books on discrete aspects of that history—focusing on research in a single prison, a single archaeological discovery of African American bones in a medical school basement, a single experiment with syphilitic men, or a single radiation experiment.

Why? "History is written by the victors," warned Churchill, and a Nigerian proverb issues a similar caveat: "Don't let the lion tell the giraffe's story." The history of medicine has been written by medical professionals and so reflects their points of view. The experimental suffering of black Americans has taken many forms: fear, profound deception, psychological trauma, pain, injection with deadly agents, disfigurement, crippling, chronic illness, undignified display, intractable pain, stolen fertility, and death. None reflect well upon their medical practitioners, so this experimental abuse often has been downplayed or misrepresented as "therapy" in the medical and popular literature. This book reveals these tendencies as well as the lack of objectivity and sensitivity with which African American fears are often greeted, and the social and cultural reasons for the lack of common ground.

The slave appropriated by physicians for experimental surgeries, the impoverished clinic patient operated upon to devise or demonstrate a surgical technique, the sharecropper whose body is spirited from the morgue for dissection, the young girl whose fertility is stolen via an untested contraceptive technique or a "Mississippi appendectomy" (involuntary sterilization), the soldiers, prisoners, and children who find themselves without options when government physicians foist novel medications and techniques upon those with little legal protection—all these African Americans, and many more, have found themselves voiceless as medical lions have chosen to present this research in a bowdlerized manner.

The oral histories of medical abuse voiced by African Americans are often dismissed as mythological, but without objective proof of this label. African Americans' personal stories and familial histories of abuse have rarely surfaced in the medical literature, or in the popular literature. This is not surprising, because African Americans were not well represented in these canons until fairly recently.

Why should we give the physicians' medical narratives more credence than the numerous contentions of slaves, sharecroppers, and contemporary African Americans that they have been subjected to abusive medical research? Until now, the discussion has suffered greatly from our Western literary bias, which encourages us to believe planters' and physicians' writings about the health and medical issues of African Americans, but to give insufficient weight to a rich oral history passed down by African Americans, a history that has preserved the memory of medical abuses. We quite logically cede medical authority to medical experts, but this book will illustrate how race, culture, and economics have trumped medical and scientific truths at every turn. It will make the case that physicians had every motive to skew narratives against their black subjects, not because they were especially racist or unfair (although many were) but because the culture of American medicine has mirrored the larger culture that encompassed enslavement, segregation, and less dramatic forms of racial inequity. The bias against African American medical narratives emanates from culture and politics, including the Western literary bias against oral history.

Because slaves were forbidden to read, and segregated educational institutions perpetrated illiteracy and undereducation, black Americans' contributions to historical understanding of their role in American medicine were dwarfed or silenced. Finally, physicians' accounts carefully inculcated beliefs about black fearfulness, credulousness, emotional instability, and a tendency toward falsehoods that helped to discount claims of abuse.

The resulting lacunae in American medical history feed erroneous assumptions about blacks' medical wariness. An almost innate resistance to all medical research is ascribed to all African Americans. Often, the fear of becoming an abused, unwitting subject is laid to one signal instance of abuse, the Tuskegee Syphilis Study, rather than to a centuries-long history of such abuse.

Fortunately, the facts recorded by researchers and scientists themselves, in medical journals, texts, speeches, and memoirs, buttress African American claims for several reasons. Until three or four decades ago, these researchers were speaking only to their like-minded peers—other whites, usually male and rarely of the lower classes. They could afford to be frank. Blacks were barred from many medical schools and training programs, and newspaper and magazine reporters rarely read the medical publications perused by specially trained medical men of means. There was very little danger any blacks would read medical accounts, because in the antebellum period black literacy was banned by law and illiteracy persisted long beyond slavery. Therefore a doctor could be open about buying slaves for experiments, or locating or moving hospitals to areas where blacks furnished bodies for experimentation and dissection. Public Health Service physician Thomas Murrell could brashly insist in the 1940s, "The future of the Negro lies more in the research laboratory than in the schools. . . . When diseased, he should be registered and forced to take treatment before he offers his diseased mind and body on the altar of academic and professional education." Even more recently, the segregated nature of U.S. medical training emboldened some physicians to speak with candor of misusing black subjects. "[It was] cheaper to use Niggers than cats because they were everywhere and cheap experimental animals," neurosurgeon Harry Bailey, M.D., reminisced in a 1960s speech he delivered while at Tulane Medical School.

But as societal attitudes changed, so did physician reticence, and most became more circumspect. However, as late as 1995, radiation scientist Clarence Lushbaugh, M.D., explained that he and his partner, Eugene Saenger, M.D., chose "slum" patients as radiation subjects because "these persons don't have any money and they're black and they're poorly washed." This book will document numerous instances of such shocking frankness on the part of white researchers and physicians when they thought that nobody outside of their peer group was listening.

In the course of explaining what constitutes exploitative experimentation, *Medical Apartheid* will explain the meaning and nature of informed consent and the differences between therapeutic and nontherapeutic research. It traces the delicate balance between experimental risk and benefit because symbiosis, not complete freedom from harm, is the therapeutic goal, a goal that often eludes African Americans. The individual chapters also supply general background on how experimental practices evolved over the periods covered in this book and how laws and institutional review boards now protect volunteers, albeit still imperfectly.

Finding the Truth in Plain Sight

It is medical researchers themselves who have documented the proof of this long, unhappy history of African Americans as research subjects. Even so, this history has been a challenge to document because it has been hidden in plain sight—widely scattered, distorted, and rendered all but unrecognizable as abuse by heavy editorializing. As I recall the years I have spent ferreting out these experiments bit by bit, examining their patterns, and probing the mind-sets that they revealed, I am put in mind of the legal discovery process. A favored ploy is to provide the opposing side with all the information it seeks—buried in towering mountains of unrelated or tangentially related documents. Similarly, I have perused dusty antebellum medical journals, the Surgeon's General's Index, its successor, the Medline database, physicians' memoirs and literary efforts, slave narratives, and painfully picked my way through foreign publications in alien tongues that are sometimes more forthcoming than domestic publications about the history of our medical treatment of minority groups. Mining the bright but thin lodes within these resources, I gradually amassed a cache of evidence.

As previously hidden experimental exploits come to light, some have challenged the characterization of such research as "secret," noting that the reports were published in medical and scientific journals that could be read by anyone. But these critics would do well to weigh Marcel Pagnol's definition of secrecy: "A secret is not something unrevealed, but told privately in a whisper." Until the past few decades, descriptions in medical publications of experimentation with African Americans were shielded from the eyes of the uninitiated. Generalized professional journals such as the *Journal of the American Medical Association* and *The New England Journal of Medicine* are not available in bookstores or on newsstands. Specialized medical journals are even less accessible, and access was even more restricted in past decades. The medical libraries that house these journals have historically been closed to the public and most remain so; indeed, I have been challenged while entering such libraries while a student or instructor at various northern universities. Moreover, physical access to such journals would constitute only the first hurdle: The medical jargon in which such research papers are couched is often impenetrable even to well-educated nonmedical people.

But some of the people central to medical research have been more generous with their knowledge. Scores of researchers, physicians, and research subjects have shared their time and expertise and added depth to my understanding of the cultural divergence that has fed this history. Often, they told me more than they realized.

For example, a duality has persisted, as I have learned from them more than the facts of scientifically questionable and ethically troubled medical research. Whether we were discussing the etiology of tuberculosis, gynecological surgery, or the implication of census health statistics, these sources have conveyed to me Rorschach-like, divergent medical worldviews. The overarching presence of two Americas, one healthy and white and the other filled with sick, disaffected people of color, has haunted our discussions.

Scientists who abuse, exploit, and lie to research subjects get more than their share of ink, but I have spent enough time among physician-scientists to believe that most American researchers, white and black, are idealistic and skilled. However, when it comes to the abuse of African Americans, a different set of ethical standards has long prevailed and abusive researchers have historically been closer to the norm than we would like to think. Conventional wisdom pins experimental abuses on the "Dr. Frankenstein" stereotype—a scientific outcast of dubious pedi-

gree who harbors blatant social or mental maladjustment. But, historically, most perpetrators of ethically troubling experiments utilizing
African Americans have been overachieving adepts with sterling reputations, impressive credentials, and social skills sufficient to secure positions of great responsibility. The stereotype of the abusive researcher as
a coolly amoral renegade is a stock figure borrowed by journalism from
science fiction: Like all stereotypes, it is one-dimensional and therefore
false. Professionally and socially, these rogue stars have much more in
common with the top strata of other successful American researchers
than they do with mythical madmen.

In fact, researchers who exploit African Americans *were* the norm
for much of our nation's history, when black patients were commonly regarded as fit subjects for nonconsensual, nontherapeutic research. This
book explores the many reasons that blacks are so vulnerable, but ultimately it is because American medical researchers remain a racially homogeneous group, and I show how the racial homogeneity of American
medical researchers lies at the very heart of the problem.

The Curious World of Medical Research

Ironically, my interest in medical research using African Americans is a
direct outgrowth of my long-standing fascination with the more noble
history of medicine. In fact, when asked to describe my work, I usually
explain that I am a medical voyeur. I am an admirer of medicine, and,
when not working alongside physicians in hospitals, I have spent decades
profiling, describing, and analyzing medical advances and the remarkable people who make them. In my many magazine and newspaper articles and in books that celebrate modern medical innovation, I have tried
to convey the achievement, mission, and wonder of healers; my greatest
challenge has usually been to avoid descending into frank hagiography.
This admiration began at age eight, when Albert Schweitzer's *Out of My
Life and Thought* became my favorite book, but it crystallized while I was
an undergraduate at the University of Rochester.

My favorite floor of the undergraduate library housed physicians'
memoirs of a medical swashbuckler genre that included such titles as *My
Patients Were Zulus* and *Burma Doctor.* These heroic reminiscences of
lands populated by African and Asians mingled adventure with medical

proselytizing and constituted a guilty pleasure for me as I pored over them when I should have been reading the assigned Chaucer or genetics. These readings also constituted a guilty pleasure because, although I originally read them as accounts of selfless physicians who cared for people of color, I soon realized that these accounts reeked of xenophobia. Most were deeply disdainful of the natives on whom physicians bestowed the blessings of Western medicine and Western civilization. Because these exploits were distant in time as well as geography, I was less critical than I should have been when they sneered at the ignorant customs of superstitious natives. It all happened so long ago, I thought: surely those colonial attitudes were dead now. I even made excuses for doctors whose disdainful observations were sprinkled with ethnic slurs, or when they congratulated themselves for conducting dramatic, not always benign, experiments upon the unwitting, I excused them on the basis that all this had taken place in the unenlightened past: How could we judge them for abuses conducted under the aegis of yesterday's morals? As the years passed, this became a progressively unsatisfying rationalization, and I eventually abandoned my medical adventurers.

Some years later, I opened a drawer and lost the remains of my innocence. I was running a modest poison-control center in a teaching hospital in upstate New York, and we poor toxicologic relations had expanded into a space that had been reluctantly yielded us by Radiology, a "real" medical department. When I opened a recalcitrant drawer of a file cabinet that had been left behind, a few forgotten medical folders from the 1970s littered its bottom. One contained the file of an older gentleman in imminent kidney failure and focused upon documenting the reams of tests and assessments entailed in finding him a matching kidney for transplant. The social history stressed his loving family and determination to live. Another file also described the plight of an older man in kidney failure, but it looked different, thinner. The first page I read documented his odyssey into sickness as his kidneys failed. It noted among other things that he was retired, insured, and "Negro." Nearly every page recorded his race and someone had underlined it on his social profile, just above the line that indicated that the medical staff's plans for him were not to secure a transplant but to help him to "prepare for his imminent demise." It was signed by a kind, erudite physician I knew and admired and who had actively encouraged my interest in medicine. I could not reconcile this signature with the man I knew, a sensitive scholar and devout Christian. Probably, I thought, I was jumping to conclusions and the patient's race had nothing to do with his failure to be considered for a lifesaving organ.

When I haltingly voiced my fears to an African American acquaintance who had worked as a ward clerk in the nephrology unit, she looked at me as if I were not too bright and minced no words. "Girl, black people don't *get* organs; they *give* organs." During our ensuing debate, she pointed out to me that the race bias in the hospital where we worked should have resolved any doubts: In the early 1980s, most of its black employees worked in housekeeping and clerical support. Blacks were noticeably scarce among the administrative and medical staffs. Why, she asked, was I naïve enough to believe racial bias stopped at the staffing roster?

This was hardly proof, but my discomfort grew as she categorized instance after instance of overt bias and finally declared, "I would never have a procedure done here: I've seen too much. To them, if you're black and poor, you're nothing but a guinea pig." I realized that my discomfort with her words went beyond the truth or falsity of her allegations: The mere fact that she believed them was unsettling, because she had worked in a hospital setting, was presumably better informed than most, yet she did not trust the medical system and seemed less likely to turn to it when ill. The perception of evil in such cases, I realized, can prove as damaging as malfeasance itself.

I finally glimpsed that understanding the true extent of unethical medical research with African Americans was more than idle curiosity or an academic exercise: It was key to removing barriers between African Americans and the bounty of the American health-care system.

In the hospital's medical library, I discovered a new genre of physician confessional literature, one that described black patients not in Africa but here in the United States. Unlike the African book-length exploits, these often consisted of a revealing passage or two in an autobiography, a few pages in a memoir, or a hoary article in a nineteenth-century medical journal. I recognized in these Western accounts of black American patients the very same stereotypes belabored in African accounts.

References in American physicians' memoirs and journal articles were studded with telling vignettes and observations of their black patients. The stories physicians told mixed stereotyped comedy with exasperation as they dismissed blacks as disease-ridden, unintelligent, fearful, distrustful, and, above all, "noncompliant" patients. By "non-compliant," doctors meant patients who could not be trusted to follow medical advice or even to act intelligently in their own best medical interests. I realized that such negative presumptions hampered physicians' ability to care for black patients or even to see them as worthy of the same excellent care rendered to others.

For their part, the black patients I met and interviewed shared their own medical lore, which warned against trusting Western medical practices and physicians, a matrix they characterized as racist, rapacious, and eager to exploit black bodies for medical gain at the cost of health. Thus the disparate narratives African Americans and physicians tell unveil a state of undeclared war or, at best, an uneasy truce between physicians and their black patients.

But I knew that analyzing the history of African Americans as research subjects would necessitate more than a familiarity with history and contemporary medical literature; a sound understanding of basic medical sciences and medical cultures, regulations, protocols, research design, and procedures would also be necessary. This would require a research plan enabling me to ferret out studies in a wide variety of disciplines and subjects. Finally, I would have to speak to medical researchers, subjects, and patients about sensitive experiences. At that time, around 1980, data on racial health disparities was sparse and anecdotal, and in any event, I felt unqualified to take on such a daunting task. I had some grounding in the basic medical sciences, but having abandoned my premedical studies, my knowledge was incomplete. However, I occupied a good vantage point from which to observe and accrue an understanding of medical research culture. I had worked in hospitals for a decade, in positions ranging from ward clerk to laboratory technician to department manager and in venues ranging from the animal laboratory to the cancer-research laboratories to the psychiatric emergency department to the poison-control center. The physicians for whom I worked openly discussed their work with me and were more forthcoming with me as a lowly clerk or technician than they would have been with a journalist.

I eventually left the hospital to work as an inner-city medical social worker ensconced in settings where I constantly talked to African American clients and their caregivers about their beliefs and behaviors concerning medical care and research.

I then worked as a journalist, most notably as a news editor and science editor at daily metropolitan newspapers for seven years, including a brief stint at *USA Today*. After that, I worked as a medical journalist, a columnist, and a contributing editor for several national magazines. My work was published by the New York Times Syndicate and appeared in popular publications as diverse as *Health, USA Today, Essence,* and *Psychology Today*. I was also published in academic publications such as the *Harvard Public Health Review, Nature,* and the *American Journal of Public Health,* and I edited the *Harvard Journal of Minority Public Health,* an especially valuable experience. A monthly medical column that I wrote for *Emerge* magazine gave me experience in framing the issues this book explores for a general audience, and it opened a conduit for numerous first-person testimonies as well.

On a parallel track, I obtained a firm scientific background by completing a premedical course and medical school courses in immunology, toxicology, and neuroscience. As I took classes with medical and doctoral students and postdocs, they became my best sources by relating contemporary research they had participated in. Often they confessed to being troubled by ethical concerns, and this validated my anxiety about some disquieting trends in the commercialization of medical care and in what I increasingly perceived as an erosion of informed consent to research.

Academic institutions, including Stanford, Maryland, and the Medical University of Lübeck, invited me to share with their scholars what I was learning about the hidden history of experimentation with African Americans. At the same time, I embarked upon a Harvard Medical School Fellowship in Medical Ethics. We addressed thorny issues in the philosophy and policy of medical research and engaged in a wealth of readings seminars with important experts. But it is my own assessments of these studies, informed by my medical ethics training, that form the basis of the ethical analyses in this work. They stand or fall on my own logic and historical knowledge.

The Scope and Structure of *Medical Apartheid*

I was determined that *Medical Apartheid* not be a simplistic "black hats, white hats" story in which African Americans are passive victims and researchers are always villains. Instead, the book takes a frank but more nuanced look at the calculus of racism's effects on experimental practice. I have attempted to write a social history that traces the key role that various researchers have played in both promulgating and refuting racism in medicine.

It was impossible and undesirable to incorporate every instance of racialized experimental abuse that I unearthed: This would have resulted in a long, dreary checklist of horrors and little useful insight. The bulk of questionable experimentation upon African Americans is not detailed here because much of it consists of aberrations in therapeutics that were ostensibly meant to cure. Attempts to heal that transgress against ethical rules by dramatically escalating dosages and techniques or that involve nonmaterial breaches of consent are still wrong and risky, but they concern me less because they are sometimes products of honest error and because the intent is still to heal or help. This book focuses more heavily upon experiments with mammoth risks, little or no therapeutic content, or no possible benefit to the subjects, and upon mere attempts at exploitation to perfect medications, procedures, and techniques.

Therefore, this book is not a complete chronology of abusive racial research; rather, it is a thematically organized collection of historical and contemporary issues in medical research with African Americans, illustrated by important cases. I also broach a discussion of such previously ignored historical themes as the fact that fraud is often a traveling partner of racially abusive research. I also explore the history of using African Americans in experimentation intended to support unflattering racial stereotypes and beliefs. African Americans have been used, for example, to perfect the IQ tests that would "prove" them inferior in intelligence, to devise the treponemal tests that would prove them ridden with a distinctive strain of syphilis, and to perform the painful skin and visceral dissection that would prove that "blackness," or negritude, is a permanent mark of biological inferiority that exists independent of skin color.

Some other important medical issues have been excluded from this work because they spill outside the strictest thematic boundaries of African Americans in medical research.

Despite the long and rich history of medical abuse in African and other Third World countries, much of it conducted by U.S. researchers, there is no chapter detailing such research in this book. In one sense, this is akin to discussing Jewish issues without discussing Israel, but the sweeping history of such research is far too extensive to address in a single chapter, especially because it is burgeoning rather than abating.

Similarly, it is impossible to capture completely the important work of African American medical researchers in a single chapter, and I have reluctantly deferred a discussion of this neglected subject both for space reasons and because black researchers have tended to engage in therapeutic research rather than in the troubled investigations that are the subject of this work.

Medical Apartheid consists of fifteen chapters organized into three parts. Part 1, "A Troubling Tradition," takes a chronological approach to the role of African Americans in early American medicine. It stresses the experimental abuse and exploitation of African Americans from the first encounters in the New World through the post–Civil War era and then up until the Tuskegee Syphilis Study, which began in 1932.

Part 2, "The Usual Subjects," covers the period from the early twentieth century to the present day in a roughly chronological manner. However, it departs from strict chronology in favor of an analysis of specific types of vulnerable subjects—children, soldiers, and hospital patients—used in research conducted by institutions ranging from the federal government to private corporations.

Part 3, "Race, Technology, and Medicine," examines contemporary research issues, including genetic research, investigations into emerging diseases, and bioterrorism.

In the epilogue, "Medical Research with Blacks Today," I discuss how the worst abuses have been replaced by more subtle threats to the rights of the individual to choose whether and when to participate in medical research.

Finally, the appendix directs readers to a wealth of guidelines and regulations to help them navigate clinical trials.

Why Research Issues Still Matter

Why do centuries of mutual distrust over medical research matter today? What does the sad history of exploitative experimentation augur for black health?

"What the French see in wine, Americans see in health care," mused Robert J. Blendon, Ph.D., professor of Health Policy and Political Analysis at the Harvard School of Public Health. Americans consider access to excellent health—and even the most expensive means of maintaining it—their birthright. Americans enjoy ever-burgeoning longevity, extravagant nutrition, and everyday access to superb medical care, including expensive high-technology interventions. From CAT scans on demand to new hips to keep us on the tennis courts and new hearts to keep us in the game, we demand the best care, including novel and experimental therapies. Our devotion to the very latest in expensive remedies for increasingly marginal medical gains has many Americans bumping up against the law of diminishing returns.

At the same time, medical experts of every persuasion agree that African Americans share the most deplorable health profile in the nation by far, one that resembles that of Third World countries. When Dr. Harold Freedman observed that the health status of Harlem men resembles that of Bangladeshis more closely than that of their Manhattan neighbors, he did not exaggerate. Twice as many African American babies as babies of other ethnic groups die before their first birthday. One and half times as many African American adults as white adults die every year. Blacks have dramatically higher rates of nearly every cancer, of AIDS, of heart disease, of diabetes, of liver disease, of infectious diseases, and they even suffer from higher rates of accidental death, homicide, and mental illness. Before they die young in droves from eminently preventable diseases, African Americans also suffer far more devastating but equally preventable disease complications, such as blindness, confinement to wheelchairs, and limb loss. Studies continue to demonstrate that, far from sharing in the bounty of American medical technology, African Americans are often bereft of high-technology care, even for life-threatening conditions such as heart disease.

The much bewailed racial health gap is not a gap, but a chasm wider and deeper than a mass grave. This gulf has riven our nation so dramatically that it appears as if we were considering the health profiles of people in two different countries—a medical *apartheid*. Researchers have proffered a cornucopia of theories for this medical divide, many of which focus upon putative biological dimorphisms, especially genetic differences.

But in dissecting this shameful medical apartheid, an important cause is usually neglected: the history of ethically flawed medical experimentation with African Americans. Such research has played a pivotal role in forging the fear of medicine that helps perpetuate our nation's racial health gulf. Historically, African Americans have been subjected to exploitative, abusive involuntary experimentation at a rate far higher than other ethnic groups. Thus, although the heightened African American wariness of medical research and institutions reflects a situational hypervigilance, it is neither a *baseless* fear of harm nor a fear of imaginary harms. A "paranoid" label is often affixed to blacks who are wary of participating in medical research. However, not only is *paranoid* a misnomer but it is also symbolic of a dangerous misunderstanding. That is why I refer to African American fears of medical professionals and institutions as iatrophobia, coined from the Greek words *iatros* ("healer") and *phobia* ("fear"). Black iatrophobia is the fear of medicine.

Even those who investigate the role of medical ethics and medical policy are trying to dissect and analyze the much decried African American aversion to medical research without understanding the history that created that aversion. The historical cause of the racial health gap has been only crudely and cursorily examined and is usually reduced to knee-jerk responses to the Tuskegee Syphilis Study, as if this were the only instance of problematic medical experimentation. But scores of historical events connected with medical research have plagued black Americans and affected their health-seeking behavior. This historical silence is a grave omission, because trying to ameliorate African American health without understanding the pertinent history of medical care is like trying to treat a patient without eliciting a thorough medical history: a hazardous, and probably futile, approach.

Kill the Messenger

In fact, some otherwise well-meaning people wish to censor any analysis of troubled research with African Americans, as I discovered firsthand, to my great surprise. I was elated when a professor at a U.S. medical school summoned me to her office, explaining that she wanted to hear all about the book I was writing. Ensconced in a chair, I eagerly began to describe my work, only to be cut off before I had completed the first sentence. Bolting upright in her chair, she vehemently informed me that the topic of this book was taboo. "It's a terrible thing that you are doing. You are going to make African Americans afraid of medical research and physicians! You cannot write this book!" As she glared at me, her face became contorted with anger, suffused with blood, and her breathing grew rapid. For a moment, I was stunned into silence, because nothing had prepared me for her reaction. After all, freedom of speech and academic freedom are sacred in this country. I was also a bit surprised that a white academic whose discussions and syllabus had evinced no interest or expertise in the matter should lecture me, an experienced African American medical writer, about health communication with African Americans.

She proceeded to inform me that there had been no medical research utilizing African Americans before the Tuskegee Syphilis Study, certainly not in the antebellum past, and when I asked her how she knew this, she countered, "Can you prove that there was?"

When I responded simply, "Yes," she disgorged a clumsy inquisition, unleashing a barrage of questions that showed she knew nothing about the subject at hand. I responded that my work was well researched and that she had raised an interesting question: Was it indeed my work that would make African Americans wary of health care and medical research? Or had the work of those whose abuses I proposed to chronicle already achieved this? The answer was all too obvious: I knew from years as a medical social worker, a medical journalist, and a researcher that black Americans did not need me or anyone else to inculcate a fear of medicine. Medical history and practices had long since done so. *Medical Apartheid* is my attempt to document—at long last and as fully as possible—how and why this has happened.

PART 1
A TROUBLING TRADITION

CHAPTER 1

SOUTHERN DISCOMFORT

Medical Exploitation on the Plantation

Celia's child, about four months old, died last Saturday the 12th.
This is two negroes and three horses I have lost this year.
—DAVID GAVIN, 1855

Frederick Gardiner, a peripatetic Mormon physician, left among his travel memoirs an impression of the nineteenth-century slave markets of Washington, D.C.:

There are a great number of Negroes, nearly all of whom are Slaves. And on different Streets are large halls occupied as Marts or stores, for the sale or purchase of Slaves. . . . While I have been looking at one of these places on Gravier Street, Two Gentlemen have arrived, one of whom I have Seen in the Saloon, he is a young Planter and come to purchase a girl to take care of his children, or whatever duties he may think proper to impose upon her. The other person is a Doctor whom he has brought with him for the purpose of examining her. They pass along the front of the row in company with the agent or Salesman. As they move forward One is called upon to stand up, then another while a passive examination is made. Then finally he discovers a bright mulatto, who appears about 16 years of age and is quite good looking. She is ushered into a private room where she is stripped to a nude condition and a careful examination is made of all parts of the body by the Dr. and is pronounced by him to be sound. The money is then paid and she is transferred to her new owner. . . . I have heard that the Masters beat and scourge them most cruelly. But I have not seen anything of the kind, nor do I believe that it occurs very often. For the

southern people as a class are Noble minded kind hearted people,
as can be found in any country. . . . And moreover it would be
against their own interests, to brutally treat their Slaves. As no
planter desired to have sick negroes on his hands. According to
my judgment so far as my experience extends, I believe that the
Negroes as a class, are far more humanely treated and taken
care of, Than are the laboring classes of European countries.[1]

Enslavement could not have existed and certainly could not have
persisted without medical science. However, physicians were also dependent upon slavery, both for economic security and for the enslaved
"clinical material" that fed the American medical research and medical
training that bolstered physicians' professional advancement. Gardiner's
vignette suggests the integral role of medicine in enslavement and repeats a key belief—that slave owners and physicians shared an interest
in preserving the slave's health, "as no planter desired to have sick negroes on his hands." But although medicine was essential to enslavement, the apparent solicitude for the health of slaves was not all it
seemed. Rather, the medical interests of the slave were often diametri-
cally opposed to the interests of his owner and of American physicians.
From the first, antagonism reigned between African Americans and
their physicians.

Between the seventeenth-century advent of African settlers to North
America and the end of the nineteenth century, the slave and the physician shared an unrecognizably primitive medical world. The "germ theory" that revealed the microbial nature of much disease and led to the
first grand waves of disease cures was still well in the future: The existence of pathogens[2] such as bacteria, viruses, and fungi was unsuspected.
Almost no effective treatments existed for prevalent diseases until the
eighteenth century. Until the late 1830s, the lack of effective anesthesia
made the few common surgical procedures horribly painful and all others impossible.

Between the seventeenth and nineteenth centuries, medicine in the
United States reflected a narrowly limited understanding of disease and
a rather cursory training of medical practitioners. Public-health institutions were few, feeble, and ephemeral, rising momentarily with epidemics of yellow fever or smallpox and subsiding from neglect after the

crisis resolved. Even the simplest public-health measures—hand washing and antiseptic techniques, clean water, sound, pathogen-free housing, an untainted food supply, sewage management, and quantitative
disease reporting were all in the future. Because there were only a few effective disease therapies and no antibiotics, epidemics of yellow fever,
malaria, tuberculosis, and other infectious diseases frequently raged
unchecked. In the early 1700s, this mirrored the situation in England and
the rest of Europe, but medicine on the Continent began to undergo
modernizing changes, although these were very slow to cross the Atlantic. Europe began to embrace public-health measures and medical advances such as widespread vaccination, scientific medical education, and
the rise of the hospital, but American progress lagged behind, especially
in the insular South.

The point of this chapter's unflattering précis of nascent American
medicine is not to castigate it for its primitivism, but to put blacks' historical aversion to medical care into context, for most antebellum blacks
were subjected to southern medicine.

The South was a particularly unhealthy region and was home to 90
percent of American blacks, the majority of whom were enslaved until
1865. The first blacks arrived in the colonies in 1619, and by 1700 there
were only about 20,000 blacks. But as the slave trade flourished, 20,000
more blacks arrived each year. Although 30 percent of transported slaves
died in the nightmare of the Middle Passage, there were 550,000 chattel
slaves in the United States by 1776, when blacks constituted 20 percent of
the U.S. population. By 1807, slave importation was legally prohibited
throughout the country, and by 1860, the nation's four million enslaved
blacks had a value equivalent to four billion dollars today. In some states,
the black population completely comprised slaves: Alabama, for example, forbade the presence of free blacks.

The South was the nadir of the American medical experience, visited
by a deadly triple confluence—the pathogens of North America, Europe,
and Africa. This unholy trinity yielded a bewildering array of unfamiliar
infectious diseases, such as hookworm, types of malaria, and yellow
fever, incubated by a subtropical climate that was hospitable year-round
to pathogens that could not thrive in the colder North. Even familiar European illnesses flared anew in strangely virulent forms, abetted by the
hot, marshy climate, poor sanitation, and a public-health vacuum. Al-

though the South harbored a highly visible affluent class, the region's relative poverty led to a dearth of medical care and a host of unrecognized nutritional-deficiency diseases. So did enslavement.

A dramatically misunderstood set of disease etiologies led to the adoption of heroic remedies calculated to kill or cure. Through the eighteenth century, Western medicine was not only misinformed but dangerously so. Caustic medicines of the period often contained metabolic poisons such as arsenic, or calomel,[3] a compound of mercury and chlorine that was used as a purgative. Many other remedies contained highly toxic substances such as mercury and addictive Schedule II narcotics, including the opiates laudanum,[4] opium, and morphine, as well as cocaine derivatives. These medicines addicted, sickened, or killed outright; they also could trigger chemical pneumonitis, or progressive lung injury, if inhaled during a bout of *iatrogenic*, or physician-triggered, vomiting. No studies seem to have been done on this point, but such lung injuries may have helped to account for slaves' higher death rate from respiratory disease.

Induced vomiting was an everyday event because the common denominator of medical techniques in this period was the violent release of bodily fluids. Copious bleeding, blistering, and the induction of violent diarrhea were standard therapies. Harsh laxatives or "draughts" such as calomel or jalap[5] produced copious diarrhea, which leached nutrients, water, and electrolytes from the body. They also invited painful bedsores, which were open to infection unchallenged by antibiotics. These crude therapies were not only unpleasant but debilitating to ill persons and even to the strong and healthy. Arsenic, for example, produced not only the intended vomiting and diarrhea but also a wide range of other problems, including fainting, heart disease, disorders of the nervous system, gangrene, and cancers.[6] Mercury's very serious effects included injury to the nervous system, profound mental deficits, hair and tooth loss, kidney and heart disease, lung injury, and respiratory distress. Mercury crossed the placental barrier and concentrated in breast milk, contributing to the high black infant-death and birth-defect rates.[7]

Such ministrations were often fatal. The 1799 death of George Washington, hastened by a copious bloodletting the debilitated former president could ill afford, is perhaps the best-known example of a patient finished off by the misguided heroics of eighteenth-century medicine.

However, whites of the slave-owning class enjoyed better initial health, better nutrition, and less exposure to environmental pathogens and parasites than did enslaved blacks. Slave owners did not suffer from overwork and exposure, so they were better able than slaves to withstand the rigors of bloodletting. Sensing this, many physicians and scientists discouraged bloodletting for slaves. Thomas Jefferson, statesman and amateur physician-scientist, wrote unequivocally, "Never bleed a negro."[8] But in their everyday practices, physicians didn't listen. Dr. Lunsford Yandell wrote, "On March 16, 1833 I was called before sunrise to visit a Negro woman. I took from her twelve ounces of blood . . . I waited about fifteen minutes when she had a severe convulsion."[9] Such techniques as cupping (the use of heated glass jars to create a partial vacuum that drew blood upward to the skin's surface or through an incision in the skin) and trephination (the therapeutic drilling of holes in the skull) were risky for pampered, well-nourished adults living in relatively healthy environments. But they were fatal attentions for sickly, undernourished, and exhausted slaves and for their children, who were at even higher risk of succumbing to anemia or dehydration.

Enslaved African Americans were more vulnerable than whites to respiratory infections, thanks to poorly constructed slave shacks that admitted winter cold and summer heat. Slaves' immune systems were unfamiliar with, or naïve to, microbes that caused various pneumonias and tuberculosis. Parasitic infections and abysmal nutrition also undermined blacks' immunological rigor. Before antibiotics and sterile technique, surgery was an often-fatal affair. Unaware of the connection between bacteria and infection, surgeons operated in their street clothes and with dirty hands in filthy environments, such as the shacks that served as "slave hospitals." Even minor incisions or injuries could proceed to life-threatening infections with frightening rapidity.

Southern medicine of the eighteenth and early nineteenth centuries was harsh, ineffective, and experimental by nature. Physicians' memoirs, medical journals, and planters' records all reveal that enslaved black Americans bore the worst abuses of these crudely empirical practices, which countenanced a hazardous degree of ad hoc experimentation in medications, dosages, and even spontaneous surgical experiments in the daily practice among slaves.

Physicians were active participants in the exploitation of African

American bodies. The records reveal that slaves were both medically neglected and abused because they were powerless and legally invisible; the courts were almost completely uninterested in the safety and health rights of the enslaved.[10] The practice of hiring slaves out further endangered enslaved workers by removing much of an employer's incentive to keep the slave healthy and safe. Some humane plantation owners were careful to choose less risky work venues, but a great danger of slave death or disability was inherent in some forms of mining, tobacco production, rice farming, and most plantation work. In these settings, the slave's possible death became part of his owner's commercial calculations.

Ominously for blacks, the owners, not the enslaved workers, determined safety and rationed medical care, deciding when and what type of care was to be given. Because professional attention was expensive, most owners dosed their own slaves as long as they could before calling in physicians, who usually saw slaves only in extremis, as a last resort. In clinical notes, medical journals, and memoirs, physicians consistently decried the planters' tendency to rely upon the cheaper ministrations of overseers, slaves, and mistresses in order to save expense. Physicians' records also expressed disgust at the conditions in which enslaved workers were kept. Historian Richard Shryock observed in 1936: "Of all critics, the Southern physician was perhaps in the best position to report on the physical and moral treatment of the slaves. When he stated, as he sometimes did, that Negroes were overworked and underfed, he can hardly be suspected of antislavery bias since he was the friend of the planter who employed him. As a matter of fact, he usually approved of the institution."[11] Planters' own records and slave narratives corroborate physicians' complaints that planters provided professional medical care only when they deemed it necessary to save the slave's life—often too late.

Owners also restricted access to medical care by routinely accusing sick blacks of malingering. Slave narratives and planters' records reveal that an owner faced with a sick slave was likely to believe the illness was feigned. In her excellent and nuanced history, *Working Cures: Healing Health and Power on Southern Slave Plantations,* Sharla Fett describes how, in 1859, slave owner William Massie resentfully recorded that his eighty-year-old slave "Patty" had just died "of I know not what disease. . . . She has been saying she was sick for near a year and always pretended to be sick." No doctor was ever summoned to investigate, and not even Patty's death seems to have exonerated her from charges of malingering.[12] The enfeebled Patty was no longer valuable in the fields or as a "breeder," so the nature of her sickness was inconsequential.

Owners relied upon doctors to tell them whether slaves were malingering, but physicians were less than objective. Dr. W. H. Taylor, called in consultation for an enslaved man, prefaced his assessment with the phrase "remembering that simulation was a characteristic of his race."[13] Doctors and owners wrote articles in which they shared medical ruses and techniques calculated to get blacks, healthy or not, back into the fields. Dr. M. L. McLoud even wrote his master's thesis on the fraudulent illnesses of slaves.[14] He shared an incident in which he had accidentally administered an overdose of ammonium carbonate,[15] a corrosive white powder that was often used as smelling salts, to a slave shamming an epileptic fit. The burning sensation shocked her into abandoning her performance, and McLoud, like many other doctors, began to advocate such veiled medical violence when confronted with questionable illness in slaves.[16] But masters also responded to suspected malingering or prolonged illness with frank abuse. Thomas Chaplin wrote in his planter's journal, "Mary came out [of the sick house] today or rather was whipped out." Owners and physicians also blurred the therapeutic line by referring jocularly to whipping as "medicine" for malingering slaves. One complaining woman was "*treated* with a cowskin or hickory switch to scourge her" [emphasis added]; other doctors recommended that an owner apply "9 drops of essence of rawhide" or "oil of hickory"[17] to the back of a sick slave.

Yet, slave narratives occasionally speak of the kindness of a sympathetic white physician. In the 1930s, former Texas slave Wes Brady told WPA interviewers how "the old white Doctor that tended to us helped them get out of work. He took a little flour and meal and water and made pills." The doctor then told the master that the slave was too sick to work. "Sometimes they stayed in bed three or four days taking flour pills."[18]

But most physicians shared the economic and political interests of slave owners and conspired with planters, their real clients, to subjugate slaves by invading their bodies. Former slave Martha Griffith Browne recalled that the kindly wife of Dr. Mandly, who sometimes was called in by her master, "did not believe in slavery, yet she dared not speak against

the 'peculiar institution' of the South. It would injure the doctor's practice, a matter about which she must be careful."[19]

The belief in the eternal malingering of slaves was only one tenet of
scientific racism, a wide body of mostly unflattering beliefs about the
bodies and minds of people of African descent. These beliefs were presented as research findings, explained by scientific theories, and promulgated by whites who were sympathetic to or were actively profiting from
the institution of enslavement, so, not surprisingly, scientific racism provided medical and scientific justifications for slavery. Southern scientists
claimed that they alone could analyze blacks with authority—after all,
they lived in proximity to blacks, had studied them, and understood
their medical and intellectual characteristics. Northern scientists tended
not to study African Americans because they were less important to the
northern economy, which was not directly based upon chattel slavery.

The care and treatment of slaves was an important aspect of southern medical regionalism, and the lack of attention to "Negro medicine"
became an increasingly bitter source of contention between northern
and southern medical schools. As a result, southerners urged their medical students to eschew the schools of the North, and when tensions
mounted on the eve of the Civil War, southern students of northern
medical schools were holding rallies in which they voted to return south
en masse. In Philadelphia alone, two hundred southern medical students withdrew from Jefferson College and another hundred withdrew
from the University of Pennsylvania during a single academic year,
1859–1860.[20]

Despite their claims of unique expertise, the shoddy research that
southern physicians conducted into black health consisted of an
untested nucleus of mythology about the biological nature of blacks.
Negative visceral reactions to blacks' appearance, historical writings,
racial descriptions from antiquity, natural scientists' endless and largely
fictional catalogs of "racial" traits, and biblical interpretations all provided a framework for "scientific" and medical theories about blacks. So
did a blame-the-victim approach to the poor health of the enslaved. The
scientific racist's emphasis was not upon fact-based theories, logical
methodologies, experimental data, control groups, and verification by
replication. There were neither checks against accepting assumptions as
facts nor any tests for confounding social factors. There certainly was no

provision for removing ethnocentric bias—this "science" was the *embodiment* of ethnocentric bias. This science also served a critical political purpose, for it provided a biological and ethical rationale for enslavement. Historical documents reveal that African Americans recognized this hazardous medical agenda and resisted when they could. Thus, medical abuse fed iatrophobia, the fear and loathing many black Americans harbor to this day toward the American medical establishment.

An exegesis of American medical literature compiled in the service of scientific racism is beyond the scope of this book, and has been ably completed elsewhere.[21] However, a description of the most pertinent beliefs will help to illuminate the atmosphere in which blacks were medically abused and in which they learned to be wary of the precepts and practices of American medicine.

The science of race has always been an amalgam of logic and culture. The nature of race itself is an important but nebulous and shifting facet of scientific medical thought. As early as A.D. 160, the Roman physician Galen (129–c. 199) described African men as possessing oversized sexual organs and inferior intelligence, but until the seventeenth century, the changing meaning of *race* had encompassed only nations and families. *Race* in the singular also denoted all of mankind, as in "the race of man."

Use of the term *race* to denote biologically different types of mankind evolved only in the eighteenth century, when the study of animal breeding gave rise to heightened awareness of animal subspecies and of the possibility of breeding animals to encourage desired traits. Not coincidentally, this period coincided with the growth of the slave trade, when the biological distinctiveness of men became economically important. Those who studied the different groups of men were called ethnologists and were the forerunners of anthropologists. Ethnologists applied the classification and categorization methods of the natural sciences, called taxonomy, to the study of man. Even after the meaning of *race* came to include subgroupings of man, it had several meanings. By *races,* some meant biological subspecies of man, analogous to the different breeds of dogs. For example, Swedish naturalist Carl von Linné—Carolus Linnaeus, the most famous of the taxonomists—categorized Africans (and, by extension, U.S. blacks) as *Homo afer,* theorizing that black men had different evolutionary forebears and had evolved along a separate evolutionary track from white men. In 1735, the first edition of his *Sys-*

tema naturae also designated the subspecies *Homo sapiens americanus* for Native Americans, whom he described as "ruled by superstition"; *Homo sapiens asiaticus,* for Asians, whom he believed were "ruled by ritual"; and *Homo sapiens europaeus* for whites, who were "ruled by intelligence." But in Linnaeus's system, *Homo sapiens afer* was "ruled by caprice." This use of the word *race* in the sense of a biologically distinct subset of *Homo sapiens* was popularized in 1749 by Georges-Louis Leclerc, comte de Buffon,[22] a wealthy French intellectual who made important contributions to medicine and natural history. Buffon notably theorized that the resemblance between apes and humans hinted at a common ancestry.

For other theorists, *race* indicated entirely different species of men, with different origins as well as different characteristics for blacks and whites. Those who believed in this theory were the polygenists. Still others believed that whites and blacks shared a common ancestral ape and a single species. These were the monogenists. Most monogenists believed that whites and blacks were originally and inherently equal but that blacks had suffered from environmental and social pressures that caused them to become inferior. Other monogenists believed that blacks' devolution had imparted permanent inferiority, although they still shared a species designation with whites.

Throughout the seventeenth century and into the early eighteenth century, the theories of scientific racism were informed by the Bible as well as by science. Monogenesis, for example, held that people of every race had originated from the biblical Adam and Eve. Gradually, blacks had taken on divergent characteristics, such as darkened skin, woolly hair, and prognathous features, dictated by their African climate. The idea that blacks' features were dictated by climate was already widespread. Shakespeare's Cleopatra, for example, is described as "burnt black by Phoebus' amorous kisses." Monogenists believed that blacks' features were inferior to those of the white man, but they also believed that they were malleable and that blacks could "catch up" to Caucasians.

But in the end, it was scientific beliefs that proved malleable, and by the late 1830s, they bent to accommodate the political reality of abolitionism. Black and white abolitionists were turning world and domestic opinion against enslavement as inhumane, unjust, and un-Christian, and pro-slavery physician-scientists such as Josiah Clark Nott, Samuel George Morton, Louis Agassiz, and George Robins Gliddon, leaders of the American school of ethnology,[23] went on the defensive. They responded by portraying the enslaved black as inherently debased and immutably so: No amount of training, education, or good treatment could make him the equal of a white man.

According to polygenists, blacks were physically inferior and were liars, malingerers, hypersexual, and indolent. In the early years of the eighteenth century, blacks were most often compared to beasts. Later in the century, comparisons to European children reigned instead—children who could never grow up, and the slave became Peter Pan in blackface. The supposed lack of adult judgment rendered blacks unable to care for themselves and gave yet another justification for slavery.

It is also important to trace the tangled distinctions between *racism* and *racialism*. Racists believe in an innate, usually immutable inferiority, but *racialist* is a confusing label, because it is applied to people holding very different beliefs. The term can denote a person who believes that race or skin color does signal inherent attributes but that the attributes in question are simply different, neither negative nor inferior.[24] But *racialist* can also mean a person who interprets the different features and qualities of blacks as superior. The word *racialist* has recently been used to describe actions taken to redress long-standing racial wrongs, such as affirmative action to bolster the fortunes of blacks. Then again, *racialist* can also be a mere synonym for *racist*, as it long was used in England and has been adopted by racial hatred groups as a euphemism for *racism*.[25]

As a result of this semantic confusion, a once-useful term has been rendered worthless by its many contradictory meanings. The awkward and pallid term *race-based* seems the closest thing we now have to a neutral racial adjective.

Whatever their pet theory, the many physical differences between blacks and whites suggested a hierarchy of humanity to scientific racists: "Different" from whites meant "inferior," and inferiority was documented in entire catalogs of black flaws that filled medical journals and textbooks. In 1839, Morton published *Crania Americana*, a book written to demonstrate how human skull measurements indicated a hierarchy of racial types. Morton determined that Caucasians had the largest skulls, and therefore the largest brains, and blacks the smallest. His tests were the forerunner of phrenology, which sought to determine character and intelligence by interpreting the shape of the skull.

By 1848, Louisiana's Samuel A. Cartwright, M.D., had gained renown by publishing a plethora of articles on Negro medicine in southern medical journals, leading the Medical Association of Louisiana to appoint him chair of its committee to investigate black health and physiology. That same year, Cartwright published his paper "The Diseases and Physical Peculiarities of the Negro Race." Cartwright augmented his scholarly work with a constant onslaught of medically based pro-slavery letters to newspapers and popular magazines. He supported his widely read claims of black inferiority with a mixture of biblical lore and scientific theories that was not unusual for his time.

Cartwright suggested that blacks' physical and mental defects made it impossible for them to survive without white supervision and care, alleging that the cranium of blacks was 10 percent smaller than that of whites, preventing full development of the brain and causing a stunting of the intellect. French scientist Louis-Pierre Gratiolet added that in the Negro "the cranium closes on the brain like a prison. It is no longer a temple divine, to use the expression of Malpighi, but a sort of helmet for resisting heavy blows."[26] Cartwright even asserted that blacks had a very different breathing apparatus and skeletal structure from that of whites.

By 1851, Cartwright had also discovered and described a host of imaginary "black" diseases, whose principal symptoms seemed to be a lack of enthusiasm for slavery. Escape might have seemed normal behavior for a slave in ancient Greece or Rome, but Cartwright medically condemned such behavior in American blacks, offering a diagnosis of drapetomania, from the Greek words for flight and insanity. Hebetude was a singular laziness or shiftlessness that caused slaves to mishandle and abuse their owners' property. Dysthesia Aethiopica was another black behavioral malady, which was characterized by a desire to destroy the property of white slave owners. Cartwright claimed that it "differs from every other species of mental disease, as it is accompanied with *physical signs or lesions of the body* discoverable to the medical observer. . . ." Struma Africana was a form of tuberculosis that physicians misdiagnosed as a peculiarly African disease. Cachexia Africana referred to blacks' supposed propensity for eating nonfood substances such as clay, chalk, and dirt.[27] Actually, this disorder, which is called pica today, is not racially specific and the cravings it inspires were probably related to the rampant malnutrition among slaves. Tellingly, Dr. Cartwright recommended that these ailments be treated with corporal punishment or with internment in "work camps": "Put the patient to some hard kind of work in the open air and sunshine. . . . The compulsory power of the white man, by making the slothful negro take active exercise, puts into active play the lungs, through whose agency the vitalized blood is sent to the brain to give *liberty* to the mind."[28]

Other medical disorders were thought to manifest differently, usually less severely, in blacks. Syphilis, for example, was held to be racially dimorphic. Physicians believed it worked its most feared damage within the neurological system of whites but that the less evolved nervous system of blacks was left relatively unimpaired. In blacks, syphilis was thought to attack the muscles, including the heart. This belief that syphilis in blacks differed dramatically from the disease in whites provided a rationale for the infamous U.S. Public Health Service's (PHS) Tuskegee Study of Syphilis in the Untreated Negro Male. Between 1932 and 1972, six hundred black men, their wives, and their children were deceived into participating in a research study that denied them treatment, so that PHS scientists could trace the progress of the disease in blacks.

In an 1850 paper, Cartwright insisted that whites and blacks differed so dramatically "that the same medical treatment which would benefit or cure a white man would often injure or kill a Negro. . . ."[29] This universal belief in uniquely "black diseases" led doctors and planters to clamor for a textbook on the medical care of blacks, but such a book was not written until almost a century later. When it appeared in 1942, it was no paean to white superiority but, rather, was entitled *The Biology of the Negro*, a text edited by African American physician Julian Herman Lewis; it was followed in 1975 by the masterwork *Textbook of Black-Related Diseases*, by Richard Allen Williams, M.D.[30]

Allegedly inferior cognition was only the tip of the iceberg. In 1854, several years after Cartwright published "Report on the Diseases and Physical Peculiarities of the Negro Race," and five years before Darwin published *On the Origin of Species*,[31] Mobile, Alabama, physician Josiah Nott, M.D., and George R. Gliddon produced an equally popular screed entitled *Types of Mankind*. In it, they claimed that blacks' physical and mental differences signaled their polygenic origins and proved black inferiority. For example, Nott theorized that the distinctive knee joint and "long heel" of the black man proved he had been created as a "submissive knee-bender"—a servant to whites. Scientists adjudged the dark skin of Africans as a biblical curse that set them aside as eternal servants to other men. Black Americans were thought of as a race that was biologically identical to the African race, and there originally was some logic to this, because 20 percent of slaves were still native Africans in 1780, although that number dropped to only 10 percent by 1830, a few decades after slave·importation officially stopped.[32] Mulattoes, the progeny of black-white matings, were considered to be a separate race. According to ethnologists of the American school, blacks' features marked them as a different species: large buttocks and genitals that indicated hypersexuality, a head covering that was not hair, but analogous to the wool of livestock, the size of the skull (determined by painstaking but rigged measurements), the "prognathous" facial angles of blacks, and thick lips that testified to their apelike nature. (Had scientists of the era more correctly noted that apes and chimpanzees have the thinnest of lips, they doubtless would have ignored this feature before they credited blacks with such an evolutionary advance.) Physicians discovered many imaginary physical differences in blacks, such as fingernail anomalies, a distinctive topography of the breasts, elongated penises, disproportionably large hands and feet, distended labia and clitorides, all of which provided scientific racists with ample evidence of black biological primitivism. In fact, few anatomical sites escaped persistent labeling as "definite" indicators of black inferiority. As late as 1903, Dr. W. T. English observed, "A careful inspection reveals the body of the negro a mass of imperfections from the crown of the head to the soles of the feet."[33] Even biological advantages were cast as racial flaws: In discussing the tendency of blacks to survive yellow fever epidemics that killed whites, one physician denounced the "inferior susceptibility" of black slaves.

Insidious Immunities

Polygenism, the belief in separately evolved species, also held that persons of one race could not survive in the climate designed for another. Whites who tried to live and work in West Africa, a climate putatively designed for blacks, died in droves, earning it the sobriquet "white man's grave" when the nineteenth-century death rate for British soldiers ranged between 483 and 668 per 1,000 soldiers in Africa, compared to the general annual death rate of 15 per 1,000. Historian Warwick Anderson,

M.D., describes how the U.S. military sought to exploit the natural affinity of black Americans for the tropics:

> In 1900, Nathaniel Southgate Shaler, the dean of Harvard's Lawrence Scientific School, proposed that the "troops which are required for Federal service in tropical lands might well be recruited from the negroes"; . . . Shaler was convinced that such "children of the tropics" would "make excellent soldiers—at least as infantry men"—because the African-American constitution was preadapted to the tropical disease environment. But in the Philippines, Shaler's distinguished advice was already redundant: during the previous two years, the United States had been using African-American and Filipino scouts to suppress the resistance to its occupation of the archipelago.[34]

Physicians claimed that whites could never work in Africa or in subtropical environments such as the U.S. South. The southern landowning class, including physicians, paid attention, because they equated disease with a sinister climate and were confronted with an oppressively hot and humid "malarious" environment that they believed to be teeming with yellow fever, smallpox, pellagra, typhoid, dysentery, and cholera. They were also faced with fertile lands that required backbreaking labor, with the attendant risks of heat prostration, sunstroke, and parasitic infestation. An "immune" population specially designed by the Creator to work long, hard, and for free as "submissive knee-benders" was the perfect answer to their dilemma. In mid-century, Samuel A. Cartwright and his medical brethren, such as Charles Lehlbach, belabored the immunities to malaria and yellow fever they claimed blacks exhibited.[35] But to fully justify enslavement, scientists such as Nott had to turn from their naturalists' texts to their Bibles, from which they deduced that blacks were the children of Ham, son of Noah, who, along with his progeny, was "marked" and condemned to be servant to his brothers for having viewed his father's nakedness. Other similar biblical justifications were found, and Nott even ventured onto a twisted ethical high road when he insisted that yellow fever and malaria were visited upon whites as divine punishment for *not* enslaving blacks. He insisted that nonslaveholding whites contracted these diseases as the result of usurping the "natural" black role as laborers in the fields. Pragmatic planters and politicians ignored the religious moralizing but embraced the useful "fact" that black slaves were the only logical medical choice for backbreaking labor in their sunny fields.

The "immunities" in question were usually partial and sometimes imaginary. Planters' own records bear the best evidence that blacks' "immunity" to heat prostration was merely a convenient myth. One Virginia owner observed in 1825, "Hotest day ever—Men gave out & some fainted."[36] The 1851 journals of K. Washington Skinner, overseer on the Gowrie plantation, noted, "On Monday last Cotta and Sarey received a stroke of the sun . . . many of the other negroes staggered about considerably. . . ."[37]

Blacks were supposed to be immune to malaria, but such immunity is complex and was poorly understood before 1900.[38] Malaria denotes a group of lingering infectious diseases marked by long cycles in which waves of utter debility alternate with periods of better health. These periodic relapses can end in death, depending upon the strain of malaria and the immunological vigor of the sufferer. The disease is spread by parasites injected by the bite of the female Anopheles mosquito, and at the time, it was widespread outside of New England, especially throughout the South. However, eighteenth- and nineteenth-century southern physicians did not understand that malaria, which they called "intermittent fever," "remittent fever," "fevers and ague," or "quotidian fever," actually has three different strains, with differing causes, symptoms, and prognoses.

Falciparum and vivax malaria are the most common North American strains. Another strain, malariae, is so rare[39] and so similar to vivax that scientists tend to consider them a single entity. Vivax/malariae, which antebellum physicians called "tertian fever," causes wracking symptoms of high fever, chills, headache, icy bone pains, anemia, profuse sweating, and exhaustion, many of which recur at forty-eight-hour intervals. It can become chronic and last for years, but it kills only 5 percent of its victims. Falciparum malaria ends more quickly, but it is much more severe and can cause a stroke by compromising the blood flow to the brain and kidneys: Forty percent of its victims die.[40]

In 1826, Dr. Philip Tidyman wrote, "Intermittent fever, so hostile to the constitution of the white inhabitants, has no terror for the negro, who when attacked, requires but little medicine to rid him of this insidious enemy, and to secure him against a return."[41] However, planters' records and physicians' journals are full of accounts of slaves laid low with or dying of malaria. It was an extremely common complaint, one that coincided inconveniently with harvest times in the late summer or the early fall, so it was a serious monetary concern to planters, who were willing to expend money on physicians to get their malaria-stricken slaves back into the fields as soon as possible.

Scientists were wrong in positing Africans' innate, absolute resistance to malaria and they were equally wrong in suggesting that whites could mount no immunity. Anyone, black or white, who grows up in a malarious area and survives repeated infections and bouts with falciparum comes to live in an uneasy truce with the parasite, becoming not quite well but not acutely ill. This state of immunological compromise misled planters into thinking that these slaves were unaffected when they were exposed to falciparum malaria and did not die. Such immunity is temporary, lasting only as long as one remains continually exposed to the falciparum parasite. Planters and physicians knew this and deliberately cultivated local malarial immunity in their newly arriving slaves by "seasoning," or allowing them to be bitten by area mosquitoes, thus infecting them with the local strain. Whites underwent seasoning, as well.

However, one type of malarial immunity *is* racially distributed in the United States. Ninety-five percent of sub-Saharan Africans and approximately 70 percent of African Americans are "Duffy-negative." This means that they lack the Duffy antigens, without which plasmodia vivax cannot penetrate red blood cells and cause illness.[42] People of any ethnic group who have sickle-cell trait (possessing a single gene for sickle-cell anemia) also enjoy a partial protection against deadly falciparum malaria. So do people with one gene for the related blood diseases, or hemoglobinopathies, thalassemia, hemoglobin S, and hemoglobin C.[43] These are not "black" immunities; they also protect Mediterranean, Middle Eastern, and Asian peoples.[44]

Interestingly, the contradiction of the black slave as both "riddled with imperfections from head to toe" and as a hardy laborer who was impervious to most illness escaped the scientific racists. Scientists expressed whichever opinion fit their political needs at the moment, as abolitionist Frederick Douglass suggested when he observed that ninety-nine of one hundred polygenists were Anglo-Saxon slave owners.[45]

Scientists also claimed that the primitive nervous systems of blacks were "immune" to physical and emotional pain and to mental illness. This belief, which will be discussed at greater length in the next chapter, released physicians and owners from the responsibility of shielding black slaves from painful medical procedures and justified torture such as branding, whipping, hobbling, and maiming.

All these precepts of scientific racism, although convenient for the slave owner and physician, were highly illogical articles of faith. So was the supposed inferior intelligence of blacks, because planters and doctors behaved in many contexts as though they held the abilities and judgment of blacks in high regard, employing slaves in responsible positions as nurses, cooks, herbalists, midwives, overseers, leaders of work gangs, accountants, and operators of farm and factory implements. Owners reaped profits from the many patents on slave inventions, and physicians used slaves as skilled apprentices, who often went on to practice independently. White households depended upon the specialized skills and discernment of slaves, not the other way around.

In descriptions of runaways, published as newspaper advertisements, a master's financial interests necessitated an honest description of his vanished slave. These are replete with references to "artful," "well-spoken," "crafty," and "intelligent" slaves who typically absconded in well-organized groups, often with a light-skinned confederate who posed as their owner until they reached freedom. Advertisements referred to some slaves not only as literate but as polyglots fluent in French, German, and Dutch; some were refined violinists and declaimers; others practiced professions such as "doctor" or "dentist." The master's plaintive wonder that an apparently docile slave should have given him the slip is a commonplace of these advertisements.[46]

The dearly held precepts of scientific racism sound nakedly racist, absurd, or both today, but in the eighteenth and nineteenth centuries, scientific racism was simply science, and it was promulgated by the very best minds at the most prestigious institutions of the nation. Other, more logical medical theories stressed the equality of Africans and laid poor black health at the feet of their abusers, but these never enjoyed the appeal of the medical philosophy that justified slavery and, along with it, our nation's profitable way of life.

Dr. Gardiner, whose slave-market narrative opened this chapter, spoke for many when he claimed that slave owners "must have" jealously guarded their slaves' health, coddling them to protect their own economic interests. In the Washington slave pen, Gardiner witnessed the physician in his role of pronouncing a slave "to be sound," yet he confused the physician's certification of the slave's soundness with concern for her health. Soundness did not speak to her welfare or happiness, but rather to the ability to extract work from her, the likelihood of fetching a good price on the market, and her breeding ability: Many common medical problems, from mental illness to chronic malaria and parasitic infection, were compatible with the demands of an enslaved laborer's work; in fact, many ailments emanated from these workloads.

Profit drove the medical treatment of slaves from their very first encounters with Western medicine. Kidnapped Africans en route to the Americas were cursorily examined by ship's surgeons in an attempt to cut losses by immediately jettisoning those with such stigmata as Winterbottom's sign, a swelling of the lymph nodes found in those who harbored trypanosomiasis, or sleeping sickness. They and others who would not survive the horrific Atlantic journey were unceremoniously thrown overboard.[47] Southern physicians engaged in a bustling "soundness practice" by guaranteeing the fitness for work of slaves who were to be bought and sold. Doctors charged as much or more for this service as they did for standard disease treatments.[48] A simple pronouncement of health, for example, could cost anywhere from two to ten dollars in 1850s Virginia. But such assessments were sometimes challenged when the slave died or became incapacitated soon after having been pronounced sound. Expert physicians' testimony commanded as much as fifty dollars—a very steep one-day fee for the times. Thus, testifying to soundness in court became an important—and lucrative—part of medical practice, and in 1858, Dr. Juriah Harris of Savannah Medical College declared the need for a manual that cataloged the chronic or debilitating diseases that rendered blacks unsound for work. He then cannily supplied the manual himself. Among the deal-breaking ailments it cited were loss of limbs, cancer, asthma, rheumatism, debilitating injury to muscles, keloid scars, and syphilis.[49]

How was this interest in fitness for work, or soundness, at odds with slave health? With the soundness rather than the welfare of the slave in mind, for example, slaves were not immunized against smallpox as whites were, because this might leave marks on their bodies that could discourage buyers. The memoirs of William Wells Brown, originally a slave and later a doctor, recount how the graying hair and beards of aging slaves were "blacked" on the auction block.[50] They were subsequently purchased by buyers who expected the toil of a young man.

But blacks countered with ruses of their own, as slavery apologist Edward A. Pollard illustrated in 1859: "Noey, on mounting the steps [to the auction block], had assumed a most drooping aspect, hanging his head and affecting the feebleness of old age. He had probably hoped to have avoided a sale by such a dodge."[51] Former slave Bethany Veney recalled in her memoirs:

> I had been told by an old negro woman certain tricks that I could resort to, when placed upon the stand, that would be likely to hinder my sale; and when the doctor, who was employed to examine the slaves on such occasions, told me to let him see my tongue, he found it coated and feverish, and, turning from me with a shiver of disgust, said he was obliged to admit that at that moment I was in a very bilious condition.

Veney did not disclose the specific advice the old woman shared, but many common therapeutics of her day, such as the emetic calomel, dramatically inflamed the tongue, gums, and salivary glands. Veney continued:

> One after another of the crowd felt of my limbs and asked me all manner of questions, to which I replied in the ugliest manner I dared; and when the auctioneer raised his hammer, and cried, "How much do I hear for this woman?" the bids were so low I was ordered down from the stand, and Eliza [a beautiful woman] was called up in my place. Poor thing! there were many eager bids for her; for, for such as she, the demands of slavery were insatiable.[52]

Soundness for women, and sometimes for men, was tied to sexual attractiveness and to reproductive ability. Thomas Jefferson declared, "I consider a slave woman who breeds once every two years as profitable as the best worker on the farm."[53] Every year from 1750 until emancipation, one of every five black women of childbearing age (between fifteen and

forty-four) gave birth. Girls were forced or enticed into sexual relationships at an unhealthily early age by owners who cited the girls' supposedly hot-blooded African nature. Sexually transmitted diseases thrived
on the plantation, notably syphilis, against which the immunologically
naïve Africans had little protection. Enslaved women's vulnerability began on the sea passage from Africa, as recorded in the 1788 memoirs of
English ship's surgeon Alexander Falconbridge: "On board some ships
the common sailors are allowed to have intercourse with such of the
black women whose consent they can procure. . . . The officers are permitted to indulge their passions among them at pleasure and sometimes
are guilty of such excesses as disgrace human nature."[54]

But whites ascribed black women's sexual availability not to their
powerlessness but to a key tenet of scientific racism: Blacks were unable
to control their powerful sexual drives, which were frequently compared
to those of rutting animals. This lack of control made black men dangerous and made black women sexually aggressive Jezebels who habitually
enticed white men into inappropriate sexual relations. Dr. Louis Agassiz,
the famous Harvard ethnologist, explained:

As soon as the sexual desires are awakening in the young men of
the South, they find it easy to gratify themselves by the readiness
with which they are met by colored [mixed-race] house
servants. . . . This blunts his better instinct in that direction and
leads him gradually to seek more spicy partners, as I have heard
the full blacks called by fast young men.[55]

This theory did not allocate any responsibility to the master as the
owner of the women and the person who decided when and with whom
she would have sexual relations. But slave narratives bemoan the rape
and sexual abuse that threatened a black woman at every turn. Mary
Reynolds, who was born on the plantation of Dr. Kilpatrick in Black
River, Louisiana, reflected, "Us niggers knowed the doctor took a black
woman quick as he did a white and took any on his place he wanted, and
he took them often." As the personal property of the master, black
women had no social or legal protection: They could not legally be
raped. Even consensual relationships had to be viewed through the lens
of enslavement. In her memoirs, former slave Harriet Jacobs sadly

mused that she eventually acquiesced to such sexual demands because it was less humiliating to give in than to be forced.[56] Once pregnant, women typically were kept at hard labor until their fifth month and re-calcitrant pregnant women were made to lie in trenches that accommo-dated their bellies so that they could be beaten without harming the unborn child. Soundness considerations also dictated levels of care, which varied according to a slave's value. Slaves who were strong, young, and valuable received a quality of care that was denied to the feeble as well as to the aged, who were often cast off the plantation or sold to physicians when the expense of their care exceeded their market value.[57] Former slave Martha Griffith Browne recalled the words in which an abusive master refused to pay a doctor to treat an elderly slave who had spent her life working on his plantation: " 'I ain't gwine fur to spend money on that old nigger, unless you cure her, and make her able to work and pay fur the money that's bin laid out fur her. . . . If she be gwine to die, why let her do it in the cheapest way.' "[58]

The Owner-Physician Pact

Southern physicians supported the slave system with racial medical the-ories and diagnoses, but the slave system also supported them. In an era when physicians enjoyed considerably fewer financial rewards and lower professional status than they do today, these physicians derived most of their income from caring for slaves.[59] As Samuel Cartwright observed in 1853, "The most profitable kind of practice is that among negroes."[60] Slavery created a medical partnership between physician and planter that eclipsed the patient-physician dyad, the traditional Western healing relationship. In the slaveholding United States, where the planter owned the slave and employed the physician, owners made their complaints or treatment wishes known to physicians and gave or withheld consent for procedures, from sterilization to amputation to autopsy. The planter, not the slave, had to be satisfied with the results. The planter, in every impor-tant sense of the word, *was* the patient. The southern relationship was a slaveholder-physician dyad, with the slave left outside, unconsulted, un-informed, and with no recourse if she or he was unsatisfied, injured, or killed—a medical nonentity.

Physicians were often slaveholders themselves. In fact, an 1847 state medical convention in Alabama issued a recommendation that doctors caring for slaves seek liens upon the human chattel if their bills were not paid.[61] Slave-owning physicians profited from their slaves in the usual ways—fieldwork, housework, concubines, rented labor, and breeders of slaves. However, doctors also bought and hired slaves on whom to conduct experiments too painful, too risky, or otherwise too objectionable to inflict upon whites. I will examine many instances of this practice in the pages that follow.

The matter of life insurance also illuminates the medical conflict between a slave's health and his master's economic interest in his soundness. Although most southern gentlemen found the prospect of insurance coverage for landowning whites and their families a distasteful parallel to insuring equipment and livestock, the practice of insuring slaves' lives escalated in the 1840s.[62] In 1858, 75 percent of the North Carolina Mutual Life Insurance Company policies were written on slaves.[63] But despite owners' assurances that their slaves were "like members of their family," insurers' research suggested that owners did not shy from maximizing the profit from their slaves, dead or alive. Even Dr. Josiah Nott, the famous defender of slavery, worried that rapacious masters would allow sick or injured slaves to die without treatment, warning, "Any man who will drive a horse cruelly, will drive a negro or operative to death, if he can gain anything by so doing." South Carolina and Virginia insurance companies eventually refused to insure a slave's life for full value for fear that owners would allow them to die of their ailments. Insurers also hedged their bets by requiring physical examinations of slaves, by charging more for slaves placed in especially hazardous assignments, and by requiring proof that the owner had had the slave treated for medical conditions as they arose.[64] Thus, companies that have lately taken heat for insuring slaves' lives also took steps that protected those lives.

I spoke in my introduction of *iatrophobia*, a term for the fear of medical care that joins the Greek words for healer and fear. Black iatrophobia has a very long history, and one of its earliest signs during slavery was that when they were not accusing slaves of malingering, overseers, planters, and physicians complained bitterly that slaves were concealing their illnesses. In this, they were often correct. Slaves avoided the ministrations of Western doctors by denying that they were sick as long as they could, even to the point of working while they were ill, discarding medications, and hiding their children's sickness. This enraged masters and physicians because they believed that blacks' failure to report illnesses and to accept white "cures" led to premature death and the loss of valuable slaves. However, slaves distrusted Western remedies as ineffectual and dangerous. They also complained that these treatments were stereotyped: The same remedies were offered for various ailments. Mary Reynolds could list her physician-owner's entire materia medica (the common term for pharmacological supplies) for slaves in one breath: "Dr. Kilpatrick give sick niggers ipecac and asafoetide and oil and turpentine and black fever pills." Work Projects Administration interviewers quoted former slave Joe Hawkins as charging, "Doctors then didn't doctor a person like they does now. No sir, he'd bleed you so many minutes while he watched his big watch he always carried. Bleed you for most any sickness."[65] Slaves knew that some of the treatments worsened problems and, perhaps most important, they realized that a master's interest in their fitness for work was sometimes inimical to their health. In short, enslaved blacks often eschewed Western medicine because they suspected their owners of a greater interest in them as capital than in their welfare. They also questioned the acumen and the motivation of the "regular" Western practitioners who, in turn, ridiculed the spiritual component of African medicine as "superstition."

Then, too, slaves had their own healers and preferred medicines that were less harsh and often more efficacious. Slave medicine, unlike the physiology-based, almost mechanical ministrations of whites, incorporated African healing philosophies and techniques, including strong psychological, social, and spiritual components. Slaves themselves illustrated this by the parallels they drew between their medical treatment and that given the livestock. Former slave Richard Toler remembers that owners were "as pa'taculah with slaves as with the stock—that was their money, you know. And if we claimed bein' sick, they'd give us a dose of castah oil and tu'pentine. That was the principal medicine cullud folks had to take. . . . And if we was real sick, they had the Doctah fo' us."[66]

Appeals to God, the importance of moral fitness, and enlisting the help of departed spirits, especially the intercession of ancestors, were all key to the African-based healing process. Ancestors who were angered by disrespect or neglect could cause illness, alienation, and other troubles for the living. This is one reason the respectful ritual treatment of the dead was so important to slaves and why they reviled Western medicine when they discovered that physicians appropriated the bodies of dead slaves for display and dissection. Western medicine was thought ineffective against spirit-caused illness, and slaves often lacked confidence in a Western doctor's ability to cure them: If a doctor did not believe that one could be cursed or "conjured," how could he remove the threat? This is a wide generalization, because some slaves mistrusted African practitioners, who sometimes used their skills to harm as well as to heal. But in planters' farm books and in medical journals, physicians and slave owners repeatedly berated the ignorance and superstition that led slaves to conceal illness and to shrink from "scientific" Western medicine in favor of conjure women and witch doctoring.

However, whites had no monopoly on science. The African tradition involved physiological as well as spiritual approaches to healing, including an encyclopedic knowledge of herbs, roots, and other natural medicaments. This detailed knowledge was continually passed down along lines of apprenticeship from wise women and male herb doctors to gifted young members of the community. Despite their characterization as primitive, African healers first employed citrus juice for scurvy and inoculation for smallpox and other viral illnesses; midwives used African techniques, herbs, and medicines so successfully—without dangerous tools of the day, such as forceps—that many white women called them to attend births.

Some whites were impressed by the success rate of Negro doctors and "doctresses," consulted them, and placed their medication recipes in the family book, and Western doctors faced brisk competition from black herb doctors. In an 1855 journal article, Dr. R. H. Whitfield of Alabama railed against "unscientific" midwives:

> [There are no practices wherein which] the female practitioners are less educated, being chiefly negresses or mulatresses, or foreigners without anatomical, physiological and obstetrical education. . . . That such uneducated persons should be generally successful is owing to the fact that [in] a great majority of cases no scientific skill is required, and thus a lucky negress become[s] the rival of the most learned obstetrician.[67]

For all their complaints, physicians in the early to mid-nineteenth century were happy to leave the business of birthing in the hands of black midwives. However, physicians wanted black healers under the scrutiny and supervision of white physicians. White doctors denigrated black midwives and healers, calling them "uneducated," but white physicians themselves usually had no academic preparation beyond a few months in proprietary medical school or a few years of apprenticeship, which many blacks also shared. So until the mid-1800s, such claims of superior education rang hollow. Also, regular medicine embraced no consistent curriculum, but roped in a motley association of disciplines. At the bedside, healers practiced a variety of Western fads such as hydrotherapy, which utilized harmless but ineffectual "water cures" for many ailments, and Thomsonism, followed by disciples of New Hampshire farmer Samuel Thomson, who, like black healers, advocated the use of milder herbal and vegetable remedies and emetics. The constant friction between white physicians and enslaved healers sometimes erupted into open hostility. Physicians denigrated black medical practice and imposed punishment, including execution, upon black healers, on the pretext of protecting the larger community from poisoning and from the evil machinations of occultists who, doctors claimed, controlled the minds and actions of superstitious blacks.

Black contributions to early American medicine included research. In fact, slave doctors sometimes developed medications that were so highly prized as to garner them fame, fortune, and their freedom. In 1729, Lieutenant Governor Gooch of Virginia authorized the payment of sixty pounds to manumit an unnamed "negro man." Gooch declared that his mixture of pharmacologically active roots and bark had proved an effective syphilis remedy. "It is well worth the price of the negro's freedom," wrote Gooch, "since it is now known how to cure negroes without mercury."[68] In 1751, a South Carolina slave doctor named Cesar developed several medical innovations, including an almost foolproof snakebite antidote. The cure featured a shrub called plantane and horehound, a plant that derived its name from Egyptian priests who called it the "seed of Horus" (the Egyptian god of the sun and virtue), mixed with sassafras, wood ashes, and tobacco. On February 25 of that year, the *South Carolina Gazette* published the recipe as a public service, and demand ran so high that it was reprinted widely and published as a monograph in 1789.[69] In 1799, it was mentioned in the text *Domestick Medi-cine*. Cesar's medical acumen earned him his freedom from the South Carolina General Assembly, which also granted him an annual pension of one hundred pounds. Primus was another slave who won fame for medical achievements, which included a rabies treatment.[70] The medical career of Wilcie Elfe of Charleston, South Carolina, benefited rather than suffered when the white pharmacist to whom he was apprenticed turned out to be incapacitated by alcoholism. Left to his own devices, Elfe for-mulated new medications, which proved so effective that his patent drugs became popular across the state. Meanwhile, Western doctors complained that overseers resorted to a standard remedy for every com-plaint: "an emetic followed by calomel and oil."[71]

This chapter has sketched the roots of the friction between medical practitioners and African Americans; the next describes how medical ex-perimentation heightened the aversion of black patients for white physi-cians.

CHAPTER 2

PROFITABLE WONDERS

Antebellum Medical Experimentation
with Slaves and Freedmen

Montgomery [Alabama] has not forgotten the heroic role of the three
slaves Anarcha, Lucy, and Betsy, who suffered, not only that they
themselves might be cured, but that women injured in childbirth in
future generations might be saved from lives of misery and invalidism.
—SEALE HARRIS, *WOMEN'S SURGEON*, 1950

A lie told often enough becomes the truth.
—LENIN

When he escaped to England in 1847, the former slave who had been
known as "Fed" claimed John Brown as his full name. Brown was a com-
pact dark-skinned man in his forties, with strong features and a dense
thatch of black hair that sprang from his crown at an angle, though it
had been brushed to either side of an indeterminate part. His body bore
the stigmata of enslavement: His hands were latticed with ropy scars
and the black iris of his bulging right eye lay off center, perpetually
looking inward. For all this, the worn collodion image gracing his memoirs shows a man of estimable appearance in a sober woolen suit and
brocade waistcoat. He is neither smiling nor frowning, but exudes a satisfied air of quiet dignity—a survivor. But of what? In 1855, Brown described his enslavement to L. A. Chamerovzow, secretary of the British
and Foreign Anti-Slavery Society, which published his memoirs as *Slave
Life in Georgia*.[1]

Among Brown's most remarkable recollections was the period he
spent with Dr. Thomas Hamilton of Clinton, Georgia, during the 1820s
and early 1830s.[2] Hamilton was not only a widely respected physician but
the very epitome of a southern gentleman.[3] He was born into wealth in
Washington, Georgia, graduated from the University of Pennsylvania

School of Medicine, and became a wealthy plantation owner, physician, politician, and trustee of the Medical Academy of Georgia.

But Hamilton had another face. Brown recalls how he fell into the doctor's hands when his master, a man named Stevens, fell ill.

> I do not know what his malady was. It must have been serious, for they called in to treat him one Doctor Hamilton who lived in Jones County, and who had a great name. He cured Stevens, who was so pleased, that he told the Doctor to ask him any favour, and it should be granted. Now it so happened that this Doctor Hamilton had been trying a great number of experiments, for the purpose of finding out the best remedies for sun-stroke. I was, it seems, a strong and likely subject to be experimented upon, and the Doctor having fixed the thing in his mind, asked Stevens to lend me to him. This he did at once, never caring to inquire what was going to be done with me. I myself did not know. Even if I had been made aware of the nature of the trials I was about to undergo, I could not have helped myself. There was nothing for it but passive resignation, and I gave myself up in ignorance and in much fear.

Hamilton had a deep pit dug, and built a fire in it that he damped so that only the burning embers remained; these were retained until the doctor, using a thermometer, ascertained that the pit was sufficiently hot. He then made Brown sit naked on a stool in the pit and covered the opening with a wet blanket to retain the heat. Only Brown's head was exposed while temperatures routinely exceeded one hundred degrees. Hamilton then administered his various heat remedies until, Brown recalls, "though I tried hard to keep up against its effects, in about half an hour I fainted. I was then lifted out and revived, the Doctor taking note of the degrees of heat when I left the pit."

After each day's work in the fields, Brown was given some nostrum and made to repeat the ordeal. But after all this "scientific" effort, Hamilton resorted to chicanery.

> He [Hamilton] found that cayenne-pepper tea accomplished his object; and a very nice thing he made of it. As soon as he got back

home, he advertised that he had discovered a remedy for sunstroke. It consisted of pills which were to be dissolved in cayenne-pepper tea without which, he said, the pills would not produce any effect. Nor do I see how they should have done so, for they were only made of common flour. However he succeeded in getting them into general use, and as he asked a good price, he soon realized a large fortune.

After a few days' rest, Brown was subjected to a new set of experiments, for which he was bled every other day. But still worse was to come: "He set to work to ascertain how deep my black skin went. This he did by applying blisters to my hands, legs and feet, which bear the scars to this day. He used to blister me at intervals of about two weeks. He also tried other experiments upon me, which I cannot dwell upon."[4]

After Brown's matter-of-fact account of being poached to the point of fainting and of his repeatedly burned and flayed skin, one wonders what other experimental horrors he "cannot dwell upon." When he could bear the surgical torture no longer, Brown fled to England.[5]

There were many people like Brown. The preceding chapter sketched how scientific racism, abusive medical attentions, and iatrophobia, the fear and loathing many black Americans harbor toward the American medical establishment, are connected. However, African Americans have also been exploited as the subjects of abusive medical experimentation, which was once standard medical practice.

More than scientific racism, more than heroic purges, bleedings, and cathartics, and more than the punitive use of therapeutics, involuntary medical experimentation was the scientific personification of enslavement. Violence, pain, and shame joined as physicians forced the enslaved body into medical service, not to cure, but for profit. Medical experimentation was profitable in terms of recovered health and life for whites, who benefited once the medical process had been perfected. It was also a profitable source of fame, and sometimes fortune, for physicians.

Owners boarded the captive bodies of sick slaves to hospitals or hired well ones to physicians for use in experiments. Sometimes they sold a slave outright for such use, particularly if she had become too old or infirm to work or to breed. Many slave owners such as Dr. Hamilton, Dr. Marion Sims, Dr. Nathaniel Bozeman, and Dr. Stillwell were them-

selves physicians who bought and raised slaves for the express purpose of
using them for experimentation Not only slaves were thus used but also
"free" persons of color.[6]

The Perilous Trial

What constitutes medical experimentation? The word *experiment* comes
from the Latin proposition *ex,* meaning "from" or "out of," and *periculum* "a (dangerous) trial." To conduct an experiment is to risk success or
failure, and when human health and lives hang in the balance, the stakes
are high indeed. However, famed French researcher Claude Bernard provided the definitive feature of scientific experimentation in 1865: ". . . an
experiment is an observation induced with the object of control."[7] Thus,
the researcher conducting an experiment does not simply *observe* a medical phenomenon; he or she induces a *change* under strictly controlled
conditions, makes observations, and then logically analyzes them.

Some medical experiments test treatments that may help the experimental subject; these are therapeutic experiments. Other experiments
involve nontherapeutic tests that are not designed to help the experimental subject. The experimental standards that govern research today
differ considerably from those physicians followed prior to the twentieth
century. Today, a matrix of legislation protects human subjects, at least
in theory, and informed consent is a necessary requirement for most experiments with human beings. Informed consent is not a signed piece of
paper but, rather, the fluid, continuous process by which a researcher informs the subject in detail of what he or she proposes to do, why it is being proposed, and what possible consequences the experiment carries.
Only then does the researcher ask the subject's permission, which must
be obtained in writing. Despite the signing of the consent form, the
process has not ended. The researcher must continue to inform the subject of developments in the experiment that could affect him and the
subject may withdraw from the experiment at any time.

To perform an experiment without informed consent is a serious
medical (and legal) abuse today. However, informed consent was not
part of the ethical mores of the eighteenth and nineteenth centuries and
was not required by law. Physicians did typically ask a patient's consent
to conduct experiments, but they did not explain their reasoning or detail their intent.

In addition, when we consider eighteenth- and nineteenth-century experimentation, it is important to keep in mind that medicine of the period countenanced a larger degree of therapeutic modification than is allowed today. By the standards of past centuries, not every spontaneous decision to try a new, untested medication or combination can be considered unethical medical experimentation.

For this reason, discussions of early medical experiments with African Americans in this chapter do not focus on lesser but still egregious ethical breaches such as dangerous therapeutic experiments without informed consent. Neither do I discuss those many "experimental" approaches that were essentially therapeutic adjustments of commonly accepted remedies and methods. Southern physicians and scientists engaged in many such hazardous experiments, such as those of T. S. Hopkins, M.D., of Waynesville, Georgia, who prescribed caustic solutions of nitric acid to five black children for asthma. Similarly, Joseph E. May, M.D., prescribed herculean doses of calomel and quinine to a slave with malaria, who, fortunately, recovered.[8] These were hazardous experiments that would not have been practiced on whites and they were done without the subjects' permission, but their end was at least partially therapeutic: The doctor was trying to effect a cure.

Instead, this chapter offers a few examples of the many experiments like those to which Brown was subjected. That is, they were involuntary, painful, dangerous, and either frankly nontherapeutic or obviously more harmful than beneficial. The experimental abuse of African Americans was not a cultural anomaly; it simply mirrored in the medical arena the economic, social, and health abuses that the larger society perpetuated against people of color, especially in the slaveholding states.

No one, white or black, would have chosen to be the subject of a dangerous experiment, but blacks were especially wary, based upon their earlier abusive experiences with Western medicine.[9] They were also wary because Western medical experimentation, with its mechanistic approach to the body, was philosophically inimical to the spiritual, community-based, and holistic African systems of healing as practiced by black healers.

Western physicians had placed African holistic plant- and spirit-centered healing systems outside the purview of medicine, relegating them to the realm of superstition, the occult, "voodoo," and old wives' tales. In the same manner, many African Americans placed the experimentation to which they were subjected outside of accepted modes of medicine and healing. Oral histories and extant writings suggest that many African Americans accepted and even incorporated some Native American and Western healing techniques but considered invasive medical experimentation a form of medical torture or even of medical cannibalism.[10]

Before the early-twentieth-century rise of the U.S. hospital movement, physicians and scientists conducted medical research in slave quarters, backyard shacks they designated as "slave hospitals," and clinic wards.[11] No organized bodies coordinated coherent research plans, and some "research" was utterly spontaneous and unrecorded.[12]

Physicians' recollections, medical journals, and institutional records limn a pattern of abusing African Americans that was supported by custom and sometimes by law. These accounts could be astonishingly frank because the authors were writing only for the eyes of other physicians—white males of their own class—who attended hospital wards and read medical journals. Moreover, African Americans were without legal protection and thus unable to hamper physicians' activities.

As a result, early medical records routinely identified African Americans as experimental subjects, especially in the slaveholding states. Half the original articles in the 1836 *Southern Medical and Surgical Journal* dealt with experiments performed upon blacks.[13] It is true that blacks constituted a significant part of the South's population—nearly 40 percent in 1860—but they were still represented far above their proportions in hospitals and clinics. For example, when Dr. James Dugas pioneered a new eye surgery, four of his five experimental subjects—80 percent—were black.[14] Slaves were used preferentially to test genitourinary surgeries. Beginning in 1830, 30 of 37 experimental cesarean sections performed by Dr. François Marie Prévost used slaves. Experimental ovariotomy and surgery for bladder stones also relied heavily upon black and mulatto subjects. In an exhaustive 1982 article detailing the antebellum experimental use of blacks, medical historian Todd Savitt summarized this risk: "Some whites took advantage of southern blacks by testing new techniques or remedies in the name of medical progress. In several instances physicians purchased blacks for the sole purpose of experimentation; in others the doctors used free blacks and slaves owned by others."[15]

Not all experimental subjects were black, of course, and in northern states, where approximately 10 percent of blacks lived, white subjects tended to outnumber black subjects, although blacks were still used out of all proportion to their numbers. White subjects typically emanated from the lowest social tiers. For example, Alexis St. Martin, a poor French-Canadian trapper, was harassed, pursued, and studied for years by a successful physician who wished to experiment on him after an unusual accident caused a permanent opening in his stomach.[16] So was Phineas Gage, a laborer who survived an industrial accident but suffered severe brain damage, which was assiduously recorded and tested by a long series of physicians.[17] White subjects, however, enjoyed some legal protection and could leave when they wished, to the frustration of medical researchers.

We have seen that scientific racists successfully promoted several necessary medical fictions that made blacks attractive as experimental subjects. Most physicians of the day also believed that blacks had low intellectual capacities and were sexually promiscuous, that diseases manifested differently in blacks, and that blacks could not be trusted to take medicine, follow treatment, or maintain basic standards of hygiene without white supervision. Finally, physicians believed that blacks naturally harbored diseases, notably syphilis, that threatened the health of whites.[18] Each of these common beliefs served as rationales for abusive medical experimentation. One of the most tenacious beliefs was that blacks did not feel pain or anxiety, which excused painful surgical explorations without anesthesia on blacks. Dr. Charles White declared that "[blacks] bear surgical operations much better than white people and what would be the cause of insupportable pain for white men, a Negro would almost disregard. . . . [I have] amputated the legs of many Negroes, who have held the upper part of the limb themselves." And when Kentucky surgeon Efraim McDowell wrote of gynecologic advances that were achieved by exquisitely painful surgeries, Dr. James Johnson, editor of the *London Medical and Chirurgical Review,* sneered, "When we come to reflect that all the women operated upon in Kentucky, except one, were Negresses and that these people will bear anything with nearly if not quite as much impunity as dogs and rabbits, our wonder is lessened."[19]

Politics in the Laboratory

Although experimentation with African Americans was the medical norm, especially in the South, some whites were deeply opposed to it. In the late eighteenth and early nineteenth centuries, abolitionists wrote exposés, and in 1839, Theodore Wright Weld uncovered the cruelty of medical experimentation in "American Slavery as It Is," declaring "Public opinion would tolerate surgical experiments, operations and processes performed upon [slaves], which it would execrate if performed upon their masters.[20]

Such pointed criticism may help to explain why some physician-scientists who spoke candidly of injecting, dosing, or performing revolutionary surgeries on their slave patients in the first half of the nineteenth century expressed their actions more guardedly in later writings. For example, Dr. James Marion Sims eventually hid his subjects' race and even illustrated reports of experiments on black slave women with illustrations of bourgeois white matrons. Journals sometimes dispensed with racial labels, although their articles still offered broad social cues about their subjects' ethnicity.

Language was often tortured to disguise the racial nature of hazardous experimentation. In the best patrician tradition of his times, Thomas Jefferson was not only a country squire and leading politician but also a scientist. Eager to make his mark, Jefferson embarked on enthusiastic adventures in vaccination by gambling with the lives of his slaves. He wished to establish that Edward Jenner's new technique of vaccination was superior to the technique of inoculation (or, as it came to be called a century later, variolation). Inoculation consisted of inserting or injecting infected material from a sick person directly into a well one to induce immunity. Vaccination, in this era, referred to the process of injecting cowpox to provide immunity to smallpox, as Jenner first described in 1796. Jefferson obtained some cowpox vaccine indirectly from Dr. Benjamin Waterhouse of Boston,[21] but it was known to be of dubious potency: The vaccine had failed to protect the subjects of an earlier trial. Jefferson spent that summer vaccinating two hundred of his family's and his neighbors' slaves. Only after they escaped illness did Jefferson inject his white family at Monticello.

The vaccinated persons remained well and the unvaccinated ones fell ill, but this did not convince Jefferson's scientific peers, so Jefferson had a vaccinated slave injected with live smallpox material. When this slave remained well, Jefferson wrote his daughter Martha to proceed in order to "place our families and neighbors in perfect security."[22]

As a seasoned politician, Jefferson knew that his experiments on slaves would be criticized and that they seemed at variance with his sympathetic statements about blacks, so he slyly used language to deflect possible criticism, referring to conducting experiments "on some of my own family," without clarifying that the "family" in question consisted of slaves owned by himself and his son.

An epidemic of typhoid fever raged in Virginia throughout the summer of 1832, and planters feared that the infected slaves would be unable to work and would endanger whites. Dr. Robert G. Jennings had no cure, but he decided to test a hunch that smallpox vaccine might protect against typhoid. He administered the vaccine to thirty blacks, slave and free, choosing them from uninfected family members of typhoid patients, in order to guarantee they would be exposed; he then withheld the vaccine from other uninfected family members.

Jennings reported that those who were vaccinated remained disease-free; the unvaccinated became ill. When Jennings then vaccinated blacks suffering from typhoid, he jubilantly recorded that they recovered more quickly. Jennings delivered the investigative coup de grâce when he decided to vaccinate eleven of twelve family members, withholding vaccine from the twelfth: Only the unvaccinated slave fell ill.

This "successful" experiment on an enslaved population defies all logic, because smallpox vaccine is not efficacious against typhoid. One cannot be certain whether serendipity or outright fraud was involved, but the mathematical odds against such results arising by luck are staggering and no one has ever successfully duplicated Jennings's experiment.[23]

Many other experiments on slaves accrued no benefit to the black subject, and white patients were not asked—and certainly were not forced—to assume these risks.

The next decade saw an escalation of sadism in experiments on slaves. The 1846 records of Dr. Walter F. Jones of Petersburg, Virginia, reveal that he experimented by pouring boiling water on naked enslaved typhoid pneumonia patients at four-hour intervals. He described one such treatment on a sick twenty-five-year-old enslaved man:

The patient was placed on the floor on his face and about five gallons of water at a temperature so near the boiling point as to barely allow immersion of the hand, was thrown immediately on the spinal column, which seemed to arouse his sensibilities somewhat, as shown by an effort to cry out . . .

Jones didn't reveal what had inspired him to try this remedy, and he offered a rather thin rationale for the treatment, suggesting only that it worked by somehow "reestablishing the capillary circulation."[24]

In June of the same year, John M. B. Harden, M.D., of Liberty County, Georgia, published an article in the *Southern Medical and Surgical Journal* that described how he had stripped blood vessels from the limbs of "a Negro" and of "three hogs." Harden then measured the width of the blood vessels "to determine the relative areas of the Trunks and Branches of arteries," with the stated intent of furthering anatomical knowledge.[25]

But none of these increasingly painful medical intrusions was as infamous as the slave experimentation conducted by James Marion Sims, M.D., of Alabama.

James Marion Sims, Savior and Sadist

James Marion Sims is an important figure in the history of experimentation with African Americans because he so well embodies the dual face of American medicine to which racial health disparities owe so much. Sims is revered as a women's benefactor, although he conducted years of nightmarishly painful and degrading experiments, without anesthesia or consent, on a group of slave women.

He was born into a struggling family of ten in Hanging Rock, near Lancasterville, South Carolina, in 1813. In his autobiography, *The Story of My Life*,[26] Sims described how, despite a career as an indifferent, mediocre student, he gained entrance first to South Carolina Medical College and then to Jefferson Medical College in Philadelphia. In the manner of the day, his medical education consisted of a year and half of instruction. Sims confessed that he initially found his medical training wanting: "When it came time to making up a prescription I had no more idea of what to do than if I had never studied medicine." But once he embarked upon practice on the plantations of Alabama, these feelings of inadequacy did not prevent him from blaming enslaved mothers for the high death rates of their infant children. He ascribed neonatal tetanus ("newborn" tetanus), or *trismus nascientium,* to the mothers' moral and intellectual failures.[27]

> Whenever there are poverty, and filth, and laziness, or where the intellectual capacity is cramped, the moral and social feelings blunted, there it will be oftener found. Wealth, a cultivated intellect, a refined mind, an affectionate heart, are comparatively exempt from the ravages of this unmercifully fatal malady. But expose this class to the same physical causes, and they become equal sufferers with the first.[28]

Neonatal tetanus is caused by a bacterial infection with *Clostridium tetani,* which emanates from animal manure and thrives in wounds such as healing umbilical stumps. Thus, Sims perceived the connection between filth and illness, which was not yet an accepted medical belief, but he blamed the wrong parties. Owners built slave shacks on inferior lands near horse stables and other quarters and as far as possible from the whites' dwellings. Antebellum doctors' disdain for hand washing, as well as the midwifery practice of swaddling the umbilical cord with rags, raised the risk of infection.[29] But by attributing tetanus to the laziness and weakness of slaves, he deflected attention from the simplest way of removing contagion—relocating and improving slave dwellings. Today, we know the deaths were probably the caregivers' fault.

As a plantation doctor, Sims attended many children, but he used only the black infants as subjects for dangerous experiments in tetany, a long-misunderstood children's neuromuscular disease characterized by convulsions and muscle spasms. The tetany that was epidemic among enslaved children was actually the result of severe calcium, magnesium, and vitamin D deficiency caused by chronic malnutrition,[30] but Sims was erroneously convinced that it was caused by the displacement of skull bones during birth. He took a sick black baby from its mother, made incisions in its scalp, then wielded a cobbler's tool to pry the skull bones into new positions: "During this time, I would occasionally puncture the scalp over the lambdoidal suture, with the point of a crooked awl, and prize out the edges of the parietal bones always, with the effect of greatly modifying the rigid fleure of the extremities. . . ."[31] Sims's attempt to "open" the skull was based upon a scientific myth that the bones of black infants' skulls, unlike white infants', grew together quickly, leaving the brain no space to grow and develop. This premature closing of the black skull was held to cause low intelligence and perpetual childishness in adult blacks. When the infants died, Sims castigated the sloth and ignorance of their mothers and the black midwives who attended them.

Sims soon acquired seventeen slaves, whom he used in his experiments and as workers in his clinic/laboratory. The first three such patients fared miserably under Sims's faltering scalpel. One nineteen-year-old enslaved man died after two heroic operations, including the unanesthetized removal of bone segments, presumably to prevent the spread of an infection. Sims's account of the surgeries glossed over the patients' deaths to dwell upon technical details of greater interest to his medical readers. Mistakes such as a patient's near suffocation from a sponge that Sims forgot to remove from his mouth after removing part of his cancerous jaw and Sims's failure to stanch a patient's bleeding from the carotid artery were also given short shrift.[32]

But these were mere prelude. On a June day in 1845, seventeen-year-old Anarcha, a slave on the Westcott plantation just outside of Montgomery, Alabama, felt the contractions that heralded the birth of her first child. Three days later, the exhausted, terrified girl still writhed in excruciating labor. Sims was called in and used obstetrical forceps, with which he admitted he had little experience. The child died, and although Anarcha seemed out of immediate danger, she soon faced another horrible trial. Her torn vagina began eroding and she was left with openings between the remains of her vagina and her bladder and rectum. She was now incontinent, and the incessantly flowing urine inflamed her ravaged tissues, triggering pain, recurrent infections, and odor.

As terrible as Anarcha's condition was, a certain hyperbole entered Sims's descriptions of it: He compared it to smallpox and stressed its unpleasantness for spectators as well as the fact that it made her unfit for work—a planter's perspective.[33]

Anarcha was far from alone in her misery. Her condition, vesicovaginal fistula, afflicted many women, black and white, who survived difficult childbirth. However, enslaved women had an especially high rate of this complication. Despite physicians' tendency to blame "the ignorance and obtrusive interference of our plantation *accoucheurs* and nigger midwives,"[34] Sims himself conceded that the rates of vesicovaginal fistula had risen when obstetricians began using forceps.

The condition may well have been due to a confluence of malnutrition, forceps use, and Anarcha's youth.[35] The vitamin D deficiency that was very common among malnourished slave women caused bone defects, including a small pelvis. This made birth difficult, especially in the underdeveloped pelvises of very young women,[36] and slave women became mothers approximately three years earlier than did white women.

Vesicovaginal fistula is emotionally and socially devastating and it condemned many a southern lady to permanent invalidism. Sims knew that curing it would make his medical fortune and he also knew that using white women to test such painful surgeries as might be effective against it was impossible.[37] Historian Walter Fisher sums it up: ". . . it is most improbable that Sims and [his assistant] Bozeman could have established so remarkable a surgical schedule without the slave system which provided the experimental subjects."[38] Slaves did not have to be recruited, persuaded, and cajoled to endure pain and indignity; they could not refuse.

Sims acquired a total of eleven women slaves with vesicovaginal fistula from their masters by promising to lodge, board, and treat them, and he built a spartan wooden building, where he conducted surgical experiments on them for the next four years.

During the Victorian period, layers of dress signaled sexual chastity, and doctors were not in the habit of viewing women's unclothed bodies; not even their professional stature gave them license to gaze at women's genitalia. When Sims undertook his fistula experiments, even the term *gynecology* was a few years in the future. Instead, "women's doctors" averted their eyes in a chivalrous fashion as they knelt to tend to the modestly clothed ladies of their class, relying upon their sense of touch beneath voluminous Victorian skirts.

However, Sims, working with enslaved blacks, was constrained by no such delicacy.[39] He made the women undress completely, then kneel on hands and knees while he and several physicians took turns inserting a special speculum[40] he had devised to open the women's vaginas fully to view. "I saw everything as no man had seen before," marveled Sims.

Montgomery physicians flocked to Sims's shack to see what no man had seen before. So did prominent citizens and local apprentices.[41]

The surgeries themselves were terribly painful. Not only had Sims to close the unnatural openings in the ravaged vaginal tissues; he had to make the edges of these openings knit together. He opted to abrade, or "scarify," the edges of the vaginal tears every time he attempted to repair an opening. He then closed them with sutures and saw them become infected and reopen, painfully, every time.

Several male doctors had initially assisted Sims by holding down the enslaved women as he made incisions, but within a year they could bear neither the bone-chilling shrieks of the women nor the lack of progress any longer. The doctors left, leaving the women to take turns restraining one another. Later, Sims recruited Dr. Nathan Bozeman as a protégé and assistant. Bozeman was a recent medical graduate of the University of Louisville and had trained with some of the best surgeons in the region, such as Professor Samuel D. Gross.

Medical journals and professional word of mouth had detailed the inhalation of ether as anesthesia since the early 1840s, and Sims knew of this, but he flatly refused to administer anesthesia to the slave women and girls. He claimed that his procedures were "not painful enough to justify the trouble and risk attending the administration," but this claim rings hollow when one learns that Sims always administered anesthesia when he performed the perfected surgery to repair the vaginas of white women in Montgomery a few years later.[42] Sims also cited the popular belief that blacks did not feel pain in the same way as whites.[43] However, Sims's own words belie him. In his memoirs, he noted that "Lucy's agony was extreme . . . she was much prostrated and I thought she was going to die." Sims further obscured the truth in 1852, when he described the first surgery on Lucy, writing, "That was before the days of anesthetics, and the poor girl, on her knees, bore the operation with great heroism and bravery."[44]

Sims's refusal to administer ether seems even less defensible in light of his willingness to administer it very freely to another group of women, without apparent regard for its "trouble and risk." In New York during the 1860s, Sims attended white women patients who suffered from vaginismus, a disorder marked by painful vaginal muscle contractions that prevent the entrance of the penis, making intercourse impossible.

Complaining husbands approached Sims, who regularly etherized their wives, rendering them unconscious so that their husbands could have sex with them.[45]

Sims's writings often utilized imprisonment as a metaphor for the control that he saw as key to restoring a woman's health.[46] His enslaved experimental subjects were the ultimate in controllable patients, and he eventually chose to control his slaves' pain in a peculiar manner: He addicted the slave women to morphine, but he gave it to them—"some form of opium in as large doses as can be borne, at least twice in 24 hours"—only *after* surgery, administering it for several weeks each time. Sims explained that opium "calms the nerves, inspires hope, relieves the scalding of the urine," and permitted "the patient doomed to a fortnight's horizontal position [to] pass the time with pleasant dreams, and delightful sensations instead of painful forebodings and intolerable sufferings." The morphine did ease recovery, but it did not allay the pain of the procedure itself, so this practice perplexed some of Sims's contemporaries.[47] The most logical explanation is that this practice had more to do with controlling the women's behavior than controlling their pain, because the addiction weakened their will to resist repeated procedures.[48]

As mentioned earlier, the medical association between assiduous cleanliness and infection had not yet been drawn, and although Sims was a man of scrupulously clean surgical habits, the constant exposure of the organic sutures to pathogens caused the women repeated infections. Sims, however, had a serendipitous inspiration: He decided to devise sutures of silver. Silver did not harbor pathogens, and the infections were finally tamed, allowing the possibility of healing. In the end, Sims triumphantly recorded closing Anarcha's largest, fingertip-size fistula.

He announced that he had perfected the vesicovaginal fistula operation in May of 1849, after scores of operations over five years—more than thirty operations on Anarcha alone. In 1852, Sims's paper on vesicovaginal fistula repair was published in the prestigious *American Journal of the Medical Sciences.* It made his national reputation.[49]

Sims became the celebrated "father of American gynecology," and as such his place in history was assured. W. J. S. McKay, M.D., spoke for his fellow surgeons in predicting that "when the history of modern gynecology is written, the work that [Dr. Ephraim] McDowell did will be represented as the dawn; and the first bright planet that appeared in the dim light of that dawn was Marion Sims. . . ."[50]

In the early 1850s, bouts with malaria forced Sims north to New York City, where he became a medical lion who built a society practice, did research with blacks and immigrant women, taught medicine, and held many influential positions in hospitals, medical societies, and in academe. He founded the New York Women's Hospital, "the first hospital for women," which was built at Park Avenue and Fiftieth Street, the present site of the Waldorf-Astoria Hotel. Beginning in 1862, he also sojourned abroad, where his medical fame gave him entrée into royal circles. He and his family became the toast of Second Empire Paris while Sims attended the Empress Eugénie and other members of the French royal family.[51] Across two continents, monuments, memorials, and clinics sprang up in his wake, including the one that now stands in New York's Central Park, all celebrating his stature as a physician "treating alike empress and slave."

Sims wrote copiously about his work and medical philosophies as well as his life. In Alabama, Sims's vigorous defense of the slavery system had been liberally seasoned with "nigger." However, once up north, he hid the ethnicity of his subjects, portraying them as white in the illustrations that accompanied his accounts of the surgery. His duplicitous praise of "the indomitable courage of these long suffering women"[52] failed to mention that it was chattel slavery and morphine, not courage, that had bound the women to his surgical table.

Sims never disclosed whether he closed the fistulae of his other slave patients, although many who have written about him seem to take it as a matter of course that he did so. However, his erstwhile colleague Bozeman insisted that "not one half" of the slave women they worked upon together were afforded relief by the years of painful surgeries.[53] Bozeman reported correcting some of the remaining fistulae himself, using a surgical innovation of "button sutures," a technique he perfected by performing this procedure on other black slave women—Kitty, Dinah, and an unnamed "mulatto girl."[54] Bozeman even described a case of vesicovaginal fistula *created* by Sims when he removed the bladder stones of a nine-year-old slave girl.[55]

Sims was not pleased and used the New York Academy of Medicine as a bully pulpit to attack Bozeman for appropriating his technique. But Bozeman was not the only challenger to Sims's primacy as inventor of vesicovaginal fistula repair. In 1838, fifteen years before Sims took up the problem, Virginia surgeon John Peter Mettauer had devised a similar procedure, using lead rather than silver sutures. Mettauer had operated on twenty-five women in Prince Edward County, Virginia "a large slave holding area,"[56] but cured only one woman. Mettauer blamed the slave women for his inability to help them: Speaking of one, he claimed, "I believe this case, nevertheless could have been cured in the process of time, especially if sexual intercourse could have been prevented, which intercourse I have no doubt, defeated several of the operations."[57]

Antebellum Ethics

Sims was widely criticized not only by today's ethicists but also by some nineteenth-century contemporaries on medical and moral grounds. An intriguing 2003 New York Times essay observed, "Living in an era that uncritically celebrated white male doctors, the historians contended, these writers had viewed Sims far too favorably."[58] But the criticism is actually as old as Sims's surgeries. Some contemporaries were quite critical of his claims, and not only Bozeman but also African American physicians characterized Sims's surgeries as abuses. Cardiac specialist Dr. Daniel Hale Williams, who successfully performed one of the first open-heart operations, was an especially vocal critic. Williams was not born until 1858, years after Sims's vaginal-repair surgeries were completed, but he studied and roundly condemned Sims and the continuing practice of performing surgery on unwilling black subjects. Williams also took Sims to task for pronouncements he continued to make about the sexual health and, by implication, the morality of black women. For example, Sims had reported that "60 percent" of Negro women had uterine cancer (a disease then associated with early and frequent sexual contact) or uterine fibroids. Williams demanded proof or at least evidence, but Sims had produced no raw data nor any investigative report to buttress this claim. Williams wondered in print how Sims could have determined this, when black women were not permitted into white hospitals.[59]

Dr. W. Montague Cobb, another illustrious African American surgeon, also vociferously opposed abusive experimentation with blacks, but he defended Sims. "To refer to Anarcha and the five other vesico-vaginal patients whom Sims treated with her, as human guinea pigs would be grossly unfair, as Sims continued to treat and provide for these girls at his own expense for three years in the little hospital in his yard, against enormous pressures from his family, the profession and the public . . . one of the great humanitarian as well as scientific landmarks of American surgery."[60] However, the women were held involuntarily for Sims's convenience, so requesting moral credit for lodging them is absurd. What's more, the women's lodging was not free: They did work, without pay, and Sims did profit from the surgeries, whereas only Anarcha seems definitely to have benefited from the four years of pain.

Moreover, was the building to which Cobb referred really a hospital, a designation that implies that Sims's primary intent was to render medical care to his slaves? Sims is widely admired as the founder of the nation's "first women's hospital," but this appellation refers to the more prepossessing structure on Park Avenue in New York City. If the New York structure housed the first women's hospital, then the Montgomery, Alabama, slave quarters must have been something else, perhaps a laboratory that confined unwilling subjects. Cobb's defense of Sims shows that social class and varying ethical perceptions, not only race, have fueled this lengthy controversy.

Whatever his true cure rate, Sims's silver sutures did help to end a real medical tragedy for many women, and some excuse the abuse of enslaved women on this basis. This essentially utilitarian argument presents an ethical balance sheet, with the savage medical abuse of captive women on one hand and countless women saved from painful invalidism on the other.[61]

However, such an argument ignores the ethical concept of social justice, and these experiments violated this essential value because the suffering and the benefits have been distributed in an unfair way, leading to distributive injustice. In this case, the most powerless group, which is also a racially distinct group *and* a captive group, is the group upon which doctors inflicted harm "for the greater good." Another, privileged group enjoys the benefits but shares neither the pain nor the risks. Thus the moral unacceptability is clear.

But the dangers of such practices are more shadowy. One danger of violating distributive justice is that this tends to perpetuate social inequities, and this is exactly what has happened with vesicovaginal fistula.

Today, as in the nineteenth century, the overwhelming majority of women who suffer from vesicovaginal fistula are poor blacks without access to quality health care—women in sub-Saharan Africa. They do so because they share the same risk factors as Lucy and Anarcha—malnutrition and poor perinatal care—and they have little access to surgeons who can repair their fistulas. The beneficiaries of the surgery today are many, but the same sort of women whose misery made the surgery possible are excluded. Sims's popular legacy reflects the face he turned to white women of his class, an image coined into enduring medical fame and gratitude. Only enslaved blacks such as Lucy and Anarcha saw the hideous obverse of that coin, and history has silenced them.

Whatever his ethical sins, Sims's surgical exploitation of enslaved blacks was consonant with the medical practice of his time. For black women, forced experimentation was the standard of care. A Donalson, Louisiana, surgeon named Dr. François Marie Prévost used enslaved black women to perfect cesarean sections, performing four such deliveries on them between 1822 and 1831.[62] In 1830, he performed his first successful cesarean on a woman Prévost described as a "fat colored primipara [a woman giving birth for the first time] with a contracted pelvis."[63] Twenty-nine of the subsequent thirty-six southern surgical cases to duplicate and perfect the procedure were performed on black women.[64] Prévost's contemporary Dr. Ephraim McDowell was the first to perform an ovariotomy (removal of an ovary) successfully, and he perfected this dangerous and excruciatingly radical surgery on his four slave women. McDowell performed his research in Kentucky, a state with very few African Americans.[65] So did Dr. P. C. Spencer of Petersburg, Virginia, who devised a novel surgical procedure for bladder stones after equally painful surgical experimentation on slaves. The discoveries of Robert Jennings, who eventually invented typhoid vaccine, were also tested first on blacks.

But what of other experimentation, that not described in professional journals and the halls of academe? African Americans have long circulated accounts of doctors who seized hapless blacks from the street to experiment on them. These accounts are usually derided as being paranoid, but consider this incident, originally described in a nineteenth-century textbook on the history of anesthesia:

In Anderson, South Carolina, in 1839 a group seized a black boy and forced him to inhale ether from a handkerchief that was held over his mouth and nose. Soon the boy became motionless and unconscious and was feared dead. However, after an hour he revived, no worse for his alarming experience.[66]

This incident convinced Dr. Crawford W. Long that ether could safely be tested as a potential anesthetic, as he did using three black slaves, followed by the amputation of an etherized boy's toe in 1842, and a man's finger in 1845.[67]

Another illuminating aspect of such incidents is how they differ from the conventional representations of experimentation. Robert Hinckley's *The First Operation Under Ether*, an oil painting that dominates one wall of Harvard's Frances A. Countway Library of Medicine, shows ether being administered to a supine white male attended by impeccably clad physicians in a theater holding tiers of enraptured doctors. This beautifully composed image evokes a sober atmosphere of reverent wonder underscored by the somber tones and formal stances of the surgeons. Its grandeur has informed many a viewer's conception of the experimental investigation of ether, but it is an idealized rendering, rife with inaccuracies. Although it purports to depict the first use of ether as an anesthetic, it does not.[68] This stately image is a beautiful fiction with a brutally factual negative: The body of a black slave seized by laughing medical thugs, forced to inhale ether, and left for dead in the road.

Some who ascribe African Americans' poor health to their wariness of the U.S. health system claim that African Americans have always opposed medical experimentation independently of any medical abuses. But from an early time, black Americans themselves have engaged in therapeutic medical experimentation. African herbalists investigated, tested, and perfected the use of plants they found in the New World for the new ailments that afflicted both blacks and whites. They adapted medicines and techniques they brought with them, such as the stimulant kola nut, which was adopted so widely that it eventually supplied the main ingredient for Coca-Cola.

In 1721, an enslaved African named Onesimus proposed a novel medical technique that saved the city of Boston from a dread smallpox epidemic and provided the first important medical advance in the New World. Onesimus, "a pretty Intelligent Fellow," had been given to Cotton Mather, the Puritan preacher and amateur scientist,[69] by a grateful congregation in 1706. Because a case of smallpox conferred complete lifelong immunity, slave dealers routinely advertised the fact (or the fiction) that a slave had survived a bout of the disease.[70] Therefore, Cotton Mather soon asked his acquisition whether he had had smallpox.

> He answered both Yes and No; and then told me that he had undergone an Operation which had given him something of the smalpox & would forever praeserve him from it; adding that it was often used among the Guaramantese & whoever had the courage to use it, was forever free from the fear of contagion.[71]

Onesimus was speaking of inoculation against smallpox, a successful preventive measure that was widely practiced throughout Africa.[72] Smallpox inoculation took various forms, but the common denominator was that a small amount of the pus in scabs or other infected matter from someone with smallpox was deliberately introduced into the broken skin of a well person. This "variolation," as Mather called it, evoked mild symptoms, followed by permanent, complete immunity, the Holy Grail of smallpox prevention for Western doctors and scientists. Onesimus showed Cotton Mather the technique used by those in his native country.[73]

When a smallpox epidemic revisited Boston in the summer of 1721, Cotton Mather and his clerical brethren called for a mass inoculation of the people of Boston.[74] However, the city's physicians, led by William Douglass, resented being told by a gaggle of ministers that Africans had devised the panacea they had long sought. Zabdiel Boylston was the only physician[75] to embrace inoculation, but not before testing it on 2 black slaves, then 248 more—as well as his own six-year-old son.[76] Boylston then proved they had achieved immunity by exposing them to cases of smallpox. The physicians' resistance turned uglier—and violent. The popular press played no small role, serving as the battleground while doctors condemned variolation because it was the laughable, "unchristian" product of occult African practices. The fact that inoculation worked seemed not to play into physicians' assessments, and their bitter attacks were not confined to the intellectual sphere: A lighted grenade was thrown into Mather's house, along with a note declaring, "Cotton Mather, You Dog, Dam You: I'll Inoculate you with this, with a pox to you."[77] This prompted him to complain, "I do not know why it is more unlawful to learn of Africans, how to help against the Poison of the Small-Pox, than it is to learn of our Indians, how to help against the Poison of a Rattle-Snake." In the end, the obvious reduction of death rates—from 14 percent to less than 2 percent—convinced doctors that inoculation was the city's savior.[78] Approximately 8,000 Bostonians became ill and 844 died; but while one in every nine untreated patients succumbed, only one in every forty-eight inoculated people was stricken.[79]

Mather made a scientific report to the Royal Society in 1722.[80] By 1750, inoculation was standard in America and Europe, as it long had been in Africa.[81] Historians hailed it as "the earliest important experiment in America in preventive medicine,"[82] but Onesimus came to share the fate of nearly every slave who contributed to medical research: facelessness.

Can we judge eighteenth-century doctors for experimenting on blacks? A common apology for experimental abuse insists that we should not apply present-day medical ethics to the medical behaviors of yesterday, which were governed by less enlightened medical standards for everyone, not just African Americans. However, ethical strictures did govern the behavior of nineteenth-century physicians. Before the mid-twentieth century, these binding ethical standards were not enforced by federal laws, but consisted of medical oaths, professional codes, and rules governing clinical conduct within medical schools, hospitals, and other institutions. These rules were carefully adhered to in cases of white patients but were routinely broken for African Americans.

The harm done to African Americans in such scenarios goes far beyond the injuries to the subjects themselves. As African Americans came to learn of the experiments that Sims and his contemporaries conducted, these experiments fed an aversion to the health system. They also harmed the community of African Americans by strengthening a perception of them as appropriate human fodder for research.

Another recurrent ethical issue was raised by researchers' contention that blacks were responsible for their own illnesses. Experimental remedies sought to correct disease caused by blacks' inherent physical flaws, so if an experimental procedure was painful or dangerous, the logic went, blacks had only themselves to blame, not the surgeon. Some, such as Dr. Mettauer of Virginia, claimed that if blacks had cooperated more fully, the procedures could have been perfected.

Researchers who exploited enslaved blacks were guilty of more than ethical blindness. These early medical investigators also practiced bad science on a very basic level: They were simply illogical. For example, many researchers argued that blacks were so different from whites—less intelligent, much less sensitive to pain, possessing numerous physical anomalies as well as markedly different patterns of disease immunity—as to constitute a separate species. Given this supposedly vast biological chasm between blacks and whites, how could scientists logically infer results of medical experiments from blacks to whites? This particular logical flaw recurred regularly in early research with African Americans.

But, logical or not, scientists' fascination with the black body as a medical entity was about to enter new arenas, from the clinic to the circus.

CHAPTER 3

CIRCUS AFRICANUS

The Popular Display of Black Bodies

The Negro "with us" is not an actual physical being of flesh and bones and blood, but a hideous monster of the mind, ugly beyond all physical portraying, so utterly and ineffably monstrous as to frighten reason from its throne, and justice from its balance, and mercy from its hallowed temple, and to blot out shame and probity, and the eternal sympathies of nature, so far as these things have presence in the breasts or being of American republicans! No sir! It is a constructive Negro—a John Roe and Richard Doe Negro, that haunts with grim presence the precincts of this republic, shaking his gory locks over legislative halls and family prayers.

—JAMES McCUNE SMITH, M.D.

By 1904, swashbuckling missionary-explorer Samuel Phillips Verner had acquired a veritable Noah's Ark of exotic fauna during three trips to the interior of the Dark Continent. The last expedition was commissioned in 1903 by the St. Louis Exposition Company, which paid the South Carolina–born Verner to hunt men instead of monkeys: He was to bring African Pygmies to America for display at the St. Louis World's Fair. Upon his return to America, Verner found himself romanticized as a reincarnation of Dr. David Livingstone, whom he claimed as his "posthumous mentor." As an ordained minister in the Presbyterian Church, Verner was also lionized in church circles as an imparter of morality to the Congo natives he doggedly hectored at the Southern Presbyterian Missionary House in Luebo, chiding them for their immodest dress and sexual behavior. His American admirers did not know that between 1895 and 1899, Verner had fathered a daughter and son on an African orphan girl there.

By 1906, the World's Fair was over and the cash-strapped Verner was selling off his animals, artifacts, and more. Upon the receipt of a financial gift, he bestowed a prized equatorial specimen upon William T. Hornaday, director of the Bronx Zoological Gardens.[1] Verner's present was twenty-three-year-old Ota Benga, an Mbuti widower from southern Africa, in what is now the Democratic Republic of Congo. Around 1903, Benga had returned from a hunting trip, only to find his village in smoking ruins and his wife, children, and entire tribe slaughtered by Force Publique thugs supported by the Belgian government. Benga himself was seized and sold into Verner's hands.

Hornaday's views about the natives of sub-Saharan Africa mirrored Verner's own, conscripting Darwin in the service of racism: He told the *New York Times* that there exists "a close analogy of the African savage to the apes."[2]

Scientific American agreed: "The Congo pygmies [are] small, apelike, elfish creatures, furtive and mischievous, they closely parallel the brownies and goblins of our fairy tales. They live in the dense tangled forests in absolute savagery . . . while they exhibit many ape-like features in their bodies."[3]

But Hornaday espoused a more progressive vision as a scientific artist, and we have him to thank for the modern American zoo. As chief taxidermist of the National Museum (the Smithsonian), a position he held until 1890, he had inherited a static mausoleum of tatty taxidermy enshrined on plaster pedestals with only laconic placards to suggest what the animal had been like in life. In 1888, Hornaday persuaded the museum to add a wing of living animals in lifelike settings, which proved so popular a revolution that it became the National Zoological Gardens. He resigned over differences of vision, but in 1896 he reemerged as the first director of the New York Zoological Gardens (known as the Bronx Zoo), the world's largest, lushest, and most varied zoo. Hornaday's passion was for colorful verisimilitude in the re-creation of his animals' natural habitats. With a verdant Bronx park as his canvas, Hormaday installed colorful exotic animals of every genus grouped with their natural companions amid native vegetation.

So when Benga was locked in the monkey house, before the staring crowd and with keepers always nearby, he was given a bow and arrow to brandish, his cage was littered with bones, and his two cage mates were Dinah, a gorilla, and an orangutan called Dohung. The placard on Benga's enclosure read, "The African Pygmy, 'Ota Benga.' Height 4 feet

11 inches. Weight 103 pounds. Brought from the Kasai River, Congo Free State, South Central Africa by Dr. Samuel P. Verner. Exhibited each afternoon during September."[4] A September 10 *New York Times* headline trumpeted, BUSHMAN SHARES A CAGE WITH THE BRONX PARK APES.[5]

Black New Yorkers were incensed, and representatives of the clergy, led by the Reverend Dr. MacArthur, pressed Mayor George B. McClellan to withdraw the city's support from the exhibit. As another minister, a Reverend Gordon, told the *New York Times;* "Our race . . . is depressed enough without exhibiting one of us with the apes. We think we are worthy of being considered human beings, with souls."[6]

The *Times* turned an unsympathetic ear to African American objections.

> One reverend colored brother objects to the curious exhibition on the grounds that it is an impious effort to lend credibility to Darwin's dreadful theories . . . the reverend colored brother should be told that evolution . . . is now taught in the textbooks of all the schools, and that it is no more debatable than the multiplication table.[7]

The swipe at creationism did not address Gordon's immediate concerns but did hit a nerve among many whites who shared Gordon's outrage. Some were angered by this inhumane insult to blacks, and others, who opposed the teaching of Darwin's theory of evolution, were afraid that Benga's dramatic presence would offer a powerful plebeian argument for the theory of evolution. The entertainment of a "monkey-man" might persuade people who were untouched by the theory's scientific merits. Mayor McClellan snubbed the black delegation, referring them to the Parks Department, and another *Times* account hinted that Benga differed little from the zoo's animals.

> Ota Benga . . . is a normal specimen of his race or tribe, with a brain as much developed as are those of its other members . . . and can be studied with profit. . . . The pygmies are an efficient people in their native forests . . . but they are very low in the human scale, and the suggestion that Benga should be in a school instead of a

cage ignores the high probability that school would be a place of torture to him and one from which he could draw no advantage whatever. . . .[8]

A lively epistolary debate ensued in the pages of the *Times,* heavily weighted in favor of retaining Benga, and many of the letters were signed by respondents with M.D. and Ph.D. degrees. One doctor suggested, "It is a pity that Dr. Hornaday does not introduce the system of short lectures or talks in connection with such exhibitions . . . [to] help our clergymen to familiarize themselves with the scientific point of view so foreign to many of them."[9]

Times journalists agreed that Benga provided a valuable tool for illustrating basic evolutionary precepts: To oppose his internment was to oppose science. These precepts included physical similarities to the lower primates that scientific racism was beginning to popularize widely. Anthropometric portraits of blacks and apes demonstrated how blacks' facial angles, stature, stance, and gait resembled those of monkeys, chimpanzees, and orangutans. Blacks' hair, or "wool," was compared to animal pelts. Such uncomplimentary images were published in scientific journals and would soon adorn children's textbooks. Scientists alleged that apes preferred to mate with black women, just as black men lusted after white women, their own evolutionary "betters."[10]

At the zoo, the *Times* revealed that Benga's situation was escalating:

There were 40,000 visitors to the park on Sunday. Nearly every man, woman and child of this crowd made for the monkey house to see the star attraction in the park, the wild man from Africa. They chased him about the grounds all day, howling, jeering, and yelling. Some of them poked him in the ribs, others tripped him up, all laughed at him.[11]

Finally, Benga retaliated by attacking visitors with a knife and a bow and arrows, and the zoo ejected him. Black New Yorkers organized a collection, which was insufficient to return him home, as he wished, but provided enough to cap his filed teeth and send him to the Virginia Theological Seminary and College, where he proved himself an able student.[12] Benga then found work in a Lynchburg, Virginia, tobacco factory, where he fit in well as an efficient worker and a beloved Pied Piper who taught local children to fish and hunt. But he spoke often and tearfully of wishing to return home to the Congo, and when he realized he could never save enough for passage, his depression became profound. In 1916, Benga committed suicide with that ubiquitous icon of Western technological achievement, a handgun.

Hornaday had the last word in his obituary of Benga, which appeared in the *Zoological Bulletin,* took a semicomic tone, and was filled with uncomplimentary untruths that fit his racist agenda.[13]

Benga's tragedy illustrates how American scientists found black bodies useful even when they were not trying new medications or surgeries. This chapter focuses upon the popular public display and imaging of black bodies, but the boundary separating popular display from medical display was a porous one, a permeable membrane with copious migration in both directions. Some medicalized freak body types were exclusive to blacks, who had a patent on "white Negroes" and, in the United States, a near monopoly on "primitive peoples." Even the black idiot savant, a perennial attraction, was considered more freakish than the white variety because his intellectual gifts offered a greater contrast to blacks' ostensibly low intelligence.

In the late eighteenth century, long before the 1859 publication of *The Origin of Species,* medical researchers had addressed scientific questions regarding human hierarchies by displaying black bodies in contexts that emphasized supposed parallels to animals and children, even as black scientists and abolitionists used the same bodies to illustrate the intimate kinship between whites and blacks. Unusual or exotic black bodies also provided wildly popular entertainment with a medical flavor. Alert entrepreneurs, from P. T. Barnum to Harvard's Louis Agassiz, exploited them for profit and fame.

Whether one was gawking at a "white Negro," a 161-year-old black wet nurse, an African giantess, or a Hottentot "missing link" in a cage, the subject was usually forced to display his body. He may have been a slave, a "freak" with an anomalous body, or a kidnapped freedman.[14] However, a few enterprising souls offered themselves up for pay, especially in the early days of quasi-scientific displays.

Advertisements for Myself: Henry Moss

Around 1790, when Henry Moss realized that his body had embarked upon a mystifying transformation into whiteness, he cut out the middleman to exhibit himself.[15] Unlike later sideshow freaks who had to remain mute while barkers trumpeted the manufactured exotica that passed for their life stories, Moss was his own barker. Proudly straddling a museum chair or slowly strolling the stage of a saloon, Moss peeled the linen from his variegated body in a tantalizing medical striptease while he unreeled his own story. From his humble but free 1754 birth in Goochland County, Virginia, to his Revolutionary War exploits as a soldier in South Carolina and Virginia, to the mysterious gradual lightening that was spreading his fame, Moss spoke for himself before enraptured crowds in Philadelphia taverns and museums, charging twenty-five cents per person—heady fees for 1796, the year he addressed the American Philosophical Society.[16]

Moss became a familiar figure even in Europe, where his piebald visage graced chocolates and German almanacs. President George Washington was a face in the throng when Moss appeared at Mr. Leech's tavern, the Sign of the Black Horse, in Philadelphia in 1796.[17] So were prominent racial theorists of the day, including the Reverend Samuel Stanhope Smith and an entranced Benjamin Rush, M.D., who is now remembered as the father of American psychiatry and who then believed that black skin was the manifestation of a type of leprosy that he called "Negritude." Calling blacks lepers certainly sounds like the pronouncement of an inveterate racist, and this is how Rush is sometimes regarded. However, Rush was not a racist, but a passionate abolitionist, and his views of black physiology were nuanced. Rush believed that blacks were diseased but that they could be cured. He welcomed the various albinos, *leucoethiopes,* and vitiligo-stricken "white Negroes" as "hopeful monsters," living proof that blacks could become healthily white. Cure was desirable, averred Rush, because eliminating black skin would eliminate the chief social and religious argument for enslavement and because he believed blacks themselves preferred white skin.[18]

Rush hungered to understand and hoped to duplicate the process by which Negro skin lost its color, and he theorized that "pressure and friction"—violent rubbing—could banish color from the rete mucosum, the fictional skin layer. Rush never took up the scalpel against Moss to test this theory, but he cataloged the methods that other physicians had used to whiten black skin and hair, including hydrochloric acid, bleeding, purging, the juice of unripe peaches, muriatic acid, and even pronounced fear.[19] Rush did experiment with sulfuric acid on black skins, probably those of cadavers.[20]

In late 1796, Rush's protégé, Dr. Charles Caldwell, acquired Henry Moss in a manner that can be read as a disquieting infringement upon Moss's freedom.

> I took him in some measure under my care, procured for him suitable lodgings and accommodation, induced many persons to visit him and kept him *under my strict and constant observation* and by his permission and *for a slight reward* [emphasis added], made on him such experiments as suited my purpose.[21]

Although Caldwell was careful to note that he obtained Moss's permission, one has only Caldwell's word that Moss willingly accepted the loss of autonomy, social status, and income in exchange for "suitable" but heavily monitored lodgings. I am not convinced, in part because this scenario evokes an eerie parallel to one of the most infamous exploitative experimental relationships in history—that between Alexis St. Martin, a poor, illiterate French-Canadian backwoods trapper, and Dr. William Beaumont, who used him as an experimental subject for eleven years, beginning in 1822.[22] St. Martin was a consistently reluctant subject, but Beaumont portrayed him as a willing one.[23] Also, Caldwell's veracity is suspect. In his 1855 memoirs, for example, he falsely claimed that Moss's skin had regained its color.

Caldwell forced Moss to exercise vigorously in order to produce perspiration, which he examined closely for exuded color.[24] Caldwell also minutely recorded the expanding area of Moss's white skin. Admitting that he could not find Moss's rete mucosum, Caldwell concluded that it "must" have retreated deeper into the body, away from the gaze of scientists. Only anatomical dissection can find it.

Henry Moss was lost to history after he left Caldwell in 1796, his appetite for self-exhibition apparently sated, and within a decade his brand of self-promotion became unthinkable. The display of black bodies was conducted in a more repressive atmosphere as black-white relations grew ever more acerbic, fed by abolitionist fervor, large-scale slave revolts, and legal challenges to slavery. In 1806, for example, a very dark-skinned male slave owned by Major Banks of Williamsburg, Virginia, began to turn white. Dr. Alexander D. Galt urged that he be displayed as a spectacle that would "excite the curiosity and wonder of everyone," but the slave remained voiceless and unnamed.[25]

Moreover, physicians and owners controlled and transformed the nature of the bodies they displayed by enhancing the distinctiveness of their appearance and by showcasing them in a propagandistic environment that emphasized freakishness, evolutionary inferiority, and bestiality. Barkers invented fictitious histories that emphasized the displayed specimens' alien nature. The features of displayed blacks were used to locate blacks' low status on a supposed evolutionary continuum between monkeys and whites.

The paying hordes of voyeurs, museum curators, medical students, researchers, and professors at such medical circuses grew progressively more intrusive as gaping, sketching, photographing, and ribald taunts led inexorably to physical violation. Spectators palpated and measured labia and penile lengths and tittered as they asked demeaning questions about subjects' personal habits and sexual prowess. This prurience reached its height in the display of the "Hottentot Venuses."

Delta of Venus: Saartjie Baartman

If one wonders how Ota Benga or anyone else could have been clapped into a zoo in twentieth-century New York City, it is important to realize that there had been precedents. The most infamous medicalized display of a captive black befell Saartjie (pronounced "SART-kay," and meaning "little Sara" in Afrikaans) Baartman, who was born in 1789, the year the French Revolution produced the Declaration of the Rights of Man. Baartman was, like Benga, a member of the Khoisan hunter-gatherers; she lived at the southeastern cape of Africa, in what is now South Africa.[26]

There, Baartman worked as a servant, perhaps an enslaved one, for Peter Cesar, a colonist who handed her over to British naval surgeon Dr. William Dunlop, who induced Baartman to sail with him to London in

1810. He assured her that she could quickly make her fortune, but Dunlop intended himself to be the beneficiary of her European debut.

Baartman did not know she was about to enter an arena where she would become an object of unbridled medical curiosity and physical lust. Since the late seventeenth century, the Khoi had been regarded as "the missing link between human and ape species."[27] Theories that ranked ethnic groups consistently placed Baartman's Khoi people, like Ota Benga's, at the bottom of the evolutionary scale.[28] On the basis of their supposedly overdeveloped genitals, Linnaeus classified the Khoi as a divergent branch of humanity, one that he named *Homo monstrosis monorchidei*, relegating them to the back alleys of evolution.[29] In 1839, Samuel Morton[30] described the Hottentot as "the nearest approximation to the lower animals." Buffon classed them with the monkeys.

Khoi women's dramatically endowed figures and especially their large, fleshy buttocks (medically termed *steatopygia)* were seen as markers for their sexual prowess.[31] Francis Galton, the father of eugenics, waxed rhapsodic about the extravagant figures of these women, declaring that they must be the envy of European belles.[32] A popular ditty observed that the black African "had not wit nor honestie to cover once his Taile," hinting how much the Victorians had inferred about morality and intelligence from the relative nakedness of Africans. Most scientists agreed that the hot, damp tropical climate created a licentiousness and sexual profligacy in African women that was unknown among European women.

The ascendance of medical theories about the "alien" attributes of black women had created a strongly sexualized interest in Khoi women. In an 1819 *Dictionary of Medical Science* essay, ethnologist J. J. Virey described black women as possessing a "voluptuousness" and "degree of lascivity" far beyond any known to whites.[33] Abetted by their knowledge that many African peoples practiced female circumcision, scientists believed that African women in general and Khoi women in particular had oversized inner labia that hung down when they stood.[34]

Dunlop had accordingly arranged to put Baartman's body under anatomical scrutiny. Men of science made pilgrimages to London's academic and medical settings to sketch, measure, and endlessly analyze her steatopygous buttocks and her extended inner labia, which they dubbed the "Hottentot apron," or the *sinus pudoris*, Latin for "veil of shame." Her body suffered regular violations that alternated between rape and the most intimate of medical examinations—one wonders whether she discerned much difference between them. She was displayed nude or bedecked in animal skins with accoutrements—spears and bones—that her handlers thought fitting for a "Hottentot," as her people were disparagingly called by Europeans. Hottentot is an onomatopoeic name invented by early Dutch colonists to describe the inimitable clicking sounds of the Khoi language, but Westerners applied the term imprecisely to all short Southern Africans.[35]

Even Baartman's name was stripped from her and replaced with the sardonic sobriquet "Hottentot Venus," and she was often portrayed with Cupid, the Western embodiment of carnal attraction, perched on her ample buttocks. Thus, in stark contrast to the "real" white Venus of sublime but unattainable beauty, Baartman embodied not only the boundary between man and animal but also the lure of the bestial, the base, and grotesquely hypersexual.

Baartman was not the only African woman to be exhibited as a Hottentot Venus, but she became an important exemplar of the medically exploitative display of black peoples. One may be tempted to think that the display of Africans such as Baartman is unconnected to the plight of their enslaved American contemporaries, but medical scientists viewed them as the same peoples. This era saw the burgeoning of academic ethnology, that branch of anthropology devoted to the study of race, and what scientists thought true of Africans was also believed of American "Negroes." There was some biological and much social basis to this belief. Although many African Americans sprang from an admixture of African, European, and Native American forebears, approximately one in ten American blacks was a native African, even after slave importation officially ended about 1810.[36] Also, exhibited "Africans" were often black Americans who had been given manufactured exotic origins. But perhaps most important was the stubborn social denial of the widespread black-white intermingling in America. Thus scientists insisted that what could be said of Baartman applied equally to her enslaved sisters in America.

Over the next five years, Baartman met with much rougher usage. She was made to stand naked at parties of the wealthy and to impersonate a chained animal in garish Piccadilly, where the mob paid a shilling a head to gape and shout vulgarities. They began by staring at her in disgust, progressed to laughing at her, and ended by being aroused by her. Because black women were considered as shameless as European women were modest and chaste, such behavior was possible even for Victorian gentlemen.

Many accounts of Baartman's life insist that she was a completely helpless victim of European impresarios. But in 1810, Robert Wedderburn of Jamaica, founder of London's African Association, complained to the authorities that Baartman was being demeaned. Interestingly, Baartman denied before an English court that she was being held against her will, and indicated that she appeared in order to earn a share of the attraction's profits.[37] However, no contract was produced and she probably received little or nothing of the hoped-for profits, so she certainly was exploited.

The next phase of her life left no room for ambiguous hopes. In 1814, London theater impresario Henry Taylor took her to Paris,[38] where he paraded her in degrading animalistic displays in circuses amid the "talking pigs, animal monsters, and human oddities."[39] Taylor sold Baartman to an animal trainer named Reaux, who provided her final descent when she was forced into a cage and made to behave like "a wild beast." In 1815, the last year of her life, Baartman began drinking heavily, which may have contributed to her death from infectious illness at twenty-seven.[40]

Western medicine was not finished with its Hottentot Venus. In 1817, Baron Georges Cuvier, the French zoologist and physiologist who founded the field of comparative anatomy, dissected her body. He was not an objective observer, having already been convinced of her people's inferiority. "Their colour is black, their hair crimped, their heads squashed and their noses flat. Their protruding mouths and thick lips are strikingly similar to those of the apes. The peoples which compose this race have always been savages."[41] Cuvier cast Baartman's body in plaster in 1817, preserved her brain, vulva, and anus in glass jars, then stripped the flesh from her skeleton and hung it on display in Paris's Musée de l'Homme.[42] He noted, "She had a way of pouting her lips exactly like that we have observed in the Orang-Outang. . . . Her lips were monstrously large; her ear was like that of many apes, being small, the tragus [the bit of cartilage that partially covers the opening of the ear] weak. . . . These are animal characters."

Cuvier had once noted that Baartman possessed a tenacious memory; she also spoke Dutch, English, and French. Yet, he left her this final assessment: "These races with depressed and compressed skulls are condemned to a never-ending inferiority."[43]

Dissecting History: Joice Heth

No discussion of racialized American circus hucksterism can ignore the legendary P. T. Barnum, who exhibited many blacks. In 1835, however, Barnum was just a twenty-five-year-old bankrupt eking out a living in a New York City dry-goods store.[44] Joice Heth catapulted Barnum to national fame after he purchased her from R. W. Lindsay, a promoter who had been unable to capitalize on the manufactured identity he had created for Heth as the superannuated "mammy" of former President George Washington, who had died in 1799 but had already achieved political deity. We do not know Heth's actual origins, and Barnum's unreliable memoirs spin an assortment of contradictory tales, but he was able to convince audiences of Heth's manufactured African origin and more.

Heth debuted on August 10, 1835, at Niblo's Garden in New York and was a huge success as Barnum barked the tale of the "Greatest Natural and National Curiosity in the World," the black woman who had held the Father of Our Country, her "dear little George," to her breast, had given him suck and who had taught him Negro spirituals. The claim that Heth had been Washington's nurse entailed an even more incredible assertion: Barnum swore that she was 161 years old, and many believed this.

Heth's unusually black body helped to deflect skeptics because it was gnarled by a breathtaking decrepitude that simultaneously thrilled and repelled. For Heth was skeletal (Barnum claimed she weighed only forty-six pounds), both legs and one arm were paralyzed, and her leathery skin was very deeply wrinkled. Her eyes were gone, the legacy of some unknown ailment, she was toothless, and her uncut horny nails curved "like talons." Confronted with this grotesque sight, even lay spectators indulged in a medical gaze, touching her systematically, feeling the depth of her wrinkles, and taking her pulse. Their descriptions consistently identified Heth both with Africa and with death. "Indeed she is a mere skeleton covered with skin and her whole appearance very much resembles a mummy of the days of the Pharoahs [sic], taken entire from the tombs of the catacombs of Egypt," declaimed one pseudonymous eyewitness.[45]

Even newspapers that avidly covered Heth's subsequent seven months of appearances throughout the southern and mid-Atlantic states gravely discussed the merits of her claim to longevity, and some mused on its medical significance. The *Evening Star,* for example, averred that such longevity as Heth enjoyed was rare among northern blacks but common in the South, their native habitat.[46] That the sensationalistic penny press should have devoted articles to the fantastic debate is unsurprising, but so did "six-penny" Whig papers that were usually inclined to greater sophistication and skepticism.

But because many viewers refused to believe she was really 161 years old, Barnum announced that upon her death, she would be publicly autopsied by a physician to determine whether she was a hoax. Of course, Barnum knew she was a hoax because she was *his* hoax; the voice spinning the fictional history was his.

> Joice Heth is unquestionably the most astonishing and interesting curiosity in the world. She was the slave of Augustine Washington (the father of Gen. Washington) and was the first person to put cloths *[sic]* on the unconscious infant who was destined to lead our heroic fathers on to glory, to victory, and to freedom. To use her own language when speaking of her young master, George Washington, SHE RAISED HIM! Joice Heth was born on the island of Madagascar on the coast of Africa in the year of 1674 and has consequently now arrived at the astonishing age of ONE HUNDRED AND SIXTY-ONE YEARS!!! . . . The appearance of this modern relic of antiquity strikes the beholder with amazement and convinces him that his eyes are resting upon the oldest specimen of mortality they ever before held.

"Mortality" was a revealing, even Freudian, choice of words, because Heth's death was eagerly awaited, for only afterward could Barnum stage her public dissection. In fact, in Barnum's bogus memoirs, he described her as a "remarkably old negro woman" who "was swindling my friend [her former owner, R. W. Lindsay] by her disgusting pertinacity to cling to life at his expense."[47]

Heth died the next year, on February 19, 1836. Barnum at first confirmed his belief in Heth's incredible age, but he soon announced that he had arranged for an autopsy in order to produce a scientific determination of the truth.

Heth guaranteed Barnum's fame and fortune when he commissioned New York City surgeon David L. Rogers, M.D., to dissect her publicly, a spectacle for which he sold fifty-cent tickets. On February 25, 1836, fifteen hundred spectators crowded New York's City Saloon, whose exhibition center had been transformed into an operating room for the occasion—her very public dissection. The autopsy's real attraction was an unstinting satisfaction of curiosity about her fantastic body, without niceties or guilt. After all, one had paid for the privilege of vicariously participating in this "scientific" investigation. Forty years earlier, Charles Caldwell's examination of Henry Moss's racial distinctiveness had been supposedly voluntary, restrained, private, and noninvasive. However, Heth's was a bloodily invasive circus, and no one even asked whether she had consented. As historian Bernard Reiss has noted, this important performance was both a titillating public entertainment and a pivotal scientific event that prefigured the dissections that would soon become commonplace with the bodies of African Americans.

In the end, Rogers declared that Heth was a fraud, because despite her physical disabilities, her relatively clear cardiac arteries proved that she could have been no more than eighty years old. Barnum reacted with an assortment of bold hoaxes. He visited *New York Herald* editor James Gordon Bennett to claim that the autopsy had been performed not upon Joice Heth, but upon an aged black Harlemite named Aunt Nelly. Barnum assured the *Herald* editors that Heth was actually alive and well and being readied for a European tour. The *Herald* took the bait, the *New York Sun* did not, and the city's newspapers endlessly discussed and debated the results and meanings of the autopsy in warring accounts, accusing one another of falsifying accounts, of misinterpreting the autopsy's evidence, and of having been duped by Barnum. Barnum finally admitted that Heth was indeed dead, but the journalistic furor took eighteen months to abate, during which time Barnum bamboozled yet another paper into publishing one of several divergent "histories" of Heth that he had fabricated. In one of these accounts, Barnum described how he had compelled Heth to masquerade as Washington's old nurse.

> I soon got Joyce [sic] into training, and from a devil of a terma-
> gant, converted into a most docile creature, as willing to do my
> bidding as the slave of the lamp was to obey Aladdin. I discovered
> her weak point . . . : WHISKEY. Her old master, of course, would
> indulge an old bed-ridden creature in no such luxury, and for a
> drop of it, I found I could mould her to anything.[48]

Among other things, Barnum related using her whiskey addiction to ine-
briate her so that he could pull all her teeth in order to make her look
older.

Moss had been a living symbol of how easily the boundaries between
white and black were traversed, but the owners of later racial exhibits
such as Heth stressed the rigidity, not the fluidity, of the barrier between
black and white by stressing (or manufacturing) the distinctly alien nature of black bodies. Around 1840, entrepreneurs realized that a market
hungered for black exotica, and they took a leaf from the physicians'
book by displaying blacks as medical curiosities.[49] Some were unquestionably enslaved, but other attractions were free blacks; all, however,
were kept in quasi-legal bondage.[50]

A few black Barnum attractions had no especially racial component,
such as Madame Abomah, the seven-foot-nine-inch "African Giantess,"
neé Ella Williams, a former domestic from Eastover, South Carolina, or
the enslaved Siamese twins known as Millie-Christine, the "two-headed
girl."[51] But for most quasi-scientific oddities, blackness was an integral
part of their significance, such as a gaggle of unkempt black slaves who
posed as "wild men of Borneo," and, of course, Heth.[52] In these cases,
medical display was more than entertainment; it was also a dramatic argument for the alien inferiority of black bodies. Anonymous "wild men"
have sometimes been surgically altered to resemble animal-human hy-
brids, such as Calvin Bird, who fled a circus and appeared at a Syracuse
hospital, asking to have his surgically implanted horns removed.[53] A supposedly mute black denizen of the wilds of South Africa with a very
small head was enigmatically labeled "Zip—the 'What-is-it?' or merely
'Zip'" He was actually the normally verbal William Henry Johnson of
Bound Brook, New Jersey. Such men were afflicted with microcephalia,
a congenital disorder with no racial element, which is typically manifested by a small misshapen head and lowered intelligence.[54] However,

according to their exhibit placards and carnival barkers, they represented the typical subhuman inhabitants of obscure African lands, some of whom did not enjoy the power of speech.[55] Circuses also displayed blacks with disfiguring medical conditions such as elephantiasis. This parasitic infection blocks the circulation of lymph, causing lymphedema, in which affected limbs and digits swell to monstrous size. Elephantiasis sometimes causes the genitalia to swell, and black men with gargantuan penises and testes could be seen not only in the pages of medical journals but also behind the veils of circus tents.

Blind Tom, a black mathematical prodigy, was exhibited by his physician owner for years and became famous for his ability to make fiendishly complex calculations more rapidly and exactly than the scholars of his time. He was, however, an idiot savant, incapable of the ordinary tasks of everyday living. Because he was black, his condition was often used to illustrate the deleterious effects of intense thought upon the inferior minds of blacks. But the intellectual histories of these exhibited subjects were often falsified, just as their life histories and bodies were. For example, Thomas Bethune, a slave born around 1850 near Columbus, Georgia, was ballyhooed as an untaught musical freak of nature. Actually, Bethune was a trained musical prodigy who gave piano concerts throughout the South as a child and had performed for President James Buchanan at age eight. Bethune was proficient in the classical repertoire and capable of complex harmonic inventions. He played popular music superbly, too, but, rather than being regarded as an American Mozart, he was relegated to circuses and minstrel shows. He enriched his owners but died penniless in 1908.

A few attractions appeared voluntarily: In the free states, some were former two-dollar-a-week roustabouts who realized that they could earn more as an exhibit than by engaging in backbreaking labor.[56]

Louis Agassiz, M.D., the Swiss-born naturalist, was, in 1850, one of the most famous scientists in America. He was also more forthright than most in describing the physical revulsion that blacks evoked in him. He was a protégé of Cuvier, and in 1846, when he immigrated to the United States and a professorship in biology at Harvard, he was immediately drawn to Philadelphia to view Dr. Samuel Morton's "American Golgotha," a collection of 660 white, Indian, Eskimo, and Negro skulls. Agassiz was opposed to enslavement and had originally believed that whites and blacks shared a species and a single origin. But upon his first encounters with blacks in Philadelphia, as he wrote to his mother,

> all the domestics in my hotel were men of color. I can scarcely express to you the painful impression that I received, especially since the feeling that they inspired in me is contrary to all our ideas about the confraternity of the human type and the unique origin of our species. . . . I experienced pity at the sight of this degraded and degenerate race. . . . It is impossible for me to repress the feeling that they are not of the same blood as us. In seeing their black faces with thick lips and grimacing teeth, the wool on their heads, their bent knees, their elongate heads, their large curved nails, and especially the livid color of their palms, I could not take my eyes off their face in order to tell them to stay far away. . . . God preserve us from such a contact![57]

Apparently spurred by his viscera, Agassiz changed his mind about the "confraternity of the human type" and decided that blacks must have evolved separately from whites—the aforementioned antebellum scientific theory called polygenism, the belief in multiple origins for different races. However, his revulsion was mixed with a fascinated attraction. How else can one explain the many beautiful, ambiguously erotic daguerreotype images Agassiz had made of nude or half-nude African Americans in Columbia, South Carolina, in 1850. The scientific rationale for these fifteen detailed images by daguerreotypist Joseph T. Zealy was the scientist's search for graphic evidence to bolster his polygenist conversion. The silver daguerreotype plates included frontal and side views of seven southern slaves, both men and women, and these did emphasize physiognomic features such as head shape, profile, and stance. However, these images also pay tribute to an undeniable beauty and celebrates the very bodies Agassiz decried as bestial.[58] Like pornography, the daguerreotype images of black women reinforced the conventional representation of the black woman as a hypersexual being under the control of a white owner. For example, the women's clothes were pulled below their waists and breasts and their nudity signaled sexual laxity and degradation, especially in contrast with copious layers of protective clothing in which white women were always depicted. Branding, lash marks, piercings, and other marks of oppression and ownership were common and served to confuse the biological and social markings of inferiority. But in addition to clear markings of ownership, subjects often assumed erotic poses indicating they were also sexually available.

Many other southern scientists and physicians, including Thomas Jefferson, wrote of their abhorrence of the black body, but their actions testified to its attractions. Some of the scientists who cataloged and gaped at black bodies enjoyed sexual relationships with their black slaves and mistresses. Their concept of the "negro freak" encapsulated simultaneous feelings of revulsion and attraction. Being men of science, they medicalized these feelings. In 1908, the *New York Medical Journal* observed:

> In most civilized countries there are now enacted laws forbidding the public exhibition of monsters and revolting deformities. . . .
> The genuine *lusus naturae* [trick of nature] is, however, always a valuable subject of study for the scientific physician, which may add to our knowledge of development of normal types and may possibly illuminate many difficult and obscure problems in pathology.[59]

Thus scientists justified in themselves the fascination they condemned in others. casting their own fascination with the black body as a medically important entity that represented the boundary between normal and abnormal, healthy and pathological, human and subhuman, and, sometimes, between black and white. But not just any black body. For exhibits, the normal bodies of healthy American blacks would not do.[60] Exotica sold, particularly bodies with grotesque anomalies and malformations.

Scientists invested heavily in public displays, too. They desired evidence to sell the larger American public on medicalized racial inferiority theories that were already well entrenched in the slaveholding South. Many scientists who were enamored of Charles Darwin's 1859 theory that posited how apes and men sprang from a common ancestor also believed in an embellishment: that a *continuous* chain of evolution linked apes and men and that the subhuman "missing link" was still extant. Scientists swarmed Africa in search of candidate subhumans.

They found them, and displayed them to the world.

World's Fairs were designed to present the exotic, to evoke wonder, and to hail scientific progress, and scientists at the 1904 St. Louis World's Fair attempted to entrance in a manner that was eccentric even for this celebration of the unusual. The fair's anthropology wing showcased hundreds of "strange persons" in the World Congress of Races who had been collected from around the world and were displayed in their natural habitats.[61] Simulated villages and huts housed Igorots and Negritos from southeastern Asia, as well as Malayans, Singalese, Pygmies, and Native Americans. These represented the human spoils of Western forced expansion into Africa, Asia, and other parts of the Third World. This human zoo of colonialism presented Westerners with dark-skinned savages as trophies of conquest and objects of scientific wonder. These people were displayed in St. Louis for the same ultimate purpose that Columbus had imported entire Native American villages to Europe—Columbus wished to show Queen Isabella where her money had gone and what peoples the empire of Spain now encompassed.

Curator W. J. McGee aimed for a panoply of evolution that was "exhaustively scientific" from the highest to the lowest forms of man. Accordingly, the "darkest Blacks" from the "lowest known culture" were contrasted to the "dominant whites" of man's "highest culmination"[62] The *St. Louis Post-Dispatch* proclaimed: "African Pygmies for the World's Fair; amazing Dwarfs of the Congo Valley to be seen in St. Louis, some red, some black. They antedate the Negro in Equatorial Africa. Fearless Midgets who boldly attack elephants with tiny lances, bows and arrows."[63]

Another group of "strange persons" was found in abundance amid the huts, adobes, and tepees—psychologists. For the World Congress of Races was also a huge testing site. Columbia University's Dr. R. S. Woodworth led researchers in administering a battery of psychometric and anthropometric examinations to 1,100 exotics.[64] Four Pygmies were among the exhibited, and rudimentary intelligence tests were administered to help quantify how far below whites they fell on the intellectual scales.[65] These exhibited test subjects must have had names, but only one name has survived: Ota Benga.

However, not every believer in a distinctive black physiology was a racist who wished to prove blacks innately and irrevocably inferior.

Like African American scientists, some eighteenth- and nineteenth-century white physicians and statesmen worked to promulgate the belief that one could look different and yet not be inferior. So did abolitionists. Abolitionist and journalist Frederick Douglass proved a brilliant social analyst, as he held his own in this scientific arena, demonstrating the illogic and manipulation in religious arguments for black inferiority while sidestepping the more reductionist (and often apocryphal) scientific details.[66] For example, he slashed the Gordian knot of comparative physiognomy by objecting to how scientists loaded the dice in making comparative images of relatively unattractive black subjects and unusually attractive whites with perfect Grecian profiles.

> It is fashionable now in our land to exaggerate the differences between the Negro and the European. The phrenologist or naturalist . . . will invariably present the highest type of the European and the lowest types of the Negro. . . . If the very best type of the European is always presented, I insist that justice in all such works demands that the very best type of the Negro should be taken. The importance of this criticism may not be apparent to all—to the black man it is very apparent.[67]

James McCune Smith, M.D., was another important critic. This brilliant African American physician and statistical scientist was superbly equipped to refute the scientific racists on their own ground and did so regularly. His 1837 lecture exposing the scientific fallacy of phrenology took on the ethnologists' essays and offered scathing criticisms of their logical sins in imputing character and intelligence from physiology.[68]

P. T. Barnum in Whiteface

Barnum, who had performed in blackface as a youth,[69] capitalized on another important fad in skin color when he began to exhibit his encyclopedic collection of "white negroes." These were African Americans suffering from albinism, vitiligo (also called leukoderma), genetic mosaicism, and other medical conditions that whiten the skin. Such "white negroes" were not unknown to Europeans, but in the mid-nineteenth century, Americans facing a profound racial crisis suddenly found them fascinating.[70] In 1846, Barnum hawked exhibits such as his "twin Caffres,"[71] with "bodies almost pure white, faces black as ebony, features perfectly human, noses, eyes, ears, etc. perfect miniatures of the negro, covered with black woolly hair." These were albinos with artificially darkened faces and hair.[72] Barnum also called them *leucoethiopes* (Greek for "white Ethiopians") or "leopard boys." Black albino women were displayed with exotic manufactured histories and names such as "the Circassian Beauty."

In August 1850, Barnum displayed a black man whose skin was gradually but perceptibly lightening and who "claimed to have discovered a weed that would gradually turn Negroes white. Barnum praised this discovery as the solution of the slavery problem, for "the problem of slavery would disappear with their color. . . ."[73] Other entrepreneurs displayed many "white negroes" the public seemed never to tire of.[74]

The medical fascination with the "white negro" reflected the belief of some scientists, who, pointing to the straight hair and finer features of property-owning free blacks and of enslaved house servants, proposed that African Americans were turning white as a response to the "civilizing" influences of Western, European cultures.[75] Of course, African Americans were acquiring European features the natural way, but many whites maintained a high level of denial about the degree of black-white mating.

On a superficial level, the spectacle of a black person turning white was simply a freakish reversal of nature, on the level of a bearded lady or a hermaphrodite. On another, deeper level he posed an implicit threat to civilization, because white skin was held to denote evolutionary advantage during this period, when most scientists insisted that whites were the superior humans or perhaps even the only true humans. If a Negro could turn white, what would become of the special evolutionary status that whites enjoyed? If a Negro's black skin could be shed so simply, what, if anything, did it mean to be a Negro? The justification for slavery and unequal treatment of all kinds evaporated with skin color. As Charles D. Martin muses in his provocative book *The White African American Body,* the white Negro was not only a "freak," but a troubling one, even if his viewers could not articulate why.

Interestingly, the circus circulars, carnival barkers, and even medical scientists who studied "white negroes" tended to observe that along with their fading skin color, they lost the flattened nose, broader lips, and woolly hair that marked the Africans. This is a perplexing claim, because the medical disorders that leach skin (and sometimes hair) color do not change the features. While one cannot be sure what motivated these extraordinary claims, the results of this irrational belief are clear: The purported loss of all external manifestations of race fueled the argument that to discover what constituted a Negro, it is necessary to go deeper, under the skin. To dissect. The collective delusion that "white negroes" were acquiring European facial features helped drive an impetus for the eventual surgical dissection of blacks to find the internal physiological markers and meaning of "blackness."

Not only did Barnum's "white negroes" intrigue the public but their exhibition also coincided with a fad in medicine. In every major city and in scores of smaller towns, physicians as well as gawkers hungrily thronged these exhibits. "White negroes" posed a challenge to physicians who strove to understand the medical reason for and the medical import of this transformation.[76] Physicians knew of albinism, a set of hereditary conditions that causes people to be born without the melanin that gives color to skin, hair, and the pupils of the eye. They had encountered a few blacks born with genetic mosaicism, which causes permanently mottled skin, with both white and black patches. Medical descriptions of black hermaphrodites and "leopard boys" appear in the literature at least as early as 1754, and Charles Darwin had once given a photograph of a such a "Leopard Boy" to the museum of the Royal College of Surgeons.[77] When a black person exhibited mosaicism or albinism, physicians wrote him up in medical journals, displayed him in hospitals, and sometimes took him on the road, displaying him for money.

However, doctors did not understand that most people who were born black but whose skin was gradually turning white suffered from vitiligo, a medical condition in which the skin's melanin-bearing cells, or melanocytes, gradually lose their color for a variety of reasons. This medical disorder affects both blacks and whites, but the darker skins of African Americans make vitiligo a very dramatic condition, whereas in whites it can be nearly imperceptible.

Of course, scientists also knew that matings between blacks and whites could produce offspring who were very light-skinned or who appeared white. Conventional wisdom denied that white men were impregnating the black women they owned, but the public display of a white child born of a black woman immediately evoked the spectral white father lurking in the background.[78] *Miscegenation* is a misnomer for the matings between blacks and whites, because the word, from the Latin *miscere*, "to mix," and *genus*, "race," refers to matings between two separate races rather than the intraspecies mating that takes place between whites and blacks in interracial relationships.[79] However, such mating was denied by physicians and carnival barkers as the genesis of "white negroes."[80]

Whatever their genesis, most scientists took a dim view of the white Negro. They perceived in him or her a variety of challenges to the primacy, status, and security of the white race and, with it, to nascent American scientific culture. This is because the scientific culture of the nineteenth century still relied upon taxonomy, or categorization. Movement within taxonomies such as Carl Linnaeus's celebrated evolutionary scheme was possible, but such transitions had to be logical, predicted by and explainable by medical theory. It would not do to have categories, schemes, and classifications of peoples called into question by such unpredicted changes as Negroes who inexplicably and illogically insisted upon turning white. They could not be explained by theory, so they contradicted and threatened the classification scheme and, therefore, the social order.

Some men of science, notably Stanhope Smith, rightly deduced that intermarriage was causing the Europeanizing of black features and that eventually skin-color distinctions could disappear if black-white unions were allowed to proceed unchecked.[81] However, most scientists of the period believed that race was deeper than skin color and that a white Negro was still a Negro.

The birth of white children from black mothers also reminded whites that untold numbers of Negroes were passing for white, a social problem whispered of in polite society and broadly lampooned in the pages of popular newspapers and political circulars. Foreign visitors to the South, who often harbored antislavery sentiments, remarked openly upon the difficulty of discerning the race of people whom they met. When the duc de La Rochefoucauld-Liancourt visited Thomas Jefferson at Monticello, he pointedly observed that his host owned many "mongrel negroes . . . who, neither in point of colour nor features, shewed the least trace of their original descent."[82]

Jefferson, statesman and scientist, found "white negroes" very disturbing. When he wrote about them at some length in his 1783 *Notes on the State of Virginia*, he took pains to banish the specter of miscegenation by recounting genealogies demonstrating that the parents of these anomalies were all unquestionably black.[83] Because DNA evidence has lent credibility to claims that he fathered children with his enslaved mistress, Sally Hemings, there may have been personal motives for Jefferson's discomfort. Many scientists also speculated uncomfortably that Negroes who were born white would gain the capability to pass ad infinitum by bestowing their acquired white skins on their progeny. Perhaps this is why Jefferson undertook a survey to reassure himself that "white negroes" were not proliferating. Such insecurities may also explain a peculiar corrective measure introduced in 1854 by a Dr. Lioburgs of Mississippi. He announced that his medical research had produced "a tincture" that would make a white man black, and would make his children black, as well. Lioburgs supplemented this discovery with a wash that would transform a white's hair into "negro wool."[84]

The fear that "white negroes" would usurp the favored evolutionary positions of whites certainly abetted the belief, promulgated by scientific racists such as Josiah Nott, that mulattoes were too frail, feeble, and infertile to reproduce their own kind for many generations.[85] In fact, the term *mulatto* comes from the Spanish word for mule, a sterile cross between a horse and a donkey.

Jefferson and other scientists who were desperately seeking distinctions between whites and "white negroes" also differentiated between the "disagreeable" pallor of "white negroes" and the healthily ruddy skins of true whites. Italian scientist Cesare Lambroso[86] took pains to observe that "authentically" white skin was always touched with red and that the Negro's inability to blush was seen as a distinctly racial characteristic that revealed a person's "savage" African race by revealing his inherent shamelessness.

Jefferson's quest to distinguish the Negro did not stop at the surface. He insisted that blackness resided not in the superficial changeable skin of the Negro but, rather, that it was a *permanent* badge of inferiority that resided deeper within the body. "Whether the black of the negro reside [sic] in the reticular membranes between the skin and the scarf-skin itself; whether it proceeds from the color of the blood, the color of the bile or from that of some other secretion, the difference is fixed in nature."[87] Jefferson and his fellow scientific racists did not know what "blackness" was, and they did not know where it was: They only knew that it simply *had* to be there. Permanently. Somewhere.

Many scientists of the era, like their forebears, devoted themselves to pursuing the elusive inner markers of "blackness." Dr. J. H. Guenebault compiled a list of forty-seven physical traits other than skin color that distinguished blacks; Josiah Nott made a list of twenty-five, from black areas of the Negro brain to darkened blood and internal organs to the "pendulous" breasts of African women: Every scientist had his pet method for revealing a Negro.

Cartwright and other early scientific racists had insisted all black "racial" attributes, visible and invisible, had one meaning: These differences indelibly marked the Negro as the inferior "submissive knee-bender" and "son of Ham" of the Bible: A change in skin color could not change this. Scientists had passed over the threshold of anatomical dissection as the popular event that Joice Heth's autopsy had portended. Jefferson insisted that scientists seeking the seat of the Negro's blackness should resort to the "Anatomical knife, to Optical glasses, to analysis by fire, or by solvents."[88]

Late-nineteenth-century scientists had grown dissatisfied with biblical injunctions, and impatient. Skin color had become a treacherous signal and whites were faced with an atmosphere of escalating social urgency: Ridiculed as barbarians by their former colonizer, England, and by most of Europe as well, Americans felt they could ill afford to be characterized as a nation of mongrels and mere pretenders to white status. Black skin could no longer consistently and reliably designate a Negro, so it was critically important to find other means of detection.

Physician-scientists felt long-delayed medical winds of change traversing the Atlantic that had made anatomical investigation with human bodies the gold standard of medical research. Driven by social changes such as the imminent failure of chattel slavery and the emergence of "white negroes," scientists were eager to delve more deeply under the skin of African Americans. They wished to discover clues to race that

were more than skin-deep, to invade the skin, to peel away the muscula-
ture, to unfurl the intestines, and to calibrate the bones. In this way, they
felt, they could understand the nature of race, and regain control over
the black bodies that were slipping from their intellectual and literal
grasp.

THE SURGICAL THEATER

Black Bodies in the Antebellum Clinic

Such [free] persons of color as may not be able to pay for Medical advice . . . [should call at the hospital]. . . . The object of the Faculty is to collect as many interesting cases, as possible, for the benefit and instruction of their pupils.

—MEDICAL COLLEGE OF SOUTH CAROLINA ADVERTISEMENT

IN THE *CHARLESTON COURIER*, NOVEMBER 16, 1837

Sam, a forty-two-year-old laborer on a plantation in rural Alabama, had become exhausted by pain and fear. For years, an incessant racking pain in his jaw had kept him distracted days and awake nights, miserable and dejected. When his owner learned of Sam's pain around 1838, he decided that Sam must have syphilis and applied a homemade concoction, whose only effect was to produce a painful boil on Sam's gums. Now Sam also found it difficult to eat. He should have been a strong, productive worker in the prime of his earning power, but Sam was finding it harder and harder to work, even in the face of cajoling and threats. By 1845, he had become worthless in the fields, and in desperation, his owner summoned a physician, who determined that Sam was suffering not from syphilis but from osteosarcoma—a cancer of his lower jawbone. The doctor turned to a surgical colleague, Dr. Marion J. Sims, who declared to Sam's owner that only an operation carried hope of a cure. But Sam vehemently and repeatedly refused, protesting that it would "hurt too bad."[1]

Today, refusing to undergo an operation for a treatable cancer is a tragic mistake, because surgery is the most curative mode of therapy for cancer. Today, anesthetics, antisepsis, and antibiotics banish or at least mitigate the twin nightmares of surgical pain and infection. However, Sam's cancer predated the common use of effective anesthesia[2] and of sterile technique. Purgatorial pain was certain and a fatal infection all too likely. What's more, the disfiguring surgery might have been futile, because only superficial, visible cancers were discovered during this era. Not until Wilhelm Roentgen discovered X rays in 1895 could physicians view the body's interior without invasive surgery. No imaging techniques allowed doctors to identify an internal cancer, and it could have spread internally through the long years when Sam was being erroneously treated for syphilis.

Sam's version of events is not recorded, so we don't know whether more than a fear of pain caused him to balk at surgery. But we do know that Sam might by this time have acquired a low opinion of Western medicine's ability to help him, thanks to the original misdiagnosis and iatrogenic injury. If Sam had gotten wind of Sims's dismal surgical statistics, his famed fondness for forced experimentation on captive patients, or of his penchant for taking shoemakers' tools to black infants' skulls, Sam's opinion of Sims's skill would have sunk low indeed. But he would not have dared to openly voice doubts about Sims's abilities, so refusing treatment because of "the pain" may have been a canny dodge.

However, Sam was enslaved, so the decision was left not to him but to his owner, who was eager to return his slave to profitable work. Sam was sent to Montgomery despite his loud and constant protests.

Sims, for his part, stonily declared himself "determined not to be foiled in the attempt" to operate. Sims had decided not only to operate upon Sam but also to perform the surgery in a teaching clinic for a medical audience of students and potential protégés. He hoped to immortalize the operation in a medical publication, and no mere slave would frustrate this bid for medical glory.

But when the two adversaries met, Sims was all smiles. He kindly inquired into the slave's health and graciously invited Sam to have a seat.

The barber's chair into which Sam had been welcomed had been surreptitiously fitted with wooden planks, and as soon as Sam was seated, five young physicians bounded forward to restrain him with straps about his thighs, knees, ankles, abdomen, chest, shoulders, arms, wrists, elbows, and head. Sam, Sims noted, "appeared to be very much alarmed!" While he was being immobilized, ten medical students and fifteen interested "others" filed in to watch as Sims operated for forty minutes to remove a large section of Sam's lower jawbone, sans anesthesia. When he finished, the surgeon noted with satisfaction that his surgical innovation had "proved its practicality . . . whether the patient is willing or not." The editors of the *New Orleans Medical and Surgical Journal* enthused that they were "pleased to record this highly creditable achievement of a Southern surgeon."[3]

After he recuperated, Sam apparently lost no time in escaping into rural Alabama again, certainly with a redoubled aversion to Western medicine. There is no evidence that Sims ever saw Sam again, but his medical report took this parting shot: "Sam's mouth is always open in a wide grin."

Staging Disease: Treatment Under the Microscope

There were many Sams. Like circuses, clinics and hospitals had an abundance of uses for the displayed African American body. After the mid-nineteenth century, a supply of black bodies was key to the primacy of the hospital as the new center for American medical instruction and treatment. African Americans filled medical school rosters as well as circus tents, because medical teaching, training, and research utilized black bodies disproportionately, and in some southern venues, they were used exclusively.

During the 1830s, a Dr. T. Stillman ran serial advertisements in the *Charleston Mercury* for his infirmary, in which he principally treated skin diseases. On October 12, 1838, he made a fascinating addendum: "Wanted: FIFTY NEGROES. Any person having sick negroes, considered incurable by their respective physicians and *wishing to dispose of them* [emphasis added] . . . the highest cash prize will be paid upon application as above."[4]

Slaves who had become too old or too sick to work supplied the bulk of hospital "clinical material." They enjoyed no legal rights and could mount no legal challenge to their incarceration and treatment.[5] Stillman advertised his desire for blacks who suffered from disorders far beyond his own specialty, such as apoplexy, kidney disease, and stomach, intestinal, bladder, liver, and spleen disorders, as well as scrofula and hypochondriasm. He wished to test new techniques and medications he had formulated on debilitated and chronically unhealthy blacks in the same institution where he treated paying whites. He then marketed the medications and techniques.

Slave owners were glad to rid themselves of old, sick, and unproductive slaves.[6] It was a sage bargain on the slave owner's part, because the hospital took over all or most of the cost of feeding, housing, and treating the unproductive slave. If the slave died, his owner was spared the inconvenience and expense of burying him, because the hospital would retain the body for dissection or experiment. If the slave recovered, the master would once again profit from his or her labor and breeding. Moreover, the slave owner could lay claim to benevolence; after all, he was sending his old or sick slaves to a hospital for expert care. Free blacks were also vulnerable because they were easily incarcerated in jails and almshouses for a variety of minor infractions of the many regulations governing free African Americans.[7]

Why were blacks the chief denizens of teaching-hospital wards? The "hospital movement" finally crossed the Atlantic from Europe; one-room, one-year medical schools based upon the stereotyped dispensing of a few dozen nostrums fell out of favor and began to close as medical training began to focus upon scientific experimentation and anatomical knowledge. The new spirit of clinical inquiry questioned heroic but ineffectual treatments such as bleeding, purging, and cupping, causing them to quickly lose their cachet.[8] Medical students were now expected to undergo training during several years, not months, on the clinical floors of hospitals.

Diseases such as yellow fever, smallpox, malaria, and tuberculosis still flared into epidemics with regularity, and the dominant class of property-owning whites still relied upon private physicians to care for them and their families. However, they increasingly expected those physicians to have the professional benefit of hands-on clinical experience.

However, acquiring such experience presented a challenge because hospitals were about as popular a destination as homeless shelters are today: No one who had a family, access to a private physician, or financial resources to rely upon was willing to enter one. American hospitals of the 1800s were very different from the antiseptic, high-tech, ethics-obsessed meccas of scientific medicine that we know today. They offered few effective medications and there were no federal agencies exerting exterior checks and balances to weigh the interests of patients against those of the hospitals' physician owners. Without the therapeutic options, patient protections, medical advances, and knowledge that we take for granted today, the hospital was less an institution for healing than a physician-centered venue for learning, training, and experimental approaches. These were conducted on black people and on other poor, desperate people without resources.

Perhaps Thomas Jefferson said it best: "It is poverty alone which peoples hospitals . . . to be exposed as a corpse, to be lectured over by a clinical professor, to be crowded and handled by his students to hear their case learnedly explained to them, its threatening symptoms developed and its probable termination foreboded. . . ."9 The best one could hope for in hospitals and "poor clinics" was shelter from the elements and a minimum of dangerous untried treatments among the infectious. One could, however, count upon exposure to a host of iatrogenic conditions and upon being regularly displayed to students and faculty. Hospital patients also risked involuntary treatment, including unnecessary surgery, often without the benefit of effective anesthesia. Yet, the doctors-to-be and their teachers needed "clinical material"—human bodies upon which they could practice diagnosis, treatment, and, finally, autopsy and dissection. Because no one entered a hospital voluntarily, this reluctant "clinical material" emanated from the lowest rungs of society. Sick or old people cast out of workhouses, almshouses—and, in the South, plantations—filled hospitals. Clinic patients were not asked for their consent, and any physician who hesitated to operate on protesting slaves found he was legally bound to follow the wishes of not the slave but the owner.10

In the South, African Americans were reluctant patients, but they outnumbered poor whites in hospitals.11 When the city of Richmond, Virginia, contemplated expending public funds to build a new almshouse, the professor owners of the Medical College of Virginia proposed a mutually beneficial alternative: They would take "all the sick and infirm paupers" into their infirmary and, in exchange, pay the city the funds it needed for a workhouse.12 In 1848, the faculty also proposed establishing a hospital solely for blacks, thereby ensuring a supply of patients for clinical instruction, although free blacks knew enough to give hospitals a wide berth when they could. Even in the North, hospitals expected blacks to submit to research as "payment" for having been treated in charity wards; yet no amount of money could buy a black patient a bed in the private ward where well-to-do whites received care. When a black patient was admitted in error to Boston's Massachusetts General

Hospital in 1829, his doctor, George W. Otis, M.D., was severely taken to task.[13]

Clinical Objects of Wonder

Clinical display, in which a person and his illness were presented to physicians as part of their education and training, took several forms. On the sick wards, the "clinical material" was subjected to medical observation, during which he was thoroughly inspected, examined, and questioned by professors or by students under the supervision of a professor. Many questions, some of them quite pointed and intimate, probed the patient's condition, lifestyle, and habits. Treatment was administered to blacks on the charity wards, but care was always secondary to practice, because the primary purpose of the clinic was the instruction, training, and experimentation for the physicians and students. Treatment took place without consent, often via unpleasant draconian measures. Publication in medical journals and texts was also a priority because it afforded physicians an opportunity to promote their academic careers and to advertise their practices by immortalizing their discoveries and surgical triumphs while sharing clinical curiosities and insights.[14]

The disrespect shown the "clinical material" often included speculation about their sexuality. Speculation on the sexual experiences of men and women were incongruously introduced into medical discussions, even those that lay far afield of sex and reproduction. In August 1846, twenty-year-old George Pray, a medical student at the University of Michigan, expressed surprise that the sixteen-year-old black girl whose body was undergoing dissection had died a virgin.[15] In an 1855 *Virginia Medical and Surgical Journal* article, Medical College of Virginia professor Theodore P. Mayo proclaimed that Roy, a twenty-four-year-old slave with bladder stones, "is reported to be a great buck among the dark damsels."[16] Because physicians shared the public's fascination with unusual bodies, many people with physical deformities were repeatedly displayed and examined. So were "idiots" and idiot savants.[17]

By 1830, southern medical schools competed hotly for students, and a key selling point for any medical school of the antebellum era was the availability of copious "clinical material." Advertisements trumpeted the prospective student's access to ample black clinical subjects in nearby hospitals, clinics, almshouses, and other institutions. For example, the *Savannah Medical Journal* boasted that the Negro patient census of the Savannah Medical College provided "abundant clinical opportunities for the studying of disease."[18]

In 1840, the Medical College of Virginia[19] publicly flourished a plan wherein it predicted, "The number of negroes employed in our factories will furnish materials for the support of an extensive hospital, and afford to the student that great desideratum—clinical instruction."[20]

Throughout the South, medical schools published circulars exhorting slave owners to send them patients. The schools established hospitals for blacks, where fees were lowered dramatically or dropped altogether, and advertisements for the free care of sick and aged slaves were placed in rural newspapers.[21]

The Medical College of South Carolina's circulars boasted that the excellence of its institution was based upon the many available cadavers and the "great opportunities for the acquisition of anatomical knowledge."[22] Its boast that "the object of the faculty is to collect as many interesting cases as possible, for the benefit and instruction of their pupils"[23] takes on special meaning when one considers that surgery at the Medical College of South Carolina was performed *only* on blacks—slave or free.

The other Charleston school, the state medical college infirmary, admitted poor whites, blacks, and slaves. However, while the whites and free blacks were charged fees for lodging and treatment, slaves were treated for free. The school openly stated that "the *sole object* [emphasis added] of the faculty is to promote the interests of the Medical education within their native state and City."[24]

In 1855, an advertisement in the *Atlanta Weekly Intelligencer* invited slave owners to send slaves to Atlanta Medical College for medical treatment.[25] The next year the Atlanta Medical College boasted to prospective students of a "case of hepatic abscess in a negro man" whose damaged liver caused him to be "lectured upon and prescribed for in the presence of the class" over the course of several weeks. A black woman with tuberculosis was kept "under observation" for student edification for an entire year.[26]

We find this open desire for black bodies to fill wards, surgical suites, operating theaters, autopsy tables, and pathology jars chilling today. However, it simply reflected the social realities of the slaveholding South.

What's more, this need persists in a more subtle form today. In the words of one physician, "Medical schools consider it a selling point when they have plenty of low-income patients for students and residents to see."[27]

We have already seen that medical researchers collected data and tested treatments pertinent to whites by using the supposedly inferior bodies of African Americans. In the same manner, clinics used supposedly anomalous black bodies and minds as exemplars of illness and as tools to assess the patients' responses to therapeutics. Blacks were believed to sleep more, feel pain less, endure heat better and cold worse, and be more prone to fevers, tetanus, syphilis, yaws, and tuberculosis but resistant to yellow fever and malaria. Their skins were thought thicker, their brains smaller; they were characterized as sexually precocious and intellectually retarded.[28] Yet in a familiar but illogical leitmotiv, treatments for whites were devised, adopted, or rejected based upon the black response to therapeutics.[29]

Most physicians chose simply to ignore these inconvenient contradictions, just as they had ignored the illogic of transposing experimental medical results from African Americans to whites. However, at least one addressed the issue head-on. In 1894, Rudolph Matas, M.D., published a 125-page surgical analysis arguing that the scientific racist could have his cake and eat it, too. Matas agreed with most contentions of black physiologic "pathology," but he presented a shotgun marriage of his argument for rampant racial physiologic differences to a dogmatic claim that these differences would make no practical difference to the surgeon who wanted to assess procedures.[30] He offered only opinion and little objective evidence to buttress his claims, so his work is less than convincing, but at least he acknowledged the fallacy. Matas addressed only surgical techniques, leaving medical doctors to resolve their own scientific discrepancies.[31]

In 1854, the *Richmond Daily Dispatch* wondered, "Among them [blacks] there prevails a superstition that when they enter the [medical college] Infirmary they never come out alive, although no where are they better treated. . . ."[32]

Events, however, reinforced black fears and outrage, which was sometimes shared by the white medical community. For example, an outraged owner solicited the opinion of an editor[33] of the Richmond, Virginia, medical journals, who agreed that therapeutically unjustified surgical procedures were being performed "wantonly" upon moribund slave patients in hospitals—and even upon relatively well ones—merely to allow doctors opportunities to practice or teach techniques. One such incident involved a slave whose master sent him to the medical school clinic for treatment of a stubborn leg ulcer. The surgeon decided to amputate the leg, surrounded by students, although no clinical indications existed for this extreme procedure. The slave complained that "his leg was cut off just to let the students see the operation and to bring the doctor as well as the medical college . . . into notice."[34] The journal editor investigated and then agreed, censuring the surgeon as a "heartless monster." However, neither the name of the surgeon nor of the medical school was revealed in the journal. The outraged editor even failed to sign his name.

When Georgia physician W. H. Robert similarly decided to amputate the leg of a fifteen-year-old slave girl without making any other attempts to treat the relatively minor injury, the surgeon told his students flatly that the decision to amputate should be weighed differently according to the person's race and class. "[Amputation] should be very differently estimated in the different classes of society." He explained that although such an extreme remedy is a "horrid deformity" that should be the last resort for a rich man, amputating the limb of a slave was "a matter of comparatively little importance." Students should "hesitate much less to remove a limb . . . , if he be slave, than if he be a free man, and especially a white man."[35] Robert supplemented his hierarchy of amputation with the familiar observation that the surgical pain felt by a slave was negligible, minor in comparison to that a white man facing the procedure would feel.

Hospitals and medical schools engaged in far more than the passive observation in the clinic or on paper. Professors operated in hospital theaters, as they do today, for the benefit of medical students. The performances also boosted their own reputations. Being compelled to undergo surgery before an audience of physicians, such as Sam suffered, was the standard of care for slaves.[36]

Throughout the nineteenth century and the first half of the twentieth, this use of blacks for clinical demonstration persisted largely unchanged, except that it eventually became a tacit, rather than an advertised, reality.[37] Because of the widespread use of blacks as teaching material, new physicians left their medical school training with a deeply ingrained habit of looking upon blacks as demonstration material and experimental subjects.

The demonstration of black bodies was not limited to the clinic. Publication was as important to a physician's career in the 1800s and 1900s as it is today, and the pages of medical journals were profitable places to display African American bodies. Then, as now, glory followed the ability to be the first to identify and treat a condition or disorder. Such publications often proposed, supported, or highlighted physical differences between blacks and whites, differences that were seldom interpreted in favor of black Americans. In that age, no journalists, curious family members, or activist patients had access to medical journals, only physicians, who were almost always male and white. As a result, these publications displayed an unself-conscious disregard for black patients' consent. For example, when a black South Carolina youth fell from a tree, injuring his genitals, the attending surgeon administered chloroform, which rendered him unconscious, then repaired the minor injury. *After* this successful repair, the physician decided to remove the boy's testicle, but he told the boy only that his injury had been sewn up. A week passed before the boy "became aware of his loss," and the surgeon recorded his achievement in an article entitled "Chloroform: Its Effects in a Case of Castration."[38]

Publication in a medical journal was also important because unless others could read of and reproduce the experiments with similarly successful results, a physician could not hope to be credited with discovery of a new therapy. Hospital and medical school records and medical journals show that aged and infirm African Americans were overwhelmingly more likely to be used for medical display and demonstration of such new procedures—including description in medical journal articles—than were native whites.[39]

Historian Todd Savitt inventoried Richmond medical journals that described procedures upon 198 patients between 1851 and 1860, and found that by the most conservative estimate blacks constituted 48.7 percent. Historian Walter Fisher suggested an even greater racial disparity. Of the seventeen cases discussed in Richmond Medical Society meetings during 1853–1854, ten were black. Thanks to the strong prejudice against medical display of the organs and bodies of whites, only the organs of blacks were displayed.[40]

When Professor Dugas of the Medical College of Georgia pioneered eye operations on slaves in 1838, he performed them before students. Three surgical cases, all upon "Negroes," were also performed by that school's Dr. Paul Eve before students as part of their training.[41]

Like the circus displays, medical journal reports reflected a fascination with unusual bodies. Not only were more of the displayed bodies those of African Americans, but the African American examples were also the most dramatically afflicted and most likely to be designated "pathological." Six of eleven accounts of unusual body types in Virginia medical journals described blacks whose deformities included hermaphrodism, precocious puberty, Siamese twinning, and birth monstrosities, including an extrauterine deformed fetus that was preserved and displayed for forty years. The white reports dwelled upon less fantastic, less "freakish" anomalies, including hydrocephalus, congenital heart displacement, and quadruplets. No white Siamese twins or hermaphrodites were ever recorded in these journals. This pattern is evident on the national level, as well. During one period, five of every nine medical journal reports of unusual bodies featured blacks, including another hermaphrodite and another forty-year-old deformed fetus.[42] Degrading medical reports that reproduced patients' bodies, faces, and even their names and that speculated upon sexuality were reserved for blacks. A white patient might sue; a black patient had no legal standing.

When an 1849 Philadelphia medical journal article reported on a black woman who gave birth to twins, one black and one pale, the physicians speculated that the "biracial" twinning was the result of sexual congress on successive days with a white man and a black one.[43] This sort of speculation would never have been offered about a white woman. Men were by no means spared sexual ridicule. Many curious physicians repeatedly examined Ned, a hermaphrodite, over the course of several years, and one doctor's medical journal report contained this passage: "[W]hether his amorous advances to the dusky maidens around him has [sic] ever resulted in any practical display of virility is unknown . . . it is fair to conclude that no seminal discharge has or ever will take place."[44] In such cases, the subject was blithely named in the journal or the exhibit, but no images of white subjects appeared and they remained anonymous.

Some displays encouraged the belief in widespread racial dimorphism. When a black American exhibited an unusual condition, physicians often took a leap of faith and racialized the condition, assigning it to all blacks or only to blacks. For example, Dr. Robert Knox published an article in an American medical journal wherein he described finding an eighth, "extra" intercostal rib in several dissected bodies, all of which were those of Africans or black Americans.[45] He conjectured that this anomaly was peculiar to blacks. Many such articles served double duty as pro-slavery propaganda because they interpreted these conditions or anomalies as evidence of racial inferiority.[46]

Similarly, anthropologist Ernst Haeckel asserted as late as 1906 that blacks retained a hand and foot morphology that was closer to that of the apes than of that of white men.

There are wild tribes of men who can oppose the first or large toe to the other four, just as if it were a thumb. They can therefore, use their "grasping foot" like the so-called "hinder hand." . . . The Negro, in whom the big toe is especially strong and freely moveable, when climbing seizes hold of the branches of the trees with it, just like the "four-handed" Apes.[47]

Such false assumptions were fueled by the difficulty of making internal observations of living persons. Scientists assumed that the skeleton, nervous system, and viscera of African Americans were quite different from those of whites, but proving this was a challenge. Because they had no internal imaging techniques, such empirical evidence for putative differences was ascertainable only through autopsy.

The consistent display of black patients as mere disease exemplars also blunted physicians' compassion. The result of exploiting the "clinical material" was a damping of sensitivity and altruism toward black patients, and this became an important but unacknowledged part of a physician's training. One powerful illustration of this process is found in the touching November 1846 memoirs of the newly minted Dr. Pray. He recounted how during his first anatomical dissection he had felt an overwhelming sympathy for the fate of the young girl under his scalpel. "Today our subject, a poor Negro girl, was brought up. Poor, despised and disregarded African, degraded and despised in life you are to be made a spectacle and subject of ridicule and obscene jest even in death." Yet, under professional pressure, he immediately launched into a detailed public surgical dissection of the girl's labia.

A year later, the same doctor laughingly wrote of his antics the night before, when he had delighted in making a group of white women of his own social class scream in horror. How? By frightening them with "a piece of dead nigar" that he has saved from the dissecting table.[48]

This sad psychological transformation suggests a possible answer to a troubling discrepancy. Most people enter medicine because they want to help others, and it is reasonable to believe that some, if not most, white physicians did intend to care for, not just to study or to display, their black patients. However, who were these sympathetic physicians of the time, as revealed by medical records? If they existed, why were they silent in the face of such egregious abuses? Slave narratives tell us that empathic physicians could be occasionally be found on plantations. But as the hospital system began to standardize the training of American physicians in the mid-nineteenth century, kindly white doctors disappeared from African American oral histories and certainly cannot be found in the southern medical journals, which were replete with disdainful, mocking depictions of African American patients who had undergone humiliating and painful involuntary procedures that no one questioned.

Those doctors who viewed blacks as persons rather than "clinical material" were often those least able to help them and least likely to record their opinions in medical journals—beginning medical students. The dehumanizing effects of their training might easily have deformed their altruism. Students such as the young George Pray were likely to be the most idealistic of caregivers, but they were also the most vulnerable to professional repercussions should they offend professors. They could not afford to criticize instructors, even obliquely, by suggesting that the clinical material should be treated as sensitively as white private patients. Eventually, students absorbed the racist values that informed their education at every turn.

Medical Fallout from Clinical Display

By the mid-nineteenth century, African Americans had already associated Western medicine with punishment, loss of control over their most intimate bodily functions, and degrading public displays. With the rise of the hospital movement, the need for living subjects forced African Americans to become objects to be studied, reproduced, written about, and practiced upon, always without consent and sometimes with brutal violence by physicians who refused to acknowledge their pain. Hospitals and medical schools became firmly cemented into the African American consciousness as places of terror, violence, and shame, not of medical care.

Moreover, clinics' use of black bodies involved far more than passive display. Medical students observed the course of illnesses in blacks for educational purposes, but clinical display grew to encompass prescribing for and treating patients in front of doctors in training.[49] Physicians demonstrated and practiced invasive and surgical procedures on interned slaves and African Americans, sometimes to pioneer a new procedure, to display surgical acumen, or to enhance the reputation of practitioners.[50]

Black physicians such as James McCune Smith and W. Montague Cobb were consistent defenders of the human rights of African Americans and were the first to object when these were violated. Unfortunately, black doctors' impact was limited because they were not yet present in large numbers and they usually were not permitted to train in the hospitals and clinics where the abuses took place. Black physicians still had to leave the South, and often the country, to obtain medical educations. Many were pressured to leave the country after obtaining an M.D. degree, and those who remained found themselves barred from necessary internship and residency training.

The white physicians who were trained by peering at, ridiculing, and practicing upon the captive bodies of African Americans had been taught to view these bodies as expendable. When loosed upon the world as practitioners, they continued to view African Americans as subjects rather than as patients. Graduate physicians utilized unwilling blacks to display their therapeutic prowess or as raw material for research papers and surgical reputations.

Medical display was not the final manner in which blacks' bodies were used against their will in the clinic. The next chapter explores how black bodies were medically exploited even after death—via autopsy and dissection.

CHAPTER 5

THE RESTLESS DEAD
Anatomical Dissection and Display

In Baltimore, the bodies of colored people exclusively are taken for dissection, because the whites do not like it and the colored people cannot resist.

—HARRIET MARTINEAU, *RETROSPECT OF WESTERN TRAVEL*

No place in the United States offers as great opportunities for the acquisition of anatomical knowledge. Subjects being obtained from among the colored population in sufficient numbers for every purpose, and proper dissection carried on without offending any individuals in our community!

—ADVERTISEMENT FOR THE SOUTH CAROLINA MEDICAL COLLEGE,

C. 1831

On September 11, 1977, Casper Yeagin, a sixty-eight-year-old retired auto mechanic, vanished. His sister Pearlie Smith, with whom he lived, contacted a police officer in the Washington, D.C., missing-persons unit, and provided the photograph he requested. "He said he would be back . . . but I didn't hear anything," Smith told the *Washington Post.* So for more than a month, Smith, Yeagin's niece Minnie Champ, and other family members made relentless inquiries of the police at the Fifth District station house. They also called area hospital emergency departments, which the officer should also have done. Everyone with whom they spoke assured them that Yeagin had never been brought into a hospital—until Champ called the police again on November 1, 1977, and reached the officer with whom Smith had first spoken. He visited them again and made several telephone calls, which revealed that his original report had never been properly filed. The police made other errors, as well: The officer had never personally checked emergency rooms, and the missing-persons unit had not followed procedure by checking Yeagin's description against a list of recently deceased unidentified patients.

When police did so, they finally found Yeagin's body—on a slab in the anatomy laboratory of Howard University Medical School, where he was on the verge of being dissected by students. While his family had searched for him and repeatedly called police, he had lain unconscious in the hospital. When he died, on November 3, "his remains were sent to the medical examiner's office . . . through some lottery or something they decided to award his body to one of the medical schools and it wound up at Howard," Dr. Linwood Rayford, then the school's assistant medical director, told the *Washington Post*.[1] On January 4, 1978, police used fingerprints to identify Yeagin.

Rayford's forthright allusion to a misplaced patient and cadaver lottery is troubling enough, but Champ nursed an even darker view of the affair. She told the *Post* her uncle had been found "up in the lab, you know [and they were] making experiments."

"We were not making any, quote, 'experiments,' " Dr. Rayford dryly demurred. Champ found it difficult to believe the hospital had made good-faith errors, but it did not help that the hospital, which insisted Yeagin had died of natural causes, was unable to tell his family from what illness he had suffered.[2] Also, Yeagin's pockets had contained the name and telephone number of a nephew, yet this man had never been called.

Yeagin's family was haunted by a plethora of unanswered questions: From what disease had Yeagin died? Why had hospital personnel failed to report his presence or to contact his nephew? They took their quest for answers and justice to the courts, suing the D.C. city government and Howard University Hospital for negligence.

Judge Nicholas Nunzio dismissed the negligence charges against the hospital, but a District of Columbia superior court jury decided against the city, awarding the family $53,000 and some answers. The ruling against the city and the award were reversed on appeal, but the answers revealed to Yeagin's family how he came to end up in the anatomy laboratory. On September 11, the police had taken an inebriated Yeagin to a detoxification center. The paper in his wallet with his nephew's name and address was ignored and placed with Yeagin's possessions in storage at the center. When he grew ill the next day, Yeagin was taken to Howard University Hospital without these items and admitted as a John Doe.

Over the next months, hospital staffers repeatedly told Yeagin's sisters that no one of his description had been admitted, even though he was the *only* unidentified patient in the hospital during this period. When Yeagin died, his body was taken to the medical examiner's office, which donated it to Howard University Medical School.

Among other things, Yeagin's story illustrates a classic discord in interpretation between many African Americans and medical personnel. Intentionally or not, Yeagin and his family were certainly abused and exploited. But like many African Americans, Minnie Champ imputed a darker motive to the hospital than was indicated by the facts. One factor feeding the friction between Yeagin's family and the hospital may have been a confusion of the concepts of experimentation, dissection, and autopsy. Human experimentation entails an induced change that is carefully controlled and monitored to reveal medical or scientific information. *Dissection,* from the Latin verb *dissecare,* means "to cut apart." This procedure is undertaken to identify and examine a body's components, during, for example, medical education. This is the surgical process that Yeagin's body had been on the verge of undergoing. *Autopsy* and *necropsy* are the terms used for an investigative dissection by physicians who are attempting to determine the cause and other circumstances of a person's death.[3]

The hospital personnel (who in this case happened to be primarily African American) cast the Yeagin incident as a regrettable fluke—rare and unlikely to be repeated. But is *this* characterization supported by the facts? How often do the bodies of the poor, the homeless, the friendless, or those who, like Yeagin, simply look that way to medical personnel, end up on anatomy tables? What role has race played in such events—yesterday and today?

The short answer is that the bodies of African Americans were once at the highest risk of being used for anatomy: In many areas, the majority of cadavers in research or dissection laboratories were black. But today, that risk has shrunk dramatically for African Americans. Experts claim that mostly white bodies are used today, but they can produce no good ethnic national data to quantify this. Because the Uniform Anatomical Gift Act of 1968 provides for the distribution of unclaimed bodies to medical schools and other public and private consumers of human cadavers and tissues, and because minority groups are overrepresented among the poor and homeless who constitute the bulk of these bodies, all indications suggest that black bodies are still more likely than whites to populate dissection laboratories.

However, the historical data are unambiguous and reveal a long-standing preference for African American bodies, which suggests that the fears of many African Americans emanate from an ugly historical tradition, not from overly fertile imaginations. Minnie Champ's fears about "experiments" may well have been misplaced, but they were not baseless. They reflected a failure to distinguish the frankly abusive dangers of yesterday from the narrower hazards of today.

Until the last century, American medical practitioners shared a deep frustration with much of Europe. Anatomical dissection had become key to physician training, but because the procurement of cadavers, and often dissection itself, was illegal and socially unacceptable, doctors and their porters had to employ a macabre creativity leavened with criminal force to secure the bodies of the recently deceased for dissection. These bodies tended to be black. "The attitudes of white southerners both toward the use of human bodies in medical education and toward blacks were silently but clearly revealed in the medical profession's heavy reliance on negro cadavers,"[4] observed Todd L. Savitt. Hospitals habitually delivered black bodies directly from the wards to the autopsy tables without asking anyone's consent. Today, the legacy of this "postmortem racism" survives in policies that continue to appropriate the bodies of "friendless paupers" such as the homeless—a disproportionate number of whom are black—for medical purposes.

Medical educators hold that dissection is necessary because students must familiarize themselves with the human body before they treat living patients. Who, they ask, would wish to be treated by a doctor who had never personally investigated and familiarized herself with a human body?[5] However, recent studies show that fewer people are donating their bodies for medical education. In a 2004 Johns Hopkins report, only 49 percent of those surveyed said they would consider donating their bodies; worse, up to 70 percent fewer African Americans said they would donate. Race and education were the most important determinants.

African American literacy was still widely outlawed and remained low in affected communities until the early twentieth century, so witnesses spread the information about this exploitation of black bodies via oral traditions that alerted others to the danger but sometimes exaggerated its extent. Word of mouth spread the reputation of hospitals and medical schools (which were not typically affiliated with hospitals until the middle of the nineteenth century) as repositories for black bodies that had been stolen under cover of darkness by "night doctors" for use in medical dissection rooms and laboratories. This oral tradition is frequently dismissed as "old wives' tales" and "superstition" because tales of the theft of black bodies sound fantastic to many whites—and to African Americans who pride themselves on their scientific sophistication. Many people assume that belief in the theft of black bodies is paranoia born of a violently racist history.

But Janie Gaines and Sarah Cox know from experience that black cadavers tend to disappear. In January 1998, the sisters frowned as they surveyed the crumbling headstones, trash, and tangled weeds strangling Greenwood, the Birmingham, Alabama, cemetery in which their family had long ago laid their sister, Addie Mae Collins. Although most Americans do not know her name, Addie Mae is a national icon of sorts. The thirteen-year-old was a martyr of the civil rights movement, one of four girls who were murdered in the 1963 bombing of Birmingham's Sixteenth Street Baptist Church a few days after the city's schools were integrated. Martin Luther King, Jr., eulogized her, and her tombstone bears the rousing inscription "She Died So Freedom Might Live."[6]

It was thirty years before her sisters could bear to visit her grave, and when they saw its neglected state, they immediately arranged to have Addie Mae moved to another, better-maintained cemetery. However, workers who opened the grave recoiled in shock: It was empty, devoid of casket and corpse. Addie Mae's body, like so many buried in black cemeteries throughout the South, is missing.[7] No one can know with certainty who took the body or why, but many are convinced that her body joined the untold thousands of anonymous black cadavers on anatomists' tables.

Skeletons in the Closet

That Addie Mae's fate is far from unique was driven home by a grisly 1989 discovery during a breathlessly hot August in Augusta, Georgia.

Construction workers renovating a stately 154-year-old Greek Revival structure that once housed the Medical College of Georgia (MCG) stumbled upon a nightmare cached beneath the building. Strewn beneath its concrete floor lay a chaos of desiccated body parts and nearly *ten thousand* human bones and skulls, many bearing the marks of nineteenth-century anatomy tools or numbered with India ink.[8]

The cool, sunless basement had preserved the remains remarkably well. Bones and human "dissected material" littered the floors, metal tubs, and even latrines. Ossified human remains spilled from broken vats that had once held cadavers preserved in alcohol. Jars held fetal organs in vanishing lakes of whiskey—an indication that scientists had displayed the purloined bodies, using the alcohol as a preservative, in addition to dissecting them. Because not only grave robbing but also anatomical dissection were illegal in Georgia until 1887, there was no legal source of such bodies: They were stolen, and in a manner that outraged decency and violated the law.

This disarticulated nightmare was all that remained of faceless people whose bodies had been dissected, then unceremoniously scattered in the basement amid a jumble of broken syringes, microscope slides, scalpels, old pill bottles, and other medical detritus. As years passed, medical personnel covered each stratum of human refuse with quicklime to quell the stench, and later the basement was cemented over. Scientists determined that most of the remains dated from the nineteenth century,[9] and detailed analyses of the bones and surrounding materials revealed that 75 percent of the bones in the basement were those of African Americans,[10] although blacks constituted only 42 percent of the area's population.[11]

The late Robert Blakeley, then chair of the Georgia State University's Department of Anthropology, gathered a multidisciplinary team, which later reported on almost every scientific and humanistic approach to analyzing the 9,800 human bones the MCG had used between 1835 and 1912. The ethnically diverse (one-third African American) scientific team included medical doctors, archaeologists, anthropologists, medical historians, anatomists, biochemists, population geneticists, nutritionists, and even folklorists who analyzed a great deal of information about the subjects' bodies, lives, and cultures from the MCG remains.[12] They determined age from the age-specific growth and fusing of bones such as sutures of the skull and wrist bones. The angle of pelvic bones and bone thicknesses and ratios revealed gender.

Many physiological and medical methods certified racial identification. The separate lives of blacks and whites in the mid-nineteenth-century South provided much of the definitive racial data. Blacks and whites ate different diets, wore different clothes, suffered from different disorders, worked at different occupations, took different medications, and died from different diseases and disorders, many of which left their marks on bones. Area residents, black and white, were also questioned about their knowledge and beliefs concerning the school's activities.[13] This inclusive approach allowed the scientists to do more than interpret medical truths; they also listened to the previously voiceless African American victims of body-stealing. Via interviews and questionnaires, blacks finally were able to contribute their perspective to the historial record.

The basement was filled with mostly black bodies not by accident, but by design. As the nineteenth century progressed, doctors' needs for cadavers for medical education and training surged, but dissection was abhorrent, a shameful fate reserved for the most heinous criminals, who received a double sentence of execution and dissection. As a result, physicians appropriated the bodies of enslaved persons with no legal rights or those of free blacks with no rights that a white man was obligated to respect.

The bodies in the basement had been spirited by night from the graveyard—but not from just any graveyard: Most were taken from Cedar Grove Cemetery, an African American burial ground.[14] We know this for several reasons. Physiological, anthropological, and nutritional assessments of the bones and other remains established that three-quarters of them came from blacks, and Cedar Grove had held black bodies exclusively since the Civil War. Since its founding, black Augusta residents had consistently complained of grave robbing there. Also, the college's four or five porters had all named the black cemetery in their periodic reports on the provenance of the cadavers they provided to students each term. In a 1908 lecture to the students, for example, porter Grandison Harris described his techniques and named Cedar Grove as his milieu.[15] Other eyewitness accounts verified this, such that of MCG Professor Eugene Murphy, M.D., whose 1938 memoirs describe how he accompanied Harris to Cedar Grove as a young medical student seeking bodies.[16] Half a century later, the MCG's scientific assessment helped to validate blacks' tales of "night doctors" who reaped grim harvests in black cemeteries. The school's dissecting tables and, finally, its basement became their victims' only resting places.

But the basement lacked even the minimal dignity of the meanest grave. It was devoid of placards, headstones, personal effects, or funerary artifacts marking the social worth, or even the very presence, of the dead. There had been no attempt to identify the bones, nor to arrange the remains in any attitude of dignity. Instead, they lay amid broken glassware, food containers, patent medicine bottles, and even the remains of vivisected animals—just another heap of discarded training material.

At first blush, robbing black graveyards to fill white anatomists' laboratories appears a purely racial issue. But men like Grandison Harris complicated the picture, because they were black. In 1852, the MCG bought the thirty-six-year-old Harris, a strapping, muscular native of the Gullah islands, on a South Carolina slave-auction block for seven hundred dollars. The school had not purchased a strong man just to clean its floors; his chief duty was to rob graves. MCG faculty taught Harris to read, which enabled him to glean details of deaths and the dates of funeral services from obituaries. He would return after nightfall to pull bodies from the fresh graves with his powerful arms. After the Civil War, the former slave became a Reconstruction judge in South Carolina, but when African Americans lost their newfound political power, the MCG offered Harris his old job at six dollars a month. Although he eventually learned some anatomy and assisted in training students, Harris remained an object of affectionate derision among faculty members, who called him "Judge" while issuing cleaning orders. But he was feared by blacks who knew that he was raiding Cedar Grove for bodies.[17] When he died in 1911 of heart failure, he was buried there, but he was the only internee whose eternal rest was assured, because his son succeeded him at the MCG.[18]

Harris is a prime example of a cadaver procurer, or "resurrectionist." Until the late 1770s, a resurrectionist meant a believer in physical or spiritual resurrection; then the term underwent a sea change, becoming an ironic label for a man who unearthed bodies for illicit dissection (the other common term was "resurrection man").[19] Many medical schools found it convenient to leave the plundering of black cemeteries to black grave robbers because the faculty tried to distance themselves from resurrectionists who were caught with the goods. But the schools were obviously providing a market for the bodies, so their claims that the porters were overzealous freelancers were rarely convincing.

To acknowledge the occasional medical victimization of blacks by blacks is considered heretical, but it is also an ugly fact. The nature of the medical abuse is racial, but class and self-interest could play pivotal roles, as with the black resurrectionists.

We can only condemn the sad horror hidden in the basement of the MCG, but it is critically important to realize that the handling of the discovery provides a hopeful note, because the MCG resisted the temptation to minimize or hide its ugly history and cooperated fully with the scientific team. Although belated, this frankness fosters an atmosphere in which it is possible to nurture trust: Augusta's African Americans may one day participate in research without fear that they may be exploited and abused.

Other construction sites throughout the country have yielded evidence of medical grave robbing. The largest and earliest African burial site in the nation was revealed in June 1991 during preparations to build on the lower Manhattan site of what is now the Foley Square Federal Office Tower Building in New York City. Construction workers unearthed 427 skeletons in what had been consecrated as the "Negros Burying Ground" in the eighteenth century. In 1992, the team of Michael Blakely, director of Howard University's W. Montague Cobb Biological Anthropology Laboratory, found widespread evidence of grave robbing, including missing coffins, as well as bodies and skulls that displayed anatomists' marks. Despite the frequent characterization of blacks as syphilitic, the team did not find the characteristic ridges caused by the disease on the cadavers' bones.[20] Smaller cadaver-disposal sites have been found on the campuses of the University of Michigan and the Medical College of Virginia, and more such remains will undoubtedly be unearthed.

Why did physicians begin amassing black bodies in the nineteenth century? Early in that century, the "Paris school," or "hospital movement," transferred the Continental focus from traditional heroic measures of dubious efficacy to clinic-based scientific medicine based upon a system of rigorous scientific education, anatomical knowledge, and experimentation-based therapeutics.[21] A detailed, systemic study of the human body began to supplement the memorization of materia medica (the formal study of therapeutics, which was the forerunner of pharmacology). It was no longer sufficient for an amphitheater of students to watch a professor perform a single anatomical dissection. The nascent physician himself required the intimate familiarity that could come only from the dissection of human cadavers.[22]

In addition to the needs of medical students, clinicians and researchers needed bodies to autopsy in order to understand the processes by which diseases ravaged the body—and to understand the real, as opposed to the supposed, causes of death. At least so medical school professors said, when urging lawmakers to give them greater access to cadavers.[23] Yet Yale historian John Harley Warner observes that it would be decades before physicians were knowledgeable enough to use the information they gleaned from autopsies to heal: At first, the anatomical course served as just another badge of professionalism. Whatever the true cause, the need for human bodies escalated sharply.

Practical or not, anatomical courses were now de rigueur in medical training, and medical school applications soared. This further fueled a hunger for corpses, which the laws of the era made very difficult to satisfy. The only legal source of bodies for dissection resulted from a double sentence of execution and dissection, which was quite rare, reserved as punishment for only the most heinous murders.[24]

Dr. A. B. Crosby described an execution-and-dissection sentence pronounced on a black man who was hung "about 1800" in Haverhill, New Hampshire. Crosby's first-person account of the subsequent autopsy evokes an appallingly circuslike atmosphere, one hard to distinguish from that characterizing a lynching:

> All the neighboring physicians were invited to be present and were requested to bring any dissecting instrument they might deem of use. Tradition says that one brought a hand-saw, another an axe, still another a butcher's cleaver and a fourth came armed with a large carving-knife and fork.
>
> . . . the cuticle of this unfortunate Ethiope was subsequently tanned and cut up into small pieces, as souvenirs . . .[25]

The invasive violation involved in the anatomical dissection of a corpse ran counter to very strong nineteenth-century sentiments regarding the sanctity of the body. Today, a dead body is an alien entity that we encounter briefly in a hospital, funeral home, or place of worship, but in the eighteenth and nineteenth centuries, people tended to die at home rather than in hospitals, and the body, imbued with religious and social significance, was lovingly cared for in a way that bound the dead person to his family and society. The corpse was carefully bathed and groomed and postmortem photographs, portraits, or other images were often created and distributed. This care of the body certified the person's meaning and status as a member of a family and community. Dissection, however, gave the corpse a very different meaning, limiting him to a bit of useful flesh, an *object* to be surgically severed from his community, treated with disdain, then discarded like trash.

For blacks, anatomical dissection meant even more: It was an extension of slavery into eternity, because it represented a profound level of white control over their bodies, illustrating that they were not free even in death.[26] Burial rituals were so psychologically important that insurance companies sold blacks a macabre "social security" by collecting relatively high weekly payments toward funeral expenses.

Physicians, however, ascribed blacks' horror of postmortem dissection to superstition, complaining that even during epidemics they avoided hospitals because they feared ending up on anatomists' slabs.[27] But whites quietly shared this revulsion, including doctors, who avoided dissecting the bodies of their colleagues.

As a result of the widespread discomfort with dissection, eighteenth-century physicians and students resorted to frenzied, surreptitious dissection of the hospital dead before family or friends could arrive to claim the body. They also preyed upon the bodies of the socially and legally powerless—black Americans. For a hundred years, young white assistant professors of anatomy and uneducated black hospital porters shared the same key responsibility: the furtive procurement of black corpses.[28]

Such exploitation of the dead was hardly limited to the South. Most of the bodies used by New York City's Columbia University and New York University were from the Negros Burying Ground.[29] In 1712 and again in 1741, New York slave rebellions were actuated in part by the refusal of slave owners to allow slaves to bury their dead.[30]

In 1788, blacks petitioned the New York City Common Council, complaining that medical students made regular Bacchanalian raids on the Negros Burial Ground when "under cover of Night and in the most wanton of sallies," they unearthed black bodies to "mangle their flesh out of a wanton curiosity and then expose it to the Beasts and Birds." The Common Council did not deign to answer the petition, and the popular press showed little sympathy. One newspaper opined that "the only subjects procured for dissection are the productions of Africa . . . if these are the only subjects of dissection, surely no one can object."[31] Some sympathetic whites, notably Quakers and abolitionists, did object, to no avail. But when emboldened medical students extended their forays into white graveyards at Trinity Church and the Brick Presbyterian Church, New Yorkers objected en masse. Blacks were among the five thousand rioters who stormed New York Hospital in the two-day Doctors' Riot of 1788, pillaging Columbia Medical School and assaulting physicians in retaliation for disturbing the eternal rest of New Yorkers.[32]

By the 1820s, instruction in anatomy was ubiquitous in medical schools, which were burgeoning. In 1810, there were five medical schools in the United States; in 1860, the nation boasted sixty-five, and by 1890 their number had doubled.[33] The demand for medical cadavers grew correspondingly, with dire consequences for black communities. In 1879, five thousand cadavers a years were procured for medical use, most of them illegally, and in the South most were those of African Americans.[34] Even in the absence of racial hatred, the bodies of blacks were preferred simply because they made easier targets.[35] No slave could withhold permission for an autopsy or dissection.[36] If a master sent a sick, elderly, or otherwise-unproductive slave to the hospital, he usually gave the institution caring for and boarding the slave carte blanche for his treatment—and for his disposal.[37]

Moreover, the least sensitive masters aggressively exploited their slaves' fear of postmortem violation. During the transatlantic slave trade, crews discouraged the frequent bloody uprisings among kidnapped Africans by dismembering their bodies "as a deterrent to other African captives who believed that the spirit of a mutilated person would not be able to return to Africa."[38] Dr. Erasmus D. Fenner also noted the effectiveness of postmortem decapitation in controlling slaves: "The negroes have the utmost horror and dread of their bodies being treated in this manner."[39]

For the resurrection man, the black cemetery was the easiest of targets. Most of the black populace could barely afford funerals, to say nothing of guards or mortsafes, cagelike arrays of vertical iron gates that were inserted over the coffin to prevent access by grave robbers.[40] In 1827, the African American newspaper *Freedom's Journal* suggested an economical defense against grave robbing:

> As soon as the corpse is deposited in the grave let a truss of long wheaten straw be opened and distributed in layers, as equally as may be with every layer of earth until the whole is filled up. By this method the corpse will be effectually secured: . . . the longest night will not afford time sufficient to empty the grave, though all the common implements of digging be used for that purpose.[41]

Whites quietly acquiesced to the violation of black bodies because they saw grave robbing as a zero-sum game. That is, whites knew that physicians' lust for cadavers would be satisfied somewhere—if not from black cemeteries, then from white ones, despite guards, mortsafes, and the wounded feelings of white families.[42]

To ensure that the anatomy laboratories in the South would continue to be peopled with black, not white, corpses, state legislatures enacted (and newspapers championed) a variety of statutes to validate the existing racial disparity with regard to dissection. In 1828, for example, the Georgia legislature considered a proposal to send the bodies of executed black felons to medical societies for anatomical dissection, expressly to ensure that white corpses would be spared. A *Statesman and Patriot* correspondent insisted:

> The bodies of colored persons, whose execution is necessary to public security, may, we think, be with equity appropriated for the benefit of a science on which so many lives depend, while the measure would in a great degree secure the sepulchral repose of those who go down into the grave amidst the lamentations of friends and the reverence of society.[43]

The *Richmond* [Virginia] *Whig* suggested in 1838 that the city's large black population made it a likely site for the establishment of a medical school that would rival those of Philadelphia because "... in Philadelphia, as every professional man versed on the subject well knows, from *the almost sole use of whites* in the labor of the city ... the supply for anatomical purposes, is totally inadequate to the wants of a large medical class." A black Richmond newspaper, *The Colored American,* quickly responded:

> ... Medical science requires "anatomical subjects;" it is not fitting the dignity nor the sensibilities of white men to use their dead bodies for such purposes; and black men are not every where to be found; but in Richmond they may be found; and as the dignity and sensibility of a black man are of no account, and the health of slaveholders requires that they should have good physicians; articles to be forthcoming only from a "Medical College" where "anatomical subjects" are abundant, *ergo* a medical college ought to be established at Richmond.
>
> ... O Slavery! Foul spirit of darkness! Not content with gorging thyself with the tears and the blood of thy living victim, thou followest him into his grave, and there tearest him limb from limb, and riotest amid the last relics of his corrupting dust, as if thou coldst be satisfied with nothing short of his annihilation!

The writings of private physicians and medical schools reveal that they freely availed themselves of the bodies of blacks who came into their care. In 1839, a Dr. Harris of Savannah lamented his failure to save a group of slave patients who had died from cholera, but within the same sentence, he comforted himself with the reflection that he "would certainly have ample material with which to investigate the anatomical characters of the disease on the following day."[44] That same year, Dr. Edward Eve went to the grave site of a slave who had died under his care, intercepted her body, and removed the stomach before her burial to study it "in a convenient place of examination."[45]

Medical journals also provide evidence of the racial disparity with regard to autopsies. Historian Todd Savitt discovered that between 1849 and 1851, fully nineteen of the twenty-four autopsies that white physicians described in the *Transylvania Journal of Medicine* and in the *Associate Sciences and the Transylvania Medical Journal* were performed upon blacks—and this transpired in Kentucky, where the white population greatly dwarfed the black. So were all three of the autopsies on Alabamans who died in an 1853 typhus fever epidemic.[46]

Around 1850, doctors' prayers for more cadavers were answered, thanks in part to Jeremy Bentham, the British apostle of utilitarianism,[47] who held that laws should be predicated upon actions that produce the greatest good for the most people. For a society that wanted superlative medical care, the greatest good lay in sacrificing the bodies of people who were dead for the well-being of the living.

Informed by Bentham's philosophical spirit, northern state legislatures began replacing absolute legal bans on dissection with colorfully nicknamed laws that sought to supply more bodies for dissection to satisfy the medical establishment. But these laws tended to protect the repose of the white middle- and upper-class populace while sacrificing the bodies of the black and poor. New York passed its "Bone Bill" in 1854, which gave anatomists legal access to the bodies of almshouse denizens and others of the "friendless poor"—who were disproportionately black. Pennsylvania's "Ghastly Act" did the same in 1867.[48] Such laws also had to address petty territoriality among various medical schools. In January 1875, an Indianapolis newspaper interviewed a resurrectionist, who confided, "Now I'm goin' to tell you about what I call a mean trick. A stiff had been raised out of grounds supposed to be the peculiar property of one of the colleges, and sold to another. It wasn't much of a stiff, a poor, miserable, emaciated Negro, that didn't weigh more'n ninety pounds. . . . But it made the faculty of ——— college madder'n hornets to think that a stiff out of their ground had been sold to a rival college. . . ."[49]

Many blacks claimed that some "night doctors" killed for anatomical specimens, and Edinburgh's 1828 Burke and Hare affair had demonstrated that this was a real risk.[50] Between Christmas 1827 and October 1828, William Burke and William Hare murdered between sixteen and twenty-three Scottish residents and sold their bodies to anatomy professor Dr. Robert Knox for from seven to ten pounds each. When they were discovered, Hare gained his freedom by turning crown's evidence against Burke, who was convicted and hanged on January 28, 1829. His legacy included the eponymous term *burking*, which denotes a murder, usually by suffocation, carried out to effectuate a sale to anatomists. Knox was acquitted, as usually happened when physicians were discovered in collusion with body snatchers: Doctors went free, while their black and lower-class confederates were punished. In America, the 1886 burking of Baltimore resident Emily Brown has been amply documented. Brown was a poor white woman who lived in a black neighborhood, and her body's sale to the University of Maryland School of Medicine for fifteen dollars by John Thomas Ross and Albert Hawkins, business associates of Anderson Perry, the school's black resurrection man, aroused suspicions.[51] There are no documented cases of burked blacks, but this may simply reflect the southern social milieu of the era: There are no legally documented rapes of black women by whites in the South during this period, either, but they occurred.

The North shared the South's dependence upon black bodies. Medical historian David Humphrey records the widespread belief that by 1788, few blacks "were permitted to remain in the grave." As in the South, northern hospitals expected blacks to submit to research, including autopsy and dissection, as "payment" for having been treated in charity wards, and all blacks were consigned to such wards. Northern schools also relied upon clandestine exports of black bodies from the South, which were only briefly interrupted by the Civil War.[52] An industry sprang up in shipping black bodies to northern medical colleges. Dr. F. C. Waite recalled that "many bodies of southern Negroes were used in northern medical colleges. . . . [A] Professor of Anatomy in a New England medical school told me . . . he had an arrangement under which he received in each session a shipment of twelve bodies of Southern Negroes. They came in barrels marked 'turpentine.' . . ."[53]

This traffic in black bodies for dissection ran in both directions. The 1841 travel memoirs of Englishman James Silk Buckingham contain this clipping:

More Pork for the South

Yesterday morning it was discovered that a barrel, which had been put into the office of the Charleston packet line . . . for the purpose of being shipped to Charleston contained ye bodies of two dead negroes. The cask and its contents were sent up to the police office and placed in the dead house for the coroner.[54]

The barrel's contents were addressed to the professors of a medical school. Buckingham added that this was the fourth such discovery that month and that "no further inquiry appears to have been made into the matter, as if it were altogether beneath the notice of white men to trace out these traders in the dead bodies of blacks."[55]

Black graveyards were the favored hunting grounds of northern body snatchers. In 1829, John D. Godman, M.D., wrote of how, on behalf of several Philadelphia medical schools, he had secretly paid the manager of a public graveyard for the privilege of "emptying the pits" of about fifty to eighty-five cadavers a month during each "dissecting season." The reference to a dissection season was pragmatic as well as academic. Before the advent of efficient preservative technology, corpses decayed quickly. Except for those corpses that were pickled in whiskey for export, bodies were exhumed during the cool of the academic year, from fall through spring. Todd Savitt explains that blacks were well aware of this morbid seasonality, as evinced by one elderly Virginia slave who, passing the medical school, shuddered and muttered, "Please God, I hope when I die, it'll be in the summertime."[56]

Newspaper descriptions of executions regularly noted that as a matter of course, the bodies of black, but not white, criminals were to be dissected. One account read, "The execution of Cook and Coppic, white men, Copeland and Green, colored, took place at Charleston [Virginia] on Friday last. . . . The bodies of Cook and Coppic were taken to Harper's Ferry in a train which was waiting at the depot. The bodies of the negroes have been given to surgeons and medical students."[57]

When Pennsylvania passed its "Ghastly Act" in 1867, it stipulated that its medical schools could use only unclaimed bodies of the poor from Philadelphia and Pittsburgh. Such laws were insufficient to protect black bodies from continuing to be seized by medical schools, simply because the laws supplied too few bodies to the schools. During the 1881–1882 academic year, Philadelphia boasted 1,493 medical students but only four hundred cadavers. Both lawfully obtained bodies and those stolen from cemeteries were likely to be those of African Americans. As David Humphrey observed, "Legalization did not substantially alter the social origins of the supply. It simply assured that cadavers would come entirely—rather than primarily—from America's lowest social strata."[58]

In 1867, an Ann Arbor newspaper reported that "two colored men were caught in Chicago on the night of the 15th with a wagon in which were five dead bodies, which they had taken from the cemetery. They claim to have been employed by the authority of Rush Medical College." Eight years later, the *Indianapolis Herald* published an interview with an unnamed resurrection man, an alcoholic physician fallen on hard times. He crowed that he sought corpses from black and pauper graveyards: "The stiffs are raised at Greenlawn Cemetery, Mt. Jackson Cemetery and the poor farm cemetery. So far as I know, Crown Hill [a private white graveyard] has never been troubled."[59]

Northern medical schools recognized that being unable to acquire sufficient cadavers to attract medical students could mean their dissolution, so they imported black corpses, and in 1933, Howard University's Dr. Montague Cobb, the first African American professor of anatomy, ironically alluded to the unconsciously egalitarian implications: "Our colleagues [in the anatomy laboratory] recognized in the Negro a perfection in human structure which they were unwilling to concede when that structure was animated by the vital spark."[60] The clandestine nature of such transactions made estimating the relative numbers of such bodies difficult, but in 1935, Cobb rose to the challenge by analyzing the 2,139 cadavers that had passed through the Laboratory of Anatomy of Western Reserve University in Cleveland, Ohio, since 1835. He showed that the bodies of whites were initially used in the Midwest but that they were rapidly replaced by imported black bodies. Cobb found that in contrast to white cadavers, which were local, "a heavy Majority" of Cleveland's Negro cadavers emanated from southern states—Georgia, Alabama, South Carolina, Tennessee, Virginia, Kentucky, Mississippi, North Carolina, and Arkansas. After the wartime exodus of blacks from the South, the imported black bodies were replaced by those of resident blacks, out of all proportion to immigration trends. "Although there were twelve times more White than Negro deaths, only twice as many Whites arrived at the laboratory *or relatively six times more of the Negro dead.* . . . In the last five years, the proportion of Negro to White *cadavera* has been much greater than would be expected from the number of city deaths."[61]

Northern medical schools also employed strategies to make the most of the black and poor-white populations they had. For example, on February 20, 1810, Dr. John Warren and Professor of Chemistry Aaron Dexter presented the president and fellows of Harvard University with a "Memorial & Petition for the Removal of Med. Lect. to Boston," in which they made their case for moving Harvard Medical School from the university's home base in Cambridge across the Charles River to Boston, where it could avail itself of cadavers from the poor black and white denizens of the almshouse. Warren successfully argued that "one of the great objects" of the school was to offer students cadavers for dissection, without which Harvard might be eclipsed by "other [medical] establishments, even in the remote areas of the country."[62] Later that year, the medical school moved to Boston.

As slavery was abolished in most of the nation, acerbic protests and occasional riots further scarred the medical establishment's relations with black communities. In December 1882, screams and curses rent the air as the Philadelphia morgue was thronged by distraught black mourners who had come to retrieve the bodies of their recently buried loved ones. They were drawn by sensationalistic newspaper accounts of an intercepted grave robbing the night before. At 11:00 P.M., newspaper reporters had stopped a wagon driven by two white men, Frank McNamee and Henry Pillet. In the back, a black man, Levi Chew, perched on an oilcloth that hid bodies uprooted from Lebanon Cemetery, Philadelphia's African American burial ground. Levi Chew was the brother of Lebanon Cemetery director Robert Chew, and the bodies were hidden in a wagon bound for Jefferson Medical College. Frank McNamee confessed that for three years he had hauled bodies from Lebanon Cemetery to Jefferson Medical College at the behest of Dr. William Forbes, Jefferson's chief anatomist, who had even given McNamee keys to the anatomy laboratory for greater convenience in completing deliveries. As gatekeeper of the cemetery and the resurrection man's brother, Robert Chew, was complicit and presumably received his share of the eight dollars that Forbes paid for each body.

Now, the intercepted bodies lay in the city morgue, awaiting identification by family members. Even allowing for the newspaper hyperbole of the era, the scene was a heartbreaking one. Distraught families vowed vengeance on the grave robbers, and sobs racked a prostrated old woman who had been able to bury her husband only after begging the requisite twenty dollars from his former co-workers at the wharves.

Utilizing a disquieting double standard, African Americans excused the resurrectionists and blamed the doctors. An African American minister raged against the doctors, saying, "They set the plot [a]foot and used the men under arrest as pliant tools!" But the law didn't agree. A jury of eleven whites and one black sentenced the three grave robbers and the cemetery director to ten-year prison terms.

On the witness stand, Dr. Forbes admitted he had paid the resurrection men for 150 bodies a year but said he enforced a strict "don't ask, don't tell" policy concerning the provenance of the bodies. Seemingly unmindful of the irony, the Philadelphia newspapers praised his subsequent acquittal with the same fervor with which they had condemned the resurrectionists. They did chide him obliquely for having perhaps acted "ignorantly or unthinkingly."

In both cases, judgments were issued along racial fault lines, not according to ethical or legal precepts. The black populace ignored the fact that the Chews were guilty of a doubly betrayed trust: to people who entrusted the cemetery owner with bodies of their loved ones and to their larger ethnic community. The racially imbalanced jury and newspaper exonerated the white physician and focused blame on the grave robbers.

Watching the Bones

For many, the final manifestation of medical racism is the postmortem display of African American bodies. Without their consent, stuffed, mummified, or skeletal black bodies have been displayed in doctor's offices, anatomy laboratories, museums, traveling sideshows, and even private businesses. Some libraries and physicians still possess books bound in the skins of African Americans, souvenirs that were typically bought from grave robbers: Even in death, African Americans were bought and sold.[63]

"They put my mother on display like a monkey in the zoo," complained retired Brooklyn teacher Frances Oglesby in 2001 as she announced her suit against the Medical College of Georgia for the return of her mother's remains and $800,000 in damages for pain and suffering.

All that remains of Oglesby's mother, Bessie Wilborn, is a skeleton that has hung on display for half a century in the pathology laboratory of the same school that hid African American bones in its basement. However Wilborn, a poor, frail African American woman who lived in Lincoln County, sixty miles northwest of Augusta, was consigned not to obscurity but to display as an object of horrible wonder. Why? She suffered from Paget's disease, a bone disorder that deformed her skeleton so monstrously that she died of the ailment in 1950, at age twenty-eight.[64] Augusta surgeon Peter B. Wright fully explored Wilborn's crippling bone deformities when he performed her autopsy, which he vividly described in a 1951 *Journal of Bone and Joint Surgery* article.[65] Wright then removed the flesh from her body and reconstructed her skeleton, which he displayed at that year's winter meeting of the American Academy of Orthopedic Surgeons in New York City. Her bizarrely arresting bony cage won Wright a medal for originality.

Wilborn's family thought she had been buried. After Oglesby sued, the MCG eventually agreed to return Wilborn's remains and pay for their burial, but on her lawyer's advice that this would destroy evidence central to her suit, she refused.[66] A Georgia court of appeals ruled against Oglesby in 2004, noting that the school had been immune from lawsuits when her mother died and that she had waited too long to sue.[67] Wilborn's skeleton still hangs in the MCG, jealously guarded from all but MCG eyes.[68]

Displaying the bodies of African Americans has helped to alienate them from the health-care system very efficiently. An incident in the life of a Dr. Simpkins of Lewisburg, West Virginia, was offered by a local biographer to illustrate that the doctor was "imbued with the spirit of research and a desire to improve his knowledge of medicine." When an enslaved African American named Tom was condemned to death for a murder in 1824, Simpkins said he obtained Tom's body by promising him all the gingerbread he could eat until his hanging.[69] After the execution, Simpkins assembled Tom's skeleton and hung it on his waiting-room door, where, the biographer explains, it terrified patients when the wind occasioned its movements. The latter detail is telling, because Tom's skeleton is no symbol of scientific illumination: It has been transformed into a sort of medical bogeyman.

Black bodies on anatomists' tables, blacks' skeletons hanging in doctors' offices, and the widespread display of purloined black body parts constituted the same kind of warning to African Americans as did the bodies of lynched men and women left hanging on trees where blacks would be sure to see them, or cut up as souvenirs of racial violence.

Yale historian John Harley Warner has observed that a symbolic parallel is also clearly visible between the formal stances in the dual tableaux of commemorative professional portraits of medical students and the commemorative portraits of whites celebrating the lynching of African American men and women. Warner has also noted that posing for professional portraits in anatomy laboratories with remains of dissected cadavers became an important professional ritual for medical students, a sort of specialized class portrait that highlighted their new professional and class standing and their completion of the anatomy course, an important medical rite of passage. Before 1920, the students were nearly always white and the cadavers often black. Images of African Americans who were lynched and dissected were treated alike in several telling ways. The dead bodies were often horribly mutilated: Body parts are excised and missing, and they are burned, castrated, or fresh wounds are visible. The bodies were also posed in undignified attitudes that accentuated whites' dominance over them: The lynched were shown handcuffed, bound, hanging, gagged, and tied to stakes, and the dissected had been flayed, propped up, with playing cards placed in their hands and cigarettes in their mouths, posed in chairs, or dressed in outlandish clothes or hats. The dead bodies were often stripped nude or partially so, while the revelers tended to be well, even festively, dressed. The white groups project an air of jubilant camaraderie and tend to look directly at the camera in an unself-conscious, even proud manner.

Souvenir images of both types were often distributed in the forms of photographs or postcards of the anatomists or lynchers with the body. Actual body parts such as fingers, ears, patches of skin, and bones were seized, sold, and collected as souvenirs. Lynched bodies and grisly human souvenirs served as warnings to blacks that whites could torture them, murder them, and defile their bodies with impunity: Any African American, literate or not, could read the same clear warnings in professional portraits of groups of jocular white physicians and physicians-to-be posing with flayed, dissected black remains.

The disrespectful use and display of black cadavers by white medical students is a recurring motif in physicians' writings. During the 1850s, Dr. Henry Lewis Clay, a southern physician with a literary bent, published many raucous accounts of medical exploits by a fictional alter ego. In one tale, Dr. Madison Tensas, Lewis's protagonist, is a medical student who is secretly enraptured with the daughter of a Kentucky scion. Tensas ventures into the basement of his school, where he spies a group of corpses, including that of a mother and infant.

> I strove to depart, but something formed a bond of association between that dead nigger baby and myself, which held me to my place, my gaze riveted upon it. I wanted just such a subject—one I could carry up in my private room and dissect whilst I was waiting for my meals—something to wile [sic] away my tedious hours with—

On impulse, he steals the body, hides it beneath his coat, and darts into the street, where he unexpectedly encounters his intended and her father and collides with him, spilling the dead black baby at their feet. "My cloak opened as I fell and the force of the fall bursting the envelope, out in all its hideous realities rolled the infernal imp of darkness upon the gaze of the laughing, but now horrified spectators."[70]

Lewis's other disturbing tales also feature medically abused black bodies, including one in which he hides the face of a harelipped albino Negro in his rooms to frighten a snooping landlady.[71] Even Mark Twain's classic *Adventures of Huckleberry Finn* includes a tale of terror in which Jim, Huck's forty-year-old black companion, is forced by his medical-student owner to warm up a corpse he cannot see on a dissecting-room table in a completely darkened room, "to git him soft so he can cut him up." Interestingly, this tale is now deleted from most editions of this book.[72]

Such narratives unveil the social acceptability of treating black bodies disrespectfully and the widespread understanding that the corpses used for anatomical dissection were black. In Dr. W. J. Mcknight's memoir *The Pioneer Doctor: Recollections of a Body Snatcher,* he regales readers with tales of his years as cadaver procurer, including a section entitled "How I Skinned the Nigger." One especially repugnant tale manages to combine racism with implied sexual aggression and actual medical cannibalism. His fellow medical students play a prank upon Mcknight by placing a cadaver in the bed of his darkened bedroom. Sliding into bed, he feels the body, turns on the light, and sees that the cadaver is that of an African American woman, whom he dubs "Black Sue."[73] "Admiring neither her color nor her temperature," he exacts his revenge by cutting flesh from her body and arranging for it to be cooked and served to his tormentors. Such cadaver stories reflect the importance of enduring anatomy and dissection as a rite of passage and bonding ritual for medical students. Medical aggression against black bodies, whether literal or literary, not only served to foster cohesion among the students but also placed blacks firmly outside the medical circle.

Old Habits Die Hard

The use of black bodies for anatomical dissection died slowly in the South.

As the twentieth century arrived and progressed, the racial disparities in cadaver use persisted. So did the threatening display of black bodies. In 1912, when embattled African American medical student Louis Tompkins Wright walked into his first day of anatomy class at Harvard, he was greeted not by his fellow students, but by a strategically placed black male cadaver swinging in the front of the room by ice tongs inserted in its ears.[74]

In 1893, only forty-nine cadavers were procured legally at seven Baltimore medical schools that served twelve hundred students. Johns Hopkins was the law-abiding exception: The school legally procured all its twelve hundred cadavers over the next six years; however, two-thirds were black.[75] In 1913, Alabama and Louisiana still lacked a legal source of cadavers. Seven years later, Tennessee grave robbers still supplied bodies for its state medical school *and* for Iowa City's school of medicine.[76]

A 1913 survey of fifty-five medical schools determined that a large majority obtained most of their bodies for dissection from almshouses; other major sources included hospitals and tuberculosis sanitaria. As late as 1933, Dr. W. Montague Cobb conducted a survey for the American Association of Physical Anthropologists which revealed that many southern medical schools of the early twentieth century still used *only* black cadavers for teaching anatomy. By about 1967, in the period during which Addie Mae Collins's body was buried, forty-seven out of eighty-seven schools received less than half of their bodies through volunteers and family donations; the rest were supplied by "entrepreneurs."[77]

Compared to the past, in which African Americans constituted the majority of such bodies, anatomists assure us that today no such ethnic disparity exists. But there is no way to prove this because no federal oversight agency exists and no ethnic data are recorded. Moreover, anatomy professors involved are reluctant to discuss the provenance of the bodies, because each time an exposé hits the newspapers, donations fall.

In 1968, the federal Uniform Anatomical Gift Act (UAGA) was implemented to modernize the distribution of cadavers for medical use, and each state has its own version of the UAGA statute.[78] Today, cadavers are used not only for medical school anatomy laboratories but also for scientific research and specialized surgical training, so the laws also govern the distribution of cadavers to mortuary schools, feet to schools of podiatry, heads to plastic surgery residency training programs, and so on. The laws that dictate the distribution of bodies still foster disparities based upon income, class, and race. In general, the bodies that are used for anatomical dissection and research without the person or his family's permission are today's version of the "friendless poor"—the homeless, and proportionately more blacks than whites are homeless. Another group whose bodies are relatively likely to be donated are poor persons whose families cannot afford to bury them. According to Todd Olson, M.D., professor of anatomy at the Albert Einstein School of Medicine, these persons are more likely to be minority-group members, but he could provide no statistics to support this. Thus the disparity still exists, but in a less dramatic form. Once, black bodies in many anatomy laboratories outnumbered white ones. Now they do not, but they remain present in numbers that are larger than their representation in the population. No one has documented how much larger, but the troubling disproportionate prevalence of black body parts such as organs, corneas, and other tissues is suggestive that blacks also make up a greatly disproportionate number of the entire bodies that are used in research. An overrepresentation of black body parts and organs in transplantation and in industry is driven by legal and medical policies such as the 1987 amendment of the UAGA, which licensed the nonconsensual retrieval of body parts.

Medical policies include bias in organ recruitment and human leukocyte antigen (HLA) matching requirements, which exclude more black than white organ recipients and thus render transplant kidneys unavailable to blacks but not to whites. Legal bias also exists in the form of presumed consent statutes, which were enacted in the 1980s to increase the number of organs donated for transplantation, and which in practice provide black body parts without the consent or knowledge of the decedents or their families. Twenty-nine states allow the coroner or his representative to collect or "harvest" tissues and organs for transplantation and research via various *presumed consent* statutes, which presume that the decedent would want to donate his body parts. However, many blacks do not wish to donate their bodies and body parts. Only 5 percent of black Americans surveyed by DePaul law professor Michele Goodwin considered presumed consent a legitimate source of organs. Eighty-six percent of the blacks she surveyed thought that presumed consent should be illegal.[79] It is blacks whose organs and tissues are most likely to be appropriated via presumed consent by coroners after autopsy, because coroners autopsy the bodies of persons who die in catastrophic accidents or homicides, and during the same period that the presumed consent statutes were enacted, the homicide rates of blacks and Latinos skyrocketed. Since 1980, black Americans have remained six to eight times more likely than whites to be murdered.

I am in no way suggesting that this predominance of black body parts was deliberately engineered, but the confluence of presumed consent statutes and the appearance of black homicide victims on coroners' tables explains why their organs and tissues dominate body-part scandals. For example, in 1997 the Los Angeles coroner's office was found to have sold more than five hundred pairs of corneas a year to the Doheny Eye & Tissue Transplant Bank: 80 percent were of blacks and Latinos whose corneas fetched a profit of *1000 percent*. Theoretically at least, persons may opt out by preventing the harvesting of their own or their loved ones' organs—if they know how and where to lodge objections before death; but few people in the affected twenty-six states know about the laws, which means that they cannot opt out. No public service announcements alert people in affected states, as they alert people of the option of organ donation and of the possibility of signing one's license in order to donate organs.

The same high rate of homicide that delivers blacks to coroners' tables can ultimately deliver them to those of anatomists, because coroners also supply medical learning institutions through the provisions of the UAGA. Today, as in the past, most people whose bodies are so used never gave their permission, because although informed consent remains the gold standard for medical research with living persons, decisions about the donation of one's body after death are made by others. Olson says that in New York State, most cadavers are donated by families.

Some schools, such as Harvard Medical School, preclude exploitation of any bodies by using only those of persons who donated their bodies before their deaths. But in most medical institutions, there are three roads to the anatomist's table. One can volunteer to be dissected or used for medical education; a family can donate the body after death; or the coroner's office can give a body to a medical school if no one with the legal right to do so claims the body and takes responsibility for the costs of disposing of it. In 1999–2000, half the bodies in New York State were donated not by family but by the coroner's office. Eight percent of the bodies used in New York schools fall into the latter category. These unclaimed bodies are more likely to be the bodies of the homeless than not; few other people remain unclaimed for the two to four months that most schools wait before using a cadaver. Estimates from anatomists leave ample grounds to suspect that African Americans still run a greater risk of having their bodies conscripted for medical demonstration, autopsy, and display.

Olson explains that there are no national data describing the proportion of unclaimed bodies to donated bodies. But the case of New York State is instructive because it distributes more bodies for scientific use than any other state. In 1999–2000, New York distributed 120 unclaimed bodies for anatomical dissection; one of every two bodies falls into this category.[80]

The racial disparity may persist, but still there is also evidence of a changed attitude toward anatomical dissection. This evidence lies not in numbers but in new medical traditions. Students no longer mock cadavers by indulging in ribald poses with them; the gruesome genre of stories medical students tell themselves about anatomy-class experiences has persisted, but no longer exclusively features disrespectfully treated blacks. Most hopeful is a new tradition, the anatomical memorial service. In the nineteenth century, the Medical College of Georgia and other schools blindly tossed the bones of African American dissection subjects into its basement, but today's medical schools provide anatomical subjects with burials. Many medical schools also hold memorial services at the conclusion of each anatomy course. Family members are invited and students offer prayers, poems, thanks, and remembrances. There are candles and tears. One would be hard-pressed to distinguish these services from the memorials for any beloved friend or family member.

CHAPTER 6

DIAGNOSIS: FREEDOM

The Civil War, Emancipation, and
Fin de Siècle Medical Research

The regular, simple life, the hygienic conditions, the freedom from dissipation and excitement, steady and healthful employment, enforced self restraint, the freedom from care and responsibility, the plain, wholesome, nourishing food, comfortable clothing, the open-air life upon the plantation, the care and treatment when sick, in those days, all acted as preventive measures against mental breakdown in the negro.

—DR. WILLIAM P. DREWRY, SUPERINTENDENT,
VIRGINIA STATE HOSPITAL FOR THE INSANE, 1908

A witty statesman said, you might prove anything by figures.
—THOMAS CARLYLE, *CHARTISM*, 1840

His medical screeds indicate that Dr. Peter Bryce, superintendent of the Alabama Insane Hospital, thought of himself as progressive. He had run the Tuscaloosa institution since its 1860 opening and prided himself on his currency with scientific advances in mental health. Unlike other institutions for lunacy, his was no human warehouse where diagnostic labels were applied intuitively and treatment was homey and futile. Bryce was scientific: He compiled carefully annotated case histories and observed patients closely before hazarding a diagnosis informed by the very latest in medical research, even research on blacks. For unlike most southern asylums, Bryce's admitted a few black patients. In 1867, he had admitted a former slave of his, and now the very next year a hypervigilant forty-five-year-old ex-slave named John Patterson had been brought for treatment. Patterson was clearly manic, possessed of an unfocused energetic furor that Bryce had encountered often. The doctor believed that, as with other blacks with this condition, the psychological pressure of caring for himself when Patterson possessed neither the intelligence nor the judgment to do had proved too great, and Patterson had sunk into madness. Hence Patterson's mania could have only one cause.

"Diagnosis: Freedom," wrote Bryce.

However, Patterson's medical history belied this diagnosis, because Bryce meticulously documented the course of Patterson's mental illness over the previous dozen years, and Patterson had been free for only five. The pressures of freedom could not have caused his illness. But even had Bryce recognized the glaring illogic of his diagnosis, he might not have been swayed: After all, he had the weight of medical research behind him.[1]

As the Civil War approached, social changes laid heavy siege to the institution of slavery. There were still far more enslaved blacks than free, yet the specter of Negro freedom haunted southern culture. In 1800, Washington, D.C., one of the most important slave markets in the country, was already thronged with 6,152 free blacks; by 1840, its 8,361 free blacks dwarfed its population of 4,694 slaves. By 1860, free blacks there outnumbered black slaves by more than three to one. There were other intimations that American slavery was doomed, such as the panic generated by the escalating slave rebellions. The deaths of fifty-seven whites in Virginia's 1831 Nat Turner revolt radiated shock waves and engendered desperately repressive legislation throughout the slaveholding South. Some states, such as Tennessee, even forced free blacks to leave.[2]

Perhaps the unkindest political blow of all was delivered by Thomas Jefferson's grandson in 1831, when he introduced a bill in the Virginia legislature to abolish slavery. It was defeated by only seven votes.[3]

By 1840, the South's grip on slavery was loosening, but its nondiversified agrarian economy, political power, and medical advances remained utterly dependent upon an unpaid labor force. However, even more was at stake, because the burgeoning ranks of free blacks upped the ante in an all-or-nothing game of social Darwinism. Without the restraining effects of white control, the pro-slavery camp argued, Negroes and mulattoes would outbreed whites in short order. Indeed, the official count of mulattoes had leaped at least 50 percent in just thirty years, and this number represented only the *acknowledged* progeny of black-white matings. Southern whites feared that a proliferation of free, pale-skinned mulattoes would soon efface the all-important social boundary between white and black, rendering "whiteness" meaningless. Years earlier, they had frequented "white negro" exhibits in circuses to experience a frisson of delicious revulsion at a distance—a Coney Island of the southern mind. Now, the threat of the "white negro" was too common and too immediate to entertain.

Scientific racists rode to the rescue by explaining that mulattoes were too weak and infertile to infiltrate and replace whites. Dr. Josiah Nott was the most oft-cited articulator of this "frail mulatto" theory. In his paper "The Mulatto a Hybrid—Probable Extermination of the Two Races if the Whites and Blacks Are Allowed to Intermarry,"[4] Nott explained that mulattoes were an infertile, weak species, who died at a younger age than did whites and whose progency were born feeble.[5] Thus, a mulatto's family line would die out long before the visible evidence of a black forebear became undetectable.[6]

Of course, slavery advocates came from disciplines other than science or medicine. Legal minds scaled the mountain of constitutional support for slavery; philosophers expounded upon the "natural law" that made blacks inherently subservient to whites; and spiritual leaders cited reams of biblical and moral sanctions for enslavement. But scientific medicine was beginning to trump other philosophies. Scientific theories of racial inferiority had strongly informed the entire nation's medical perception of African Americans as befitted for slavery, if only because few scientists outside the South troubled themselves to investigate.

However, by the 1840s, the larger American social climate was inimical to slavery. The North's industrialized economy no longer depended upon cheap southern labor, and the rest of the nation had grown jealous of the political power that the "three-fifths clause"[7] imparted to the South: Its slave population allowed southerners to control Congress.[8] International opposition to slavery had made it an institution truly peculiar to the United States. The nation had become a lonely Western trafficker in human chattel. The medical rationale for slavery—that inferior and feeble blacks were simply unable to govern and care for themselves—was derided as insular and self-serving, and counted few active sympathizers outside the South.

In this contentious climate, the sixth U.S. census (of 1840) began enumerating whites and free and enslaved blacks. For the first time, the census also undertook to count the "insane and idiots"—nineteenth-century argot for the mentally ill and intellectually challenged.[9]

Racism by Numbers

When the census was completed, no one was prepared for its revelations. It enumerated seventeen million Americans, of whom three million were black.[10] But far more important, it revealed that free blacks suffered far worse health, especially far worse mental health, than did enslaved blacks, who enjoyed low rates of disease[11] and suffered almost no mental illness.[12]

These data bolstered pro-slavery arguments by providing copious statistical "proof" that slavery was essential to preserve the health of blacks. Printed in 1841 under the aegis of the U.S. Department of State, the document seemed the very model of objectivity, offering dense or-derly rows and columns of numbers collected by census takers without salient bias.

Census data consistently documented how free blacks died sooner and suffered dramatically higher rates from every known disease, includ-ing tuberculosis, malaria, pellagra, and the final stages of syphilis.[13] The census also revealed high rates of miscarriage and infant mortality among free blacks that in turn were ascribed to blacks' higher rate of sex-ual immorality and sexually transmitted disease.[14]

The census data posited madness as the most dramatic indicator of black helplessness. The North and South held equivalent rates of "insane and idiot" whites[15] but not of mentally defective blacks. One out of every 1,558 blacks in the South was an "idiot or insane"; but 1 out of every 144 northern blacks had similar mental problems.[16] Thus, mental defects were *eleven times* more common among free blacks in the North than among slaves.[17] Even the northern state with the *lowest* percentage of in-sane blacks, New Jersey, had twice the black insanity rate of Delaware, the southern state with the *highest* rate.[18]

This powerful scientific argument for slavery was fed by research conducted by the presumably disinterested federal government, not by southern slavery apologists. Slavery's defenders quickly roused them-selves to explain to naïve northerners the dangers of freedom for the "sickly freedmen" of the North, who sank into debilitating insanity when faced with having to provide for themselves or indeed to undergo any of the pressures of daily life that whites managed as a matter of course. They claimed that blacks lacked the mature judgment of whites and were unable to resist the allure of liquor, indiscriminate sex, constant dancing, and frequent fighting. Medical case histories described how blacks almost starved after spending their money on wine and tobacco or fell ill with tuberculosis after buying flashy clothes that were completely unsuitable for cold northern weather. Moreover, blacks' probable doom was not ascribed simply to lower intelligence, because their profoundly defective bodies were prey to a host of diseases that never plagued whites: The conditions Cachexia Africana ("dirt eating," or pica), hebetude, pellagra, and Dysthesia Aethiopica, which have been discussed earlier, were just a few examples, and new "black" diseases still were being discovered.

Blacks' fertility had also fallen, allegedly because they were murderously indifferent mothers and absent fathers in the best of circumstances: Without white intervention, black children had even less of a chance at life than their parents.

Slavery was also thought necessary to protect whites, because freely roaming sick blacks were perceived as vectors of infectious disease. The supposed concern for the health of blacks and alarm for the safety of whites provided a welcome dual rationale for enslavement and it justified draconian public-health methods such as racial segregation to contain the contagion of freed blacks.

"So little trouble do men take in search for the truth," Thucydides once observed, "so readily do they accept whatever comes first to hand." The behavior of the U.S. intellectual elite validated his centuries-old lament. Powerful statistical arguments for slavery were widely accepted in the corridors of power, and census data spiced many a fiery political speech delivered by powerful politicians. The message found an especially vociferous champion in Secretary of State John C. Calhoun, a former medical student and an inveterate southern advocate of slavery. Calhoun used the data to rebuff criticisms of slavery at home and abroad—on a U.S. government letterhead.

The shocked political opponents of slavery, intimidated by the statistical weight of the numbers and by the impeccable prestige of the U.S. census, never mounted a coordinated refutation of the census. Although it probably could not have prevented emancipation, the census research did contribute to a revitalization of slavery until the early 1860s.[19]

However, the celebrated census data were deeply flawed, as was revealed when serendipity, in the form of a broken leg, drew one of the finest statistical minds of the era into the fray. Dr. Edward Jarvis,[20] a Concord, Massachusetts, physician, was specially trained both in mental illness and in statistics and helped found the American Statistical Association in 1839. But the next year, the peripatetic physician was ordered to bed with a fractured leg, and, bored, he began to peruse the census report. He was instantly galvanized by what he saw, because he was familiar with northern health statistics and realized at a glance that the census was riddled with serious numerical errors. Jarvis investigated and found that the census was a "fallacious and self-condemning document," a mixture of accidental and intentional falsehoods.[21]

Jarvis, who was white, sagely refused to be drawn into debates about the merits or logic of scientific racism. Instead, he spent months analyzing the enumeration of black and white inhabitants and their health status. Jarvis compared these to independently verified data describing northern towns, their inhabitants, and the mental health profiles.

He emerged with a catalog of misinformed calculations and the deliberate insertions of hosts of fictitious numbers. Some northern towns that had no black residents at all were credited by the census with "insane negroes." For example Scarboro, Massachusetts, which "had a lily-white population" was mysteriously endowed by the census with six insane Negroes; Dresden, Maine, which had three black inhabitants, was also invested with six insane Negroes. The 1840 census indicated that the town of Worcester, Massachusetts, was the home of "133 colored lunatics and idiots," but this was actually the number of *white* patients in Worcester's State Hospital for the Insane.[22]

The mysterious appearance of these imaginary black insane was only the beginning of the census duplicity. When Jarvis compared the numbers in the federal census, which was still being refined, with the accurate, verified state censuses, the numbers for blacks and whites were erroneous. Even the numbers in the four printings of the 1840 census differed, without explanation.

His damning indictment of the census criticized only the northern data. But even before Jarvis had completed his attack of the northern data, Dr. James McCune Smith of Harvard had deftly analyzed both the northern and southern numbers. Smith, an African American physician, scientist, and social theorist, had earned an M.D. from Scotland's University of Glasgow in 1837 after American schools barred his entry on racial grounds.[23] Like Jarvis, Smith was a statistical expert and member of the American Statistical Association. His clear analysis addressed the flaws in the southern data,[24] revealing that the census's methodology was so deeply flawed that it was tantamount to libel regarding the health and mental status of African Americans.

Smith understood that black mental illness was destined to be under-enumerated in the South, where there was almost no accommodation for the diagnosis and mental health treatment.[25] Blacks were typically barred from mental hospitals, and those too deranged to work were dumped into almshouses or jails,[26] into which census marshals did not venture. Enumerators took an owner's word that his slaves were healthy, by which owners meant not emotionally healthy but simply fit to work.

Making the all-important racial assessments was a quixotic task. Census marshals had been told to go from house to house and to make note of every occupant to determine his or her race (either "white" or "colored"[27]) and health status. Such a simplistic assessment of people who were varying mixtures of Native American, African, and European was a herculean task in itself and determining race was made futile by such laws as the "one-eighth rule" or the "one-drop rule," which tended to assign a "colored" label to anyone with discernible or known African heritage. Although race was hard to gauge visually,[28] census takers accepted a neighbor's assessment or simply glanced at a member of a family to determine its race, with predictable results.[29] Take Jack Coon of Alabama. A federal census marshal had listed him as white in 1850, but that year's state census recorded him as a mulatto freeman. In the 1860 U.S. census, Coon was listed as "Indian."

It was similarly difficult to determine health status.[30] Diseases such as syphilis, cholera, and pellagra were largely racialized, and whites who suffered from them were loath to admit it. Meanwhile, diseases such as syphilis were ascribed to blacks en masse. An owner's complaint that all his slaves were sexually immoderate and syphilitic was taken literally. Even legal status could deceive: Some planters misrepresented their slaves as free persons to avoid taxes. Census takers were duped by the ruse, or were complicit.

On May 3, 1844, Smith submitted to the United States Senate a "memorial," a shrewd analysis of the census document, denuding its many fallacies and reducing it to an absurdity.[31] His paper "Comparative Anatomy and Physiology of the Races," delivered before New York City's intellectual elite, also painstakingly refuted the science that sought to explain the excess insanity among free blacks, including the popular theory that the Negro's arrested cranial development resulted in a smaller brain and lessened intelligence.

That year, Jarvis published a similar refutation with this editorial comment:

> Here is proof to force upon us the lamentable conclusion that the sixth census has contributed nothing in the statistical nosology[32] of the free blacks, . . . such a document as we have described heavy with its errors and misstatements. . . . So far from being an aid to medical science, it had thrown a stumbling block in its ways, which will require years to remove.[33]

His last sentence proved prescient.

Congressman and former President John Quincy Adams propelled a resolution through the House of Representatives to compel Secretary of State Calhoun to reexamine the census for "gross errors."[34] But Calhoun appointed his friend William A. Weaver, the originator of the deeply flawed census, to examine it for intentional errors. Weaver pronounced the census flawless. Calhoun reported this to the House of Representatives, permitting himself a bit of triumphant sermonizing on the dangers of black freedom: ". . . so far from bettering the condition of the Negro or African race, by changing the relationship with the European in the slaveholding states, it would render it far worse. It would indeed, to him, be a curse rather than a blessing."

This manipulation of public-health data specifically in furtherance of a racial agenda illustrates that public health and medical research are not mutually exclusive. Worse, the erroneous figures and conclusions persisted in medical journals. In 1851, the august *American Journal of Insanity* reprinted without comment an article asserting the following: "It is obvious taken from the following schedule [taken from the 1840 census] that there is an awful prevalence of idiocy and insanity among the free blacks over the whites, and especially over the slaves. Who would have believed without the fact in black and white before his own eyes, that [e]very fourteenth colored person in the state of Main[e] is an idiot or lunatic?"[35]

But finally war achieved what science would not: It doomed slavery.

Without Sanctuary

Military medicine proved inadequate in the face of the legendary carnage wrought by the War Between the States. Eighty-eight of every 1,000 white volunteer soldiers in the Union army died, but proportionally one and half times more black Union soldiers—148 per 1,000—succumbed.[36] One Northern officer declared, "You can't replace these white boys, but if a nigger dies, all you have to do is send out and get another one."

Still, it was much safer and healthier to be a black soldier than a black civilian. Most slaves fled the plantations when the war began and most free blacks fled the South. This internal nation of homeless roamed northward, hungry, tattered, sick, and penniless, seeking safe harbor.

As the Union army drove back the boundaries of the Confederacy, it initially took control of 750,000 black people. The government assigned responsibility for their care to the reluctant Union army, which argued that it had neither the resources nor the expertise to give the refugee blacks the care they needed. Nevertheless, during its peak year, 1866,[37] the army's Freedmen's Bureau health system comprised forty-six field hospitals, fifty-two colonies, asylums, and dispensaries (smaller clinics), 118 physicians, and 406 hospital attendants.[38] Waves of sick blacks were herded into camps without adequate nutrition, sanitation, or medical care.[39] Only 138 physicians ever cared for the 1.1 million freemen who eventually lived in the camps, and many of these doctors expressed disdain for the black "animals," as at least one doctor called the contraband in front of relief workers.[40] Some flatly refused to care for them.

The results were predictable: One out of every four freemen died in the camps. Many died of rampant infectious disease, especially tuberculosis. Infant mortality, which had always run high among enslaved blacks, swelled exponentially. The African American refugees themselves staffed and ran the camps, but always under the Argus eyes of paid white administrators. The high disease and death rate, primitive medical conditions, and callous attitudes of some camp physicians further fed African American distrust of medicine.

When the war ended, Martin L. Delany, M.D., who had distinguished himself as an officer and surgeon during the war, headed the Freedmen's Bureau, but its medical services were sabotaged by a lack of financial support. When the freemen's camps dissolved, no public-health support replaced them. Poverty and desperation trapped southern blacks into an insidiously indirect new form of slavery—sharecropping. The exploitative, abusive medical care of slave owners was replaced by no medical care at all for most poor blacks, and disease and death ran rampant through black populations.

However, nineteenth-century scientific medicine, bolstered by census data, perpetuated the belief that blacks' inherent inferiorities, not exposure, starvation, and neglect catalyzed by wartime privation, caused their public-health disaster.

The censuses of the postbellum decades not only perpetuated but also expanded upon the racial libels of the 1840 documents. However, their principal foci were physical illnesses, not mental. By the time of the eighth census, that of 1860, superintendent Joseph C. G. Kennedy was predicting the certain demise of black Americans. By the census of 1890, the black birth rate had fallen in relation to that of whites. Life-insurance companies considered blacks uninsurable and black extinction was actually predicted for the year 2000. These predictions dwelled upon the inherent and immutable physical inferiority that doomed the Negro and offered frequent predictions of his extinction. Census analyses ignored many environmental and external causes of illness among blacks, and blacks were held to be inherently susceptible to venereal diseases and to such "black diseases" as pellagra and imaginary diseases, such as hebetude, drapetomania, and Struma Africana.

The theories promulgated by the census takers were essentially updates of the old polygenist view that held such diseases to be immutable elements of blacks' evolutionary lot and maintained that races could not survive outside their climates of origin. For example, the British anthropologist James Hunt claimed in 1863 that blacks could not live north of the fortieth longitude and that death would ensue "at such a rapid rate that they would perish like monkeys and lions in a zoo."[41]

Therefore, the census apologists saw preventive and corrective measures such as better housing, health care, and nutrition as futile. This tendency to see environmentally and socially triggered illnesses as inherent defects of blacks is a troublingly persistent trend in American medical research.

One of the delicious paradoxes of quantum physics is the Heisenberg uncertainty principle, which warns that the very act of measurement changes the entity being measured, destroying the accuracy of the data. Similarly, the census's methodological clumsiness, accidental and intentional, horribly distorted the image of the African American for decades. Yet the chief distortions of the census were *intentional* falsehoods, and these constitute yet another powerful example of how scientific fraud and abuse have often been traveling partners when it comes to research into African American health.

A successive assortment of mental health and intelligence theories were adopted, "proved," and then discarded through the end of the century. These theories shared two constants: They were all detailed numerical assessments that indicated the lower intelligence of blacks and they all measured a fixed attribute that could never be improved. Phrenology, for example, involved determining personality (including a propensity to violence) by interpreting the shape of the head. Intelligence was gauged by measuring the size of the brain, either directly or by measuring the cranial capacity of a skull. Scientists compared the values for various races and each "found" the lowest intelligence in blacks. Furthermore, each detailed numeric was determined to be static and immutable.

The same arguments for black mental inferiority that had kept slavery on life support were now applied to support claims of innate black physical inferiority. Blacks were also seen as a danger to whites and a vector of infectious disease because more blacks were now living in cities. In 1890, 12 percent of the 7.5 million African Americans lived in cities, although only 4 percent had been urban in 1860.[42] Many spent most of their time in white households as domestic servants.

Thus, the advent of the twentieth century saw a complete reversal of a basic mantra of scientific racism. Medicine had once justified slavery on the basis that blacks were hardier than whites and so were ideally suited to survive and to work in harsh climates that would have meant death to more delicate whites. Now, it was African Americans who were adjudged too delicate to survive. A familiar theme of medical journals and popular magazine articles alike became "Would blacks survive the new century?"[43]

Burgeoning Black Diseases

Turn-of-the-century research into the once rampant disorder pellagra illustrates the tenacity of the identification of disease with inherent black frailty. Pellagra is marked by a constellation of symptoms, as deep skin eruptions are followed by diarrhea, dementia, and, in 40 percent of cases, death. Many survivors were relegated to mental institutions. It was long considered a black infectious disease caused by poor hygiene and was called the "sharecropper's scourge."

Pellagra was actually neither a black disease nor infectious, but a deficiency disease caused by poor blacks' sparse and monotonous diet of white corn and inferior fatty pork, which was severely deficient in niacin, an essential amino acid.

But after 1906, economic downturns and changes in processing corn that removed remaining traces of niacin fueled a more widespread nutritional deficiency among white southerners, as well, and pellagra was now recognized as a public-health emergency.

In 1914, the United States Marine Hospital Service (USMHS), forerunner of the U.S. Public Health Service, assigned Joseph Goldberger, M.D., to investigate. Goldberger, the industrious son of Jewish immigrants and an 1895 honors graduate of Bellevue Hospital Medical School, doubted that pellagra was a black disease; in addition, he did not believe it was infectious, because he had noted that the patients but not the staff of institutions tended to contract it, and infections tend to be more democratic. He decided that the ultimate proof of the disease's noninfectious, nonracial nature would lie in inducing pellagra in healthy white people.

He did this by limiting a group of white jail inmates to a strict diet, one similar to that on which poor blacks had subsisted for centuries. Because they developed the disease, Goldberger was able to demonstrate that pellagra was not infectious, but a deficiency disease that affected blacks and whites alike.[44] Goldberger had divorced pellagra from race, but unfortunately, this revelation was resented and ignored. The nutritional, nonracial nature of pellagra became forbidden knowledge, just as the refutation of the 1840 census had been. As a result, this easily preventable disease remained epidemic until 1940.

Pellagra was but one of many diseases that fed the early-twentieth-century black health crisis. The next important "black disease" to be discovered was more demonstrably "racial" than pellagra.

In the 1870s, scattered reports had appeared of black patients who suffered from a constellation of mystifying symptoms that included excruciating pain, bruising, mysterious strokes, anemia, and extensive sores. In late 1904, Walter Clement Noel, a wealthy black first-year student at the Chicago College of Dental Surgery from Grenada, was admitted to the Presbyterian Hospital. Dr. Ernest E. Irons, the intern who cared for him, obtained a medical history and performed routine physical, blood, and urine examinations. In the blood smear, Irons saw that Noel's blood contained "many pear-shaped and elongated forms." Enraptured, Irons sketched them, suspecting that they held the key to Noel's symptoms. He also alerted cardiologist James B. Herrick, his attending physician. Together, Herrick and Irons cared for Noel over the next two and a half years, but when Herrick wrote up the case for publication in 1910, including their opinion that Noel's was a disease that struck only blacks, he excluded Irons from the publication and so received sole credit for the discovery of Herrick's anemia, which is now called sickle-cell anemia, because of the "elongated forms" that Irons first recognized.

Noel returned to Grenada to practice dentistry, dying only nine years later, at age thirty-two. Many blacks had been treated for the severe pain and mysterious injuries of sickle-cell anemia, even during slavery. But Noel's was the first case to receive such intensive attention and investigation, perhaps because as a wealthy foreign dental student, he was a medical insider and class peer of his physicians.[45]

Today, most of the 72,000 Americans with sickle-cell disease are descended from Northern Africans or sub-Saharan Africans. One out of every five hundred African Americans and one in every one thousand to fourteen hundred Hispanic Americans suffer from sickle-cell anemia. Yet the disorder also affects millions of people of nearly every ethnicity in South America, Cuba, Central America, Saudi Arabia, India, Turkey, Greece, and Italy—in fact, almost anywhere malaria is found. For the common denominator of sickle-cell disease is not race, but living in proximity to the malaria-bearing Anopheles mosquito. Possessing a gene for sickle-cell disease affords protection against some strains of malaria and so people with this gene have an evolutionary advantage in areas where malaria is prevalent. U.S. whites suffer from sickle-cell anemia as well, but it is often misdiagnosed as a related blood disease, and when the occasional white person is accurately diagnosed with sickle-cell anemia, this is still presumed tantamount to the discovery of an occult black biological heritage rather than simply a case of the disease in a white person. However, within a decade of its identification, the erroneous belief that sickle-cell anemia strikes only blacks became firmly entrenched, thus reinforcing belief in the inherent inferiority of African Americans.

African American physicians did not passively accept damning indictments of black physiology. The slowly increasing number of black physicians, among others, rose to the challenge by establishing hospitals where blacks could obtain medical care. Daniel Hale Williams, who performed the first successful open-heart operation, founded Provident Hospital in 1893. In 1897 Dr. Alonzo McClennan opened a hospital and nurse training school and, by 1916, Dr. Matilda Evans of South Carolina had opened three different hospitals there. Eventually, seven African American medical schools joined these to provide the long awaited entrée to medical education for African Americans. But in 1910, a single research report felled the schools. In 1908, the Carnegie Foundation for the Advancement of Teaching invited the influential Dr. Abraham Flexner to critique the nation's 147 medical schools. When Flexner's report was published two years later, it damned all but two black medical schools—Howard and Meharry—as substandard, sounding the death knell for the others, which subsequently found it impossible to attract funding. By 1924 only Howard and Meharry remained open.

Even in the midst of doomed black hospitals and shuttered medical schools, these medical guardians actively refuted the allegations of inherent physical and mental inferiority. The story of how such African American healers and researchers affected the trajectory of American medical research with blacks is related in several works, such as *A Century of Black Surgeons, The History of the Negro in Medicine,* and *Making a Place for Ourselves.* An important group of socially conscious white Americans made promising overtures as well, including physicians; leaders of institutions such as Metropolitan Life and North Carolina Life, which supported black health programs; and private philanthropies, such as the Rockefeller Foundation and the Julius Rosenwald Fund.

The Rosenwald Fund would soon turn its attention to infectious disease among blacks by initiating a fateful syphilis-control program in Macon County, Alabama, the home of Tuskegee University.

CHAPTER 7

"A NOTORIOUSLY SYPHILIS-SOAKED RACE"

What *Really* Happened at Tuskegee?

*The future of the Negro lies more in the research laboratory than in
the schools. . . . When diseased, he should be registered and forced to
take treatment before he offers his diseased mind and body on the
altar of academic and professional education.*

—THOMAS MURRELL, M.D., U.S. PUBLIC HEALTH SERVICE, 1910

*We now know, where we could only surmise before, that we have
contributed to their ailments and shortened their lives.*

—OLIVER CLARENCE WENGER, M.D., U.S. PUBLIC HEALTH SERVICE, 1950

n 1932, the U.S. Public Health Service inaugurated its Study of Syphilis in
the Untreated Negro Male ("Tuskegee Syphilis Study"), which promised
free medical care to about six hundred sick, desperately poor sharecroppers in Macon County, Alabama. The study was designed, the PHS explained, to study the progression of syphilis in black men. Scientists had
long claimed that the venereal disease manifested differently in blacks
than in whites, and PHS scientists decided to document this by finding a
pool of infected black men, withholding treatment from them, and then
charting the progression of symptoms and disorders. But the PHS lied to
the subjects, convincing them that they were being treated, not studied.
When the men died, the physician-researchers determined to autopsy
them in order to trace precisely the ravages of the disease in their bodies.
Among other things, the PHS expected to validate its belief in a specific
racial dimorphism of syphilis: Whereas the disease was thought to do its
worst damage to the neurological systems and brains of whites, it was
thought to wreak its worst havoc on the cardiovascular systems of blacks,
sparing their relatively primitive and "underdeveloped" brains.

The Best Intentions

The origin of the Tuskegee Study was a benign one, however. In 1898, when Booker T. Washington, founder of Tuskegee Institute,[1] met wealthy philanthropist Julius Rosenwald, founder of Sears, Roebuck & Company, they were mutually impressed. The head of the Rosenwald Foundation, who had a history of initiating self-sustaining black economic programs, had already generously supported beneficent research and self-sustaining industrial initiatives among black southerners. He recognized in Tuskegee Institute a potential center of black industry and in Washington the man who could realize this potential.

Rosenwald also realized that Tuskegee's promise was surrounded by the grinding poverty, public-health vacuum, poor health, and rampant infectious disease of Macon County, and that this dreary indigence would stifle its potential workforce and limit its industrial growth. Together, he and Washington planned a Tuskegee-based program to provide medical treatment for Macon County, a system that began in earnest in the late 1920s.

By that time, slavery had ended in Macon County nearly seventy years earlier, but in name only. Except for the staff and students of Tuskegee Institute (later to be Tuskegee University), most of the county's 27,000 blacks lived the same lives as had their enslaved forebears. In 1932, 82 percent of its residents were black, and half of these lived far below the poverty line: Their median income was a dollar a day. But like their enslaved forebears, they never saw a dollar from one year to the next. Trapped in the usurious cycle of tenant cotton farming, they were chained by debt and forced to work the same land as had their enslaved grandparents, and, like Alabama's slaves, they owned nothing, not even the crumbling shacks they lived in. These sharecroppers, including children, were weighed down by hundred-pound bags of cotton, living and working under the orders of white landowners who kept them in economic thralldom by paying low prices for their crops and charging inflated prices for food, seed, and other necessities. Those blacks who tried to flee the land were arrested, punished, and returned—or worse—just as their enslaved grandparents would have been. Beatings, lynchings, and murders that were never investigated enforced black serfdom. The strictly segregated schools were poorly equipped and sparsely staffed, and in any event, few families could spare children from the fields long enough for them to learn to read and write well. The only thing blacks had was a great deal of illness. But medical care did not exist for most of them. Fifteen of the sixteen doctors practicing in the county were white, and although the overworked black doctor would see patients for "trade"—a chicken, some greens, whatever the patients could spare—the rest wanted their fee in cash, plus a dollar a mile. The four doctors of the John A. Andrew Veterans Hospital tried to care for the sick blacks who appeared at its doors, but they could help only a fraction of them, for their job was to care for the staff and students of Tuskegee Institute.[2]

Poor nutrition, a lack of decent housing, and rampant infectious diseases, from malaria to tuberculosis to syphilis, haunted the sharecroppers of Macon County. The 1929 syphilis survey of black Alabama residents commissioned by Dr. Taliaferro Clark, chief of the PHS Venereal Disease Division, determined a high rate of 36 percent in Macon County. However, some other Alabama counties had higher rates, so this could not have been the chief impetus for the study. It is more likely that the presence of Tuskegee Institute, and later the John A. Andrew Veterans Hospital, made the site a scientifically attractive one. The survey also suggested that although treatment could eradicate the disease, 99 percent of the cases in blacks had never been treated.[3]

Syphilis was indeed a serious threat to health and productivity. The disease is caused by a type of bacterial organism named *Spirochaeta pallida,* or, more specifically, *Treponema pallidum,* a spirochete. Spirochetes are named for their spiral shape: Under a microscope, the wormlike bacteria wiggle furiously. *T. pallidum* can be acquired through sexual activity or congenitally, from an infected mother. In the initial stage of sexually transmitted syphilis, a chancre, or hard, painless sore, appears on the genitals or other point of entry, followed by flulike symptoms. If the disease is not treated, it enters a long latent secondary stage before emerging to inflict an assortment of skin growths, running sores, gumma, bone decay, and heart damage. The final, tertiary, stage of syphilis may erupt several decades later, causing profound neurological damage—blindness, insanity (paresis), paralysis, and death.[4] Because thirty years or more can intervene between the onset of syphilis and the dramatic mental symptoms of paresis, or tertiary syphilis, it was thought to be a separate mental disease until the mid-1940s, when an-

tibiotics, particularly penicillin, were discovered to cure it and it was belatedly recognized as the final stage of an infectious illness—syphilis.

Rosenwald responded by earmarking money for syphilis-treatment
programs. Unfortunately, his wealth was consumed in the stock market
crash of 1929, and with it vanished the support for Macon County's economic and disease-treatment programs.

The U.S. Public Health Service stepped in. But PHS physicians never
shared Rosenwald's goal of black self-sufficiency. The writings of its doctors reveal a lack of faith in African Americans' ability to manage their
own economic and health issues.

PHS physician Thomas W. Murrell, M.D., expressed ambivalence
about the possibility and even the advisability of eradicating syphilis
among black Americans.

> So the scourge sweeps among them. Those that are treated are only
> half cured, and the effort to assimilate a complex civilization drives
> their diseased minds until the results are criminal records. Perhaps
> here, in conjunction with tuberculosis, will be the end of the negro
> problem. Disease will accomplish what man cannot do.

PHS doctors portrayed black Alabamans as resistant to health measures, intellectually inferior, impetuous, degenerate, and, above all, at the
mercy of frighteningly powerful sexual drives. "Morality among these
people is almost a joke and only assumed as a matter of convenience,"
sneered Murrell.[5] Such medical speculation fostered an image of African
Americans as sexually promiscuous and infected with syphilis, an impression that doctors reinforced with pithy sayings. "Virtue in the negro
race is like angels' visits—few and far between. In a practice of sixteen
years in the South I have never examined a virgin over fourteen years of
age,"[6] alleged Dr. Daniel D. Quillen of Athens, Georgia. Their point was
that such sexual irresponsibility doomed blacks to chronic syphilitic infection.

The PHS castigated blacks as "a notoriously syphilis-soaked race,"
and Murrell predicted, "Another fifty years will find an unsyphilitic negro a freak; unless some such procedure as vaccination comes to the relief of the race and that in the hands of a compelling law."[7] Dr. Frank
Lydston theorized that black men were more likely than white men to

spread venereal diseases: "The negro's well-known sexual impetuosity may account for more abrasions of the integument of the sexual organs and therefore more frequent infections than are found in the white race."[8] With imagination rather than evidence as his guide, Dr. S. S. Hindman estimated the national prevalence of syphilis among blacks at 95 percent. But because clinical examinations did not support such widespread infection among blacks, Dr. Joseph Moore militated for Wassermann tests on all black men, opining that "a mere history of a penile sore only would not be adequate, inasmuch as the average Negro has as many penile sores as a rabbit has offspring."[9]

Despite the PHS physicians' cracker-barrel wisdom, family histories and clinical assessments revealed that 61 percent of the true syphilis cases in Macon County were not contracted through sexual activity but were congenital, nonvenereal syphilis. Medical researchers consistently ignored this fact in their publications and in their investigations; they persistently characterized syphilis in blacks as due to sexual profligacy.[10]

However, not all the men who tested positive for syphilis via the Wassermann test really had the disease. The test was notoriously nonspecific, and men who suffered from related illnesses such as yaws also tested positive, because yaws, a common nonvenereal infectious disease endemic to West Africa, is caused by a subspecies of the *Treponema pallidum* bacterium that causes syphilis. In 1932, yaws was prevalent in the South, especially among blacks, not for racial reasons but because it is abetted by conditions of poverty: People who were malnourished and exposed to the elements, went shoeless, and were prone to frequent injuries that broke the skin (the sort that cotton pickers experienced daily) were vulnerable to infections by pathogens that caused yaws. Unlike syphilis, yaws causes no long-term cardiovascular or neuronal damage.

Macon County's high prevalence of syphilis, coupled with a nearly perfect treatment vacuum, suggested to Taliaferro Clark not a need for treatment, but an opportunity for experimentation. In 1932, the Tuskegee Syphilis Study officially began when he suggested that the PHS save the expense of treatment by merely observing the course of the disease in blacks and publishing the data.[11]

PHS doctors frequently defended their failure to offer therapy by insisting that blacks with syphilis would never voluntarily seek treatment.

However, this does not explain why they enticed study subjects by disguising the experiment as the treatment program promised by Rosenwald. The PHS doctors knew that being cared for by a physician who professed himself devoted to restoring their health would be a godsend to the sick, forgotten blacks of Macon County. Accordingly, the PHS announced a day of free health assessments and screening tests that would be performed in Macon County.

PHS nurse Eunice Rivers remembers that the clinic was "overflooded with people coming in to get their blood drawn." Oliver Clarence ("O.C.") Wenger, M.D., wrote, "Of course the crowd milled around like so many sheep," adding that 316 were given treatment before 2:00 P.M. Most had never seen a doctor before.[12]

The physicians ran various tests while telling the men that they were being treated for the nebulous disorder "bad blood," which commonly referred to a wide array of symptoms from anemic blood to muscle aches, general malaise, disorders such as parasitic infections, gonorrhea, syphilis, and other venereal diseases. Doctors dispensed "treatment" in the form of vitamins, ineffectual doses of arsenic, and worse-than-useless mercury salve to those they suspected of having syphilis.[13] Mercury had been used to treat syphilis for centuries, but, as described in chapter 1, it was ineffectual and caused devastating side effects such as injury to the nervous system, profound mental deficits, hair and tooth loss, kidney and heart disease, and lung injury. However, doctors withheld the state-of-the-art treatment for syphilis, which in 1932 consisted of arsenic compounds such as arsphenamine and neoarsphenamine, also known by their trade names Salvarsan or 606.[14] These were developed by German biochemist Paul Ehrlich in 1910 and were typically partnered with mercury ointments as adjuvant therapy.

After the first clinics enabled doctors to identify syphilitics, they selected study participants. They wanted only men, whose signs and symptoms were on the exterior genitalia and therefore easier to identify than lesions hidden within the genitalia of women. They also wanted to exclude men whose syphilis was the result of a recent infection, because doctors could be surer of choosing sick men if they chose those in the secondary or later stages of infection. Identifying such study candidates entailed taking painstaking medical histories and performing painful, medically risky spinal taps, ostensibly to determine the extent of syphilis's neurological involvement. When the PHS sent out notices to invite subjects for spinal taps, the wording clearly indicated that participants were recruited under the guise of treatment.

> Some time ago you were given a thorough examination and since that time we hope that you have gotten a great deal of treatment for bad blood. You will now be given your last chance to get a second examination. This examination is a very special one and after it is finished you will be given a special treatment if its [sic] believed that you are in a condition to stand it. REMEMBER THIS IS YOUR LAST CHANCE FOR SPECIAL FREE TREATMENT. BE SURE TO MEET THE NURSE.[15]

When another throng appeared seeking the second examination, the PHS ran the spinal taps and selected 399 men with syphilis as subjects to observe. Again, doctors dispensed inadequate medications such as aspirin, which was craved as a miracle drug by the overworked, sickly men, who marveled at how it assuaged their omnipresent aches and pains. Raymond Vonderlehr, M.D., Taliaferro Clark's successor, later added a control group of two hundred uninfected men, who also were wooed with medications. When a dozen of these men developed syphilis over the forty-year course of the experiment, they were simply transferred to the infected group, a blatant violation of experimental design.[16] Perfect separation of infected and control groups was necessary for any accurate and truly objective comparison of their health states. By switching a man from the control group to the infected group, the physicians falsified data, because they reported an event, in this case a syphilis infection and its concomitant symptoms, as transpiring in an *infected* member, while, in fact, it actually happened to be a control-group member. This switching also artificially reduced the number of men in the relatively small control group who went on to contract syphilis. The comparison over the entire course of the disease, which was the ostensible purpose of the study, was made impossible when someone was switched from active to the control group after the disease had been progressing for some time before diagnosis.

Vonderlehr confessed in a letter to Clark, "It is my desire to keep the main purpose of the work from the negroes in the county and to continue their interest in treatment." But there was no treatment. The next year, 1933, the PHS doctors went on to write of "bringing these cases to autopsy." If any doubts lingered about the PHS physicians' intention to withhold treatment, O. C. Wenger, the PHS senior officer for its syphilis programs, swept them aside that year: "As I see it, we have no further interest in these patients *until they die.*" Like Joice Heth, the aged black woman who was displayed, then dissected, for profit by P. T. Barnum, these men were regarded by an impatient PHS as living cadavers, more valuable to American medicine dead than alive. Wenger, who has been portrayed as a public-health hero in Paul de Kruif's 1938 book, *The Fight for Life,* eagerly awaited the men's deaths because autopsies would be necessary to confirm the diagnosis and the extent of injury caused by their untreated disease. These reports would be compared with those on the bodies of control subjects to characterize in terrible detail the ravages of syphilis. However, the physicians anticipated difficulty in obtaining the men's bodies for autopsy, largely because, as was discussed in chapter 5, African Americans bitterly resented the fact that their bodies were often stolen and exploited for anatomical examination. Wenger wrote Vonderlehr:

> There is one danger in the latter plan and that is if the colored
> population becomes aware that accepting free hospital care means
> a post-mortem, every darkey will leave Macon County. . . . The
> only way we are going to get post-mortems is to have the demise
> take place in Dibble's [Eugene Dibble, M.D., the African American
> director of the Tuskegee medical center] hospital and when these
> colored folk are told that Doctor Dibble is now a Government
> doctor too they will have more confidence.[17]

The surgeon general enlisted the Tuskegee Hospitals to provide a site for spinal taps and autopsies and he accordingly gave Dibble a PHS appointment. But because they feared losing track of the men before autopsy, the PHS doctors added inducements that maintained the treatment fiction. Eunice Rivers, the eldest daughter of a Georgia farmer and one of only four black public-health nurses in the state of Alabama, was recruited from her dispiriting job as a night nurse at the John A. Andrew Hospital to serve as a "scientific assistant" to assist in procedures and examinations and to keep track of the men.

Rivers looked in on the men periodically and dispensed the medicines, mostly aspirin, iron tonic, and vitamins, that made them believe they were in treatment.[18] Rivers injected a bit of variety into their lives of drudgery and dispiriting poverty when she drove them into town for their doctors' appointments in a shiny black car and distributed the occasional inducements of a dollar or two. She waited while they visited friends and marveled at the manicured university lawns and the painted shops on the city streets. She listened sympathetically to the litany of sicknesses, deaths, and family woes and helped when she could. She interceded on their behalf when the doctors were especially brusque or derisive. She was their friend.

However, the men did not know that Rivers was also charged with tracking their movements, ultimately to ensure their presence at autopsy, which she didn't mention to the men but would describe to their survivors as an "operation" to gain their assent. The PHS doctors still feared that the men would evade the hospital and die at home, cheating the researchers of the chance to autopsy them, so they offered "free burials" as an inducement. The Milbank Fund, an organization with strong eugenic leanings, agreed to pay the fifty-dollar fee, which was split by the funeral parlor and the physician who performed the autopsy.[19] The men had the peace of mind of knowing they would not end up unburied or in a potter's field. But this reassurance was illusory, because the chief reason they feared indigent burial was their fear of being autopsied first—and this was to be their precise medical fate.

The syphilitic men were monitored so well that most received no treatment for forty years, despite the myriad dramatic changes in the medical landscape between 1932 and 1972. In 1934, PHS doctors met with local black doctors and asked them not to treat the men who were receiving care in the research study; the black doctors agreed. In 1941, the PHS circulated a list of subjects' names to the draft board, instructing military physicians not to treat any men who were inducted. When the United States entered World War II, Tuskegee Syphilis Study subjects were exempted from the draft because the PHS feared that they would be treated for syphilis in the military. In the early 1940s, some study participants made their way to the PHS's "fast track" VD-treatment clinics, which were vociferously dedicated to the eradication of syphilis. But a list of their names had preceded them and most were physically removed.

When penicillin proved an effective and safe cure for syphilis in 1943, a vigorous national program of treatment ensued and some determined subjects did succeed in circumventing the government dragnet to obtain treatment. Thirty men, 7.5 percent of the infected study participants, managed to obtain an effective degree of treatment, prompting Vonder-lehr to worry that the treatment might interfere with the study data. "I hope that the availability of antibiotics has not interfered too much with this project," he wrote to scientist Stanley H. Schuman early in 1952.[20] PHS doctors knew that this degree of treatment hopelessly polluted any data that they might salvage from the study. So they later put a fictitious spin on the numbers of participants who had received adequate treat-ment, bolstered by the oft-repeated fiction that the blacks did not want or seek out medical care: "These men . . . still regard hospitals and med-icine with suspicion and prefer an occasional dose of time-honored herbs or tonics to modern drugs."[21]

As men began to die, the PHS performed autopsies and regularly published the results in medical journals. They even shared study results at a 1936 American Medical Association meeting, which means many white physicians were informed of the study's details—but not African American physicians, who were largely barred from AMA membership.[22]

The 1936 AMA report revealed that 84 percent of the infected sub-jects showed signs of illness. A decade later, the death rate of the infected men was twice that of the control subjects, prompting Wenger to boast smugly in 1950, "We now know, where we could only surmise before, that we have contributed to their ailments and shortened their lives." By 1955, nearly one-third of the autopsied men had died directly of syphilis, and many of the survivors were suffering its deadliest complications. Forty wives were infected and at least nineteen children were born with syph-ilitic birth defects.

In 1958, the PHS awarded a certificate of appreciation, signed by the surgeon general and replete with a gold seal, to each infected man, along with twenty-five dollars—a dollar for each year of the study.

A Magic Bullet Withheld

Imagine the global jubilation that would greet the announcement of a simple injection to cure AIDS. This kind of exuberance accompanied the discovery of penicillin, a "magic bullet," with which scientists believed they would finally tame syphilis, a plague with which medicine had wrestled for centuries. In 1943, the PHS's network of clinics triumphantly dispensed penicillin nationally, to the deep satisfaction of Surgeon General Thomas Parran, who had adopted syphilis eradication as a personal and professional crusade.[23] In his 1937 book, *Shadow on the Land,* Parran had bemoaned the high rates of syphilis in black and poor populations and now he could lay claim to having orchestrated its demise. But even Parran, when presented with this antibiotic Holy Grail, opted for continued experimentation with the black men of Macon County. He explained that the availability of penicillin meant the "opportunity" represented by the Tuskegee Syphilis Study's pool of syphilitic patients would never come again, and must be exploited.[24]

Thirty-three years after the study began social changes eclipsed the moral question posed by penicillin, a question that the PHS had dismissed so blithely. The nation that had passively accepted medical apartheid and sharecropper slavery in 1932 was wracked by constant ethnic tension and racial warfare by the 1960s. Deadly racial repression with dogs, guns, lynchings, and bombings reigned in the defiant South, and in the North, murderous street brawls erupted over voting rights, school desegregation, de facto segregation, and conflicts with police. National Guard troops enforced integration as urban riots consumed northern and southern cities alike in blood and fire.

But these events were tangential to the shabby, tightly circumscribed lives of the weary, destitute sharecroppers in the rural study, whose median age was now seventy-four. They were enfeebled beyond their years by poverty, prostrating labor, and syphilis, and the PHS physicians were deeply concerned, because three men had already been lost to autopsy when they died without the researchers learning of it in time to obtain the bodies.[25] In order to assure the needed autopsies, it was essential for the PHS to track closely the aged men's serious illnesses and hospitalizations, any one of which could end in death. However, Eunice Rivers was aging, too, and becoming too old to track them. She was given the Department of Health, Education, and Welfare's highest honor, the Oveta Gulp Hobby Award, for "25 years during which through selfless devotion and skillful human relations, she has sustained the interest and cooperation of the subjects of a venereal disease control program in Macon County, Alabama," then retired. The black nurse who replaced her was told to be sure to visit any seriously ill or hospi-talized man frequently.

Suddenly, in 1965, the nation's civil rights drama played out in the medical sphere as the PHS found its ethics assailed from many direc-tions. The radical leftist group Students for a Democratic Society (SDS) discovered the Tuskegee Syphilis Study and held rallies urging that it be ended, but they were easily dismissed as a fringe group given to counter-culture hyperbole. However, the question of racism in the study also sur-faced within the medical fold, as Allan Brandt discovered when he found the minutes of a 1965 meeting at the Centers for Disease Control (CDC). An excerpt is illuminating: "Racial issue was mentioned briefly. Will not affect the study. Any questions can be handled by saying that these peo-ple were at the point that therapy would no longer help them. They are getting better medical care than they would under any other circum-stances."[26]

The same year, a white physician, Dr. Irwin J. Schatz of the Henry Ford Hospital in Detroit, wrote the PHS after reading a medical paper on the Tuskegee Syphilis Study in the *Archives of Internal Medicine*. His let-ter began, "I am utterly astounded by the fact that physicians allow pa-tients with potentially fatal disease to remain untreated when effective therapy is available." His letter was never answered.[27]

By the year's end, the study was dealt what would eventually prove a fatal blow by Peter Buxtun, a young Polish immigrant who worked as a venereal disease interviewer for the PHS. He learned of the study and immediately risked his job by writing his superiors to ask that it be stopped. A handful of PHS physicians responded by holding meetings, at which they lectured Buxtun on the scientific merits of their work and de-cided to continue the study.[28] In 1967, Buxtun left the agency to attend law school, but he occasionally wrote the PHS to renew his complaints, to no avail.

By 1969, physical examinations and autopsies revealed that as many as one hundred of the men had died of syphilis and its complications and others had died of heart disease that researchers ascribed to syphilis.[29] In 1972, Buxtun, exasperated by seven years of PHS inaction, told a journalist friend about the study. On July 25 of that year, Jean Heller broke the story for the Associated Press.

Shocked PHS officials denied any knowledge of human-rights

abuses. However, they also deftly defended their work by explaining how the syphilis treatment available in 1933, arsphenamine, would have been worthless and possibly too dangerous to give the men. They added that treating the men now would risk their health. None of these claims was true. Arsphenamine had been the standard of care when the study began and treating the men now would imperil only the study's data.

The news media, physicians, politicians, and ordinary citizenry, black and white, expressed horrified anger and demanded an explanation from the government and some sort of assurance that such cruelty would never again be sanctioned by the PHS. The government promised to conduct an internal review, but when it became evident that this would neither mollify the press nor appease public outrage, Senator Ted Kennedy held hearings and a Department of Health, Education, and Welfare (HEW) official, Assistant Secretary for Health and Scientific Affairs Merlin K. DuVal, M.D., announced an investigation on August 24, 1972.[30] DuVal appointed a nine-member panel of esteemed professionals whose dissection of the study quickly degenerated into inefficiency, shouting matches, political infighting, accusations of a government cover-up, and the appalling destruction of key evidence—a grimly self-destructive brawl that has never before been made public.

Cover-up? The Ad Hoc Panel

Because the government-appointed ad hoc panel to the Tuskegee Syphilis Study did indeed end the study and also provided the impetus for important new laws that still regulate U.S. human medical experimentation, it is widely assumed to have done its job. But interviews I conducted with its surviving members suggest that the ad hoc panel also suffered miserable failures.

The group of academic, political, and economic leaders was chaired by Dillard University president Broadus Butler, Ph.D., an illustrious educator and Tuskegee Airman. The other members included Jay Katz, M.D., a Yale University psychiatrist and professor of law; Ron Brown, the general counsel of the National Urban League and future U.S. secretary of commerce; and Vernal Cave, M.D., director of the Bureau of Venereal Disease Control for the New York City Health Department.[31]

After sanctioning the most lengthy instance of experimental abuse in Western history, Secretary DuVal petulantly cast himself in the role of masochistic victim, declaring, "I wanted a panel that would be sympathetic to the public point of view rather than to the scientific or factual point of view, so I loaded it with angry blacks . . . that way there could be no criticism." The panel was not "loaded" with blacks—five members were black, including Chairman Butler, Vernal Cave, and Ron Brown, and four were white, including Jay Katz. Although nearly all the panel members expressed deep anger as they learned details of the study, they were also seasoned thinkers familiar with ethics, medical issues, or both. Because the black panelists included physicians, scientists, lawyers, and a university president, they presumably were able to grasp the scientific point of view. But the panel had no historian.

The panelists' clamor for the truth was muted by the narrowness of the charge DuVal gave them. The committee was to "determine whether the study was justified in 1932 and whether it should have been continued when penicillin became available"; to "recommend whether the study should be continued at this point in time and if not, how it should be terminated in a way consistent with the rights and health needs of its remaining participants"; and, finally, to "determine whether existing policies to protect the rights of patients participating in health research conducted or supported by the Department of Health, Education, and Welfare are adequate and effective and to recommend improvements in these policies, if needed."

The second charge was the easiest. The panelists decided that the study should be terminated immediately and that the men and their families should be given medical care and compensatory funds. On the first charge, the panel determined that the study was ethically unjustified both when it was initiated and after the discovery that penicillin was a safe and effective treatment that might have saved the lives and health of the subjects. On the third charge, the panel determined that there were inadequate provisions regarding the protection of human subjects of research. It mandated that a formal department be instituted for regulation of human-subjects research—a national human-subjects investigation board.

However, the panel's charge excluded some of the most important ethical questions, skirting the critical issue of the initial 1932 decision to withhold treatment in the form of bismuth and therapeutic dosages of arsphenamine even before penicillin became available. These were imperfect medications, but they were the standard of care in the 1930s. Panel member Fred Speaker, a lawyer, complained, "I thought at the beginning that we were asked to do something by these people that was inappropriate. . . . The scope we were given was too limited."[32]

The panel also had far too little time—just twelve meetings over seven months to analyze a forty-year experiment.[33] "We asked for an extension," says Katz, "and they begrudgingly gave us three additional months. Many of us felt that it was impossible to complete the work in that time. When we asked for another extension, it was denied."

The committee's report determined that the men may have submitted voluntarily but that this did not constitute informed consent. However, the panel addressed the wrong ethical question. The pertinent issue was not whether the men had been duly informed of the experiment's danger, but that the men had never been informed that they were in an experiment at all. They thought they were only receiving treatment, yet the committee seemed not to understand this.[34]

Why? Because there was no historian on the panel, it was hampered in discerning and interpreting the veins of truth trickling through the heaps of documents the government provided and in seeking out other crucial information. Yet, despite DuVal's claim that he had selected "angry blacks," the report did not condemn the racist mentality that informed the study.

Why not? Some members pointed to panel chairperson Dr. Broadus Butler, insisting that he had been charged with engineering a government whitewash, and this suspicion generated friction from the very first meeting. In 1994, Dr. Vernal Cave said, "He [Butler] spent the whole meeting telling us how important it was to keep an open mind, to look at the facts and not to jump to conclusions. He said how important it was not to have an opinion until all the information was in. As a result, most of the meeting was spent on that—getting lectured. No one else had anything to say. Then it turned out that he was the only one that came there with a closed mind."[35]

Dr. Katz agrees: "I believe that for whatever reason, Butler was beholden to HEW at the time. I don't know what his relationship was with them prior to his appointment as chair. He insisted that our charge was more limited than the interpretations some of us gave to our mission. He constantly slowed us down and forced us to go through maneuvers to get him to do certain things he thought were beyond the mandate given to us." Fred Speaker adds, "As things developed, I just felt that we couldn't just let it go on. Butler, I think, wanted to keep things *status quo*. . . . He was not the kind of guy to make demands on the administration or to say things that would embarrass the administration."

For example, Speaker recalls, "At some point, we learned that although we had given instructions to stop the experiment, HEW had not done anything yet and the experiment was still being conducted. That's when we had our mini-revolt. What I remember saying is 'Stop fucking around: let's *do* something!' Butler had a serious discussion with [future U.S. commerce secretary] Brown, who was very forceful. Ron Brown was a hell of a guy. He deserves a great deal of credit. I'm sure the four of us on the committee forced HEW to stop it immediately."[36] Katz adds, "By October or November, it became clear that we had to challenge the chairman as a group and not accept how he wanted to proceed. An alliance formed between me and Vernal Cave and we were quickly joined by Fred Speaker and by a Princeton theologian [Dr. Seward Hiltner] who had knowledge about the problems of human experimentation. Ron Brown was . . . chair of the Urban League. He was involved in national affairs and reluctant to get involved in what would soon become a controversial study. He was concerned about how it would affect his future position in government. But he was on our side. We could count on him."[37]

Not everyone blames Dr. Butler for the group's failures. One panel member, who spoke on condition of anonymity, said, "I think that there was a great deal of guilt and frustration about the members' inability to do what they felt they were there to do; to some extent, Dr. Butler became a focus for that frustration." Another panel member, the late Dr. Jean Louise Harris, denied perceiving any friction between Dr. Butler and his colleagues until the *Final Report* was submitted, when "we all became very angry."

In the end, the panel wrote a strongly worded report that was critical of the government and the PHS. However, all the interviewed panel members agree that Butler refused to sign it or even to chair the meeting at which it was discussed. The surviving panelists say they felt it critically important to present a unanimous report, so they argued long and bitterly until, at Butler's urging, they adopted a softer version whose language was less critical. Among other changes, the less confrontational new version deleted references to intentional racism and removed complaints that the panelists were afforded insufficient time and resources to thoroughly investigate the study's issues.

When the panelists received their copies of the final report in the mail, however, they were stunned by its cover letter, which read, "The final report of the Tuskegee Syphilis Study Ad Hoc Advisory Board is transmitted herewith. The Chairman specifically abstains from concurrence in this final report but recognizes his responsibility to submit it." Butler had induced them to "water down" the report, they say, then distanced himself from it.[38]

In late December 1995, Dr. Butler agreed to discuss the ad hoc panel with me, but, tragically, he fell ill shortly thereafter and died before we could do so.[39] He almost certainly would have given a very different account of his role and of the group's dynamics, and his passing leaves a vacuum in this story that no one else can fill.

Conspiracy Theory

DuVal spoke of censure at the hands of "angry blacks," but perhaps he should have worried about angry doctors instead. Most of the panelists believed that the government had hobbled their panel to preclude any real expression of outrage.

However, the most painful revelation was yet to come.

After the panel issued its report, Allan Brandt, who was then still a Columbia University graduate student, tracked down boxes of documents in the National Archives that fleshed out the full history and rationale of the Tuskegee Syphilis Study. Upon reading these, he realized that the panel had completely misunderstood the study's nature. He then wrote a paper, clearly tracing the study's history and criticizing the panel for having failed to obtain the historical information necessary to judge the study for what it was—experimental exploitation of the unwitting.

Brandt's work made it painfully clear, says Katz, that the panel had been sabotaged by the government staff they relied upon for information. "It was the first time I had heard about them [the documents]. We had asked the staff repeatedly to find these documents and they always came up empty-handed. Allan discovered the documents in the National

Archives. I felt very foolish and am sure my fellow committee members felt foolish for not having known about the National Archives repository for documents of this kind. My speculation is that several staff members must have known about the National Archives and should have looked there. . . . They [HEW] minimized what emerged later—particularly the deceptive aspects of the study.

"I wrote a letter of complaint to Senator Kennedy and said I thought there was a cover-up. I urged him to investigate."

Kennedy's office determined that there had been no cover-up, but Katz disagreed, and he was determined to enlist the panelists' help in demanding that the government admit how it had sabotaged their investigation. He says that "with the exception of Vern [Cave], I didn't get a response from anyone. All of them had guilt feelings—including myself—that we hadn't done enough. . . . I felt guilty that I let academic work and family life and other considerations influence me to do less."

The remorse may be appropriate, but so much was arrayed against the panel. The tangential charges, the failure to include a historian in the investigation of medical abuse that spanned four decades, the likely withholding of key documents, the impossibly short time frame, and, possibly, the manipulations of government sympathizers all ensured that truth would be the first casualty of the Tuskegee Syphilis Study investigation.

However, the panel engaged in a cover-up of its own.

Cave recalled, "We went there [to Tuskegee], we interviewed the victims, Nurse Rivers, the sociologists, everyone . . . we had them all on tape. When we got back, at the next meeting, Broadus Butler said, 'The first item on the agenda is whether we should keep the tape.' I was amazed, the others were amazed and we spent the whole session talking about the tape. I'm going to confess that during that session I thought of the fact that Nurse Rivers was an innocent person in this whole thing. In a moment of weakness, I said to myself, 'It would be a shame to have this woman put in court, put on the stand, pilloried.' She was an innocent victim, so I went along with destroying the tape."

"It was terrible thing," Katz sadly muses. "He, the chair [Dr. Broadus Butler], made the recommendation. He said it was to protect Rivers and I unfortunately went along with it. I wish we hadn't done so. I wish I had been more alert to make the tape under seal, not to destroy it. . . . We hadn't done our job well."[40]

The group burned the tape, and with it were lost first-person accounts from scientists and staffers who are now dead. Moreover, in trying to protect the reputation of Eunice Rivers, the panel may have damned it by robbing her of her voice. This was a shocking act for which I have found no parallel in contemporary committees, and had there been a historian on the panel, it would not have taken place.

After the panel's recommendation ended the study in 1972, its participants and their families began to receive medical treatment. Macon County attorney Fred Gray filed a $1.8 billion class-action civil lawsuit on July 23, 1973, which named as defendants HEW, the PHS, the CDC, the state of Alabama, and the Milbank Fund, as well as several individual PHS officers and a few John Does to cover any unknown malefactors. The suit resulted in a 1974 out-of-court settlement for more than $10 million. It yielded a mere $37,500 for each living study participant, $15,000 for his heirs, and nearly $1 million in legal fees for Gray, which was deducted from the payments made to the men. The living control-group members received even less.[41]

Black Antiheroes in White

The Tuskegee Syphilis Study compromised the reputations not only of white but also of many black caregivers by alerting the nation to the possibility that they were directly responsible for this notorious medical abuse of black patients.

But the roles of some key African Americans in the study have been exaggerated. In 1995, Dr. Henry Foster's nomination as surgeon general was derailed by accusations, which he denies, that he attended a meeting where the Tuskegee Syphilis Study was discussed and the resultant media uproar castigated Foster for failing to denounce or to end the study. Foster denied knowing anything about the study before the news media exposed it in 1972. Even though no one could demonstrate that he had been present, the very accusation was enough to end his hopes for appointment. By contrast, no news accounts have censured or even identified the scores of white AMA members at a 1965 meeting where the Tuskegee Syphilis Study was reported upon in great detail. For that matter, the PHS physicians responsible for the study have never been charged or punished.

Eunice Rivers, a modestly educated black nurse in the profoundly segregated rural Alabama of the 1940s, occupied the lowest rung in the medical hierarchy. Hers was an era when a nurse was a "handmaiden" trained to assist, not to question, the physician, and a black nurse occupied an even lower professional stratum than a white one. Yet Rivers came to shoulder the burden of America's most infamous instance of medical research abuse. She has been accused of retaining men in an experiment that she knew could only harm them, but all her spontaneous statements focus proudly upon the care and protection that she provided them. She categorically denied ever seeking out and removing subjects from syphilis clinics, as she has been accused of doing by her superiors, the doctors who engineered and controlled the study. In 1953, Rivers, whose role was that of a caretaker and tracker, not of a research analyst, was listed in the coveted position of first author of a *Public Health Reports* paper defending the study.[42] Was this an earned scientific laurel or a cynical ploy to portray the study as one planned and analyzed by a racially mixed group of researchers rather than by a group of white male scientists? Her role and her own statements suggest the latter. When she was first recruited to enter the study as a scientific assistant, her response had been, "You know I don't know a thing about it," and this was likely frankness, not false modesty: As a night nurse at the Andrew Hospital, she had little scientific training: Her forte was caring for people.

When she is asked about the study details, Rivers's responses are inchoate and echo the cant with which the PHS researchers have agreed to defend themselves, which suggests that Rivers never understood the science behind the study. Her crime was believing the PHS doctors who told her that theirs was beneficent work.[43]

However, I cannot completely excuse her, as much as I long to. I wish that she had asked more questions, and once the question of whether the study was ethical had been openly raised in 1965, I wish that she had demanded reassurance on that point or left the study. Instead, she compounded her error by her continued blind faith in the researchers she had been trained to serve. She failed to see that she had been used as a Judas goat to lure the men into completing their research roles and as a shield to deflect charges of racism. But how do these pallid failings of omission compare to the sinister machinations of PHS officials who deliberately lied, plotted, abused, then deflected blame onto the powerless?

Perhaps we should ask ourselves why the name of Nurse Rivers is so closely associated with the Tuskegee Syphilis Study but the names of Taliaferro Clark, Thomas Murrell, Raymond Vonderlehr, and Oliver C. Wenger remain all but unknown.

Although at least four full-length books, two feature films, a handful of documentaries, plays, and hundreds of medical, newspaper, and magazine articles have been written about the Tuskegee Syphilis Study, there are still aspects of the study about which we know little. For example, the interpretations of the study have focused upon the monitoring of the disease's course in the untreated black men, but Benjamin Roy, M.D., an Atlanta psychoneuroimmunologist, has proposed another experimental agenda for the Tuskegee Syphilis Study. More than a decade ago, Roy discovered that PHS scientists may have used the men to develop a reliable syphilis test and vaccine. The unwitting subjects may have served American laboratories as a reservoir of *T. pallidum* bacterium: They were human incubators of the bacterium that causes syphilis.

A 1995 *Harvard Journal of Minority Public Health* article by Roy proposes that the experiment's chief medical importance was in providing a reservoir of infected men who could be used to develop new, more reliable, and profitable tests for syphilis. Roy points out that the Public Health Service's study of the men at Tuskegee was only one of a related group of research studies called the Cooperative Clinical Groups.[44] The Tuskegee Syphilis Study began in 1932, twenty years before scientists learned to culture cells in which to grow pathogens such as the syphilis bacterium. Thus, the development of a sensitive, specific test for syphilis required a constant supply of syphilis, which could not be cultured in the laboratory. This constant need for fresh supplies of blood products that contained the syphilis bacterium explains, among other things, why the study subjects were routinely administered spinal taps and had their blood drawn regularly.

PHS documents verify that the sera of the infected Tuskegee subjects was used to develop more reliable tests for syphilis, including the fluorescent treponemal antibody absorption (FTA-ABS) test and the Venereal Disease Research Laboratory (VDRL) test. In 1970, Dr. James B. Lucas, of the PHS's Venereal Disease branch, conceded, "Probably the greatest contribution that the Tuskegee Study has made and can continue to provide has been documented sera for study in our laboratory. . . . In a great measure the development and our endorsement of the FTA-ABS test rested on Tuskegee sera."[45]

The tests were marketed globally and became quite profitable for the U.S. government because its contract with Alabama's Department of Health specified that any invention arising from the Tuskegee Syphilis Study would become the sole property of the United States.[46]

Among the ruins left in the wake of the Tuskegee Syphilis Study were the blighted lives and early deaths of hundreds of subjects and their families, but this was only the beginning. The proud good name of our nation's premier African American research institution has been forever besmirched. The residual faith in medical science to which communities of disadvantaged black people clung has been blasted so fiercely that physicians and researchers are still dodging the fallout. The health of thirty million African Americans is continually imperiled, partly because many eschew effective care rather than risk the tender mercies of government-sponsored medicine. Although many studies and abuses contributed to this iatrophobia, Tuskegee remains the iconic symbol of racialized medical abuse.

The study also left a rich mythical legacy that reveals much about the cultural consequences of the study. But it is essential to separate fact from fiction, because the false beliefs generate false fears that exacerbate black aversion to medical treatment.

Perhaps the most persistent myth holds that the PHS actively injected the subjects with syphilis. This falsehood emanated not from overheated African American imaginations but from the *Congressional Record* and erroneous newspaper accounts.[47] Furthermore, this was an erroneous but not an unrealistic belief, because, as historian Susan E. Lederer reminds us, researchers have injected Americans with gonorrhea, syphilis, and other venereal diseases on at least forty occasions since 1892, most of which took place in the twentieth century.[48] In 1892, Albert Neisser intentionally infected women with syphilis by injecting them with serum from syphilitic patients. Groups consisting only of African Americans have been injected with diseases such as granuloma inguinale and falciparum malaria.[49] J. A. Macintosh of Memphis, Tennessee, boasted in 1926 that he had achieved the first instance of successful experimental transmission of granuloma inguinale from one individual to another, a black man who was "not previously exposed in any way to the possibility of spontaneously contracting this disease."[50]

Another popular myth holds that the study's infected men were soldiers, or were Tuskegee Airmen, which seems a simple erroneous association of the Tuskegee Airmen with Tuskegee Institute. This myth was reinforced when actor Laurence Fishburne played the lead role in both *Miss Evers' Boys*, the irresponsibly fictionalized HBO feature based upon the Tuskegee Syphilis Study, and the television film *The Tuskegee Airmen*. Yet this myth also reflects a sad acknowledgment that the honor of Tuskegee University, a proud scientific bastion once celebrated as the "Black Harvard," also fell victim to this shameful perversion of medical research.

Still, it is a mistake to attribute African Americans' medical reluctance to simple fear generated by the Tuskegee Syphilis Study, because this study is not an aberration that single-handedly transformed African American perceptions of the health-care system. The study is part of a pattern of experimental abuse, and many African Americans understand it as such, because a rich oral tradition has sustained remembrances of pain, abuse, and humiliation at the hands of physicians. We should remember that, as Vanessa Northington Gamble, M.D., director of Tuskegee University's National Center for Bioethics in Research and Health Care, averred, "many African Americans fear and distrust Western medicine who have never heard of Tuskegee." In 2004, Dr. Stephen Sodeke, assistant director of the Tuskegee Bioethics Center, remarked, "One of the huge challenges we have is recruitment of African Americans into clinical trials, and the Tuskegee Syphilis Study is always cited as one of the reasons why African Americans are reluctant to participate." Too many researchers and social scientists still attribute all African Americans' fears of medical abuse to the Tuskegee Syphilis Study. Their surveys often frame questions that are limited to this one study. News accounts follow suit, usually attributing all black iatrophobia to Tuskegee. Consider these newspaper and journal excerpts:

> Congress is posed to consider ill-advised legislation introduced by Rep. Gary Ackerman (D-N.Y.) that would bar the blind HIV testing of blood samples taken from newborns, writes Ronald Bayer in *The Washington Post*. According to Bayer, the specter of the Tuskegee

syphilis study—the federal experiment that traced the course of the disease in African American men, who were not informed that they had a treatable sexually transmitted disease—surrounds the debate.

—"IT'S NOT 'TUSKEGEE' REVISITED," *WASHINGTON POST,* MAY 26, 1995

Dr. Arthur Ammann, a specialist in pediatric AIDS, compared the anonymous testing of infants in New York to the Tuskegee experiment, in which black men with syphilis were observed, but not treated, in a government study.

—"THE NEW TUSKEGEE EXPERIMENT," *THE VILLAGE VOICE,* OCTOBER 14, 1996

The impact of the Tuskegee Study, in which blacks in the South were not treated for syphilis as part of a government study, continues to be felt as the mistrust it generated interferes with attempts to combat AIDS in certain black areas. . . . AIDS education programs in black communities have often prompted the topic of Tuskegee.

—"TUSKEGEE'S LONG ARM STILL TOUCHES A NERVE," *NEW YORK TIMES,* APRIL 13, 1997

The Tuskegee Syphilis Study ended a quarter of a century ago, but its effects can still be felt. . . . "Many African Americans' distrust in today's medical establishment can be attributed to Tuskegee," says Dr. Carl C. Bell, executive director of Chicago's Community Mental Health Council.

—"MISTRUST OF DOCTORS LINGERS AFTER TUSKEGEE," *WASHINGTON POST,* APRIL 15, 1997

The assumed one-to-one correspondence between this study and black distrust is chronicled in hundreds of articles with headlines such as THE GHOST OF TUSKEGEE; CLOSE-UP: TUSKEGEE EXPERIMENT'S LEGACY IS THE SPREAD OF SUSPICION; SOUR LEGACY OF TUSKEGEE SYPHILIS STUDY LINGERS; TUSKEGEE EXPERIMENT'S LEGACY: LACK OF TRUST; SYPHILIS STUDY LEAVES LEGACY OF MISTRUST; AND CLINICAL TRIALS, HEALTH CARE, AND THE TUSKEGEE LEGACY. But it is important to look beyond this one study in examining African Americans' aversion to the health-care system. By focusing upon the single event of the Tuskegee Syphilis Study rather than examining a centuries-old pattern of experimental abuse, recent investigations tend to distort the problem, casting African Americans' wariness as an overreaction to a single event rather than an understandable, reasonable reaction to the persistent experimental abuse that has characterized American medicine's interaction with African Americans.

As early as 1997, a few especially perceptive biomedical researchers placed black iatrophobia in the context of a longer history of research abuse and neglect. That year, Emory University's Otis Brawley, M.D., told the *Journal of Blacks in Higher Education* that many researchers believe that because of Tuskegee "it will be so difficult and even impossible to recruit blacks that we shouldn't waste our time," but researchers use Tuskegee as "an excuse for laziness."[51] Fortunately, more investigations with fewer leading questions are now being launched, and they will allow us to learn more about the extent of African Americans' awareness concerning the long, unhappy history of medicalized abuse and experimentation.

The Tuskegee Syphilis Study is the longest and the most infamous—but hardly the worst—experimental abuse of African Americans. It has been eclipsed in both numbers and egregiousness by other abusive medical studies, and the balance of this book tells these stories. Subsequent chapters will relate how after the Tuskegee Syphilis Study, African Americans' illnesses were not simply observed but were also induced when subjects were administered toxic substances or deliberately exposed to a wide range of biological hazards, including lethal radiation doses, hazardous experimental technologies, a wide range of untested chemical products, risky nontherapeutic vaccines, and injection with infectious agents.

In fact, in the late 1920s and 1930s, the very period when the Tuskegee Syphilis Study lost its therapeutic arm and mutated into exploitation, an experiment in malaria therapy, conducted under the auspices of the Rockefeller Foundation, was doing worse than allowing black men with syphilis to die: Researchers were killing black syphilitics outright in order to test a theory of treatment.

In 1910, New York City was home to the only hospital in the nation that was devoted exclusively to research—the Rockefeller Institute. As mentioned earlier in this chapter, neurosyphilis, or paresis, occurs in late-stage syphilis, affecting the nervous system and causing insanity. In

1910, it was long thought to be a mental ailment, not an infectious one. Dr. Mark Boyd, a researcher funded by the Rockefeller Institute, was testing a novel treatment for neurosyphilis—malaria therapy. Boyd deliberately infected both black and white people suffering from neurosyphilis with malaria in order to generate high fevers, which he hoped would kill the syphilis spirochete. But the blacks in his experiment seemed to resist infection by the relatively benign plasmodia strain of malaria, so Boyd infected 470 of the syphilitic blacks—but no whites—with the deadly falciparum strain instead, killing some of the black subjects.[52] Boyd did not stop the experiments when blacks began dying. Instead, he resorted to deceit: In his notes, he disguised their causes of death and distorted the death rate of blacks to shroud the fact that they were dying from deliberate infection with falciparum.[53]

However, the decision not to treat the sick men of the Tuskegee Study is a different crime, a crime of omission, and it illustrates several of the important patterns explored in this book. These include the selection of blacks for the riskiest studies; their disproportionate selection for nontherapeutic experimentation; the myth of medical distinctiveness (which held that syphilis was manifested differently in blacks); and the myth of hypersexed blacks as "incorrigible" vectors of sexual disease and dysfunction. The use of men as reservoirs of syphilis reinforced the familiar use of black bodies to generate the profitable wonders of new disease approaches (to which the subjects are rarely privy), and the clinical display of disease in the clinic and in medical journals.

The defenses of the study all rest upon carefully engineered fictions. Its apologists have claimed that the study was merely a passive observation, a "study in nature," but it was not, because researchers actively designed it, and lied to participants, promising treatment but actively withholding it. The study cannot be defended on a utilitarian basis because PHS physicians admitted, years before it was ended, that it imparted no new clinical knowledge that would allow them to help future patients. By 1970, James Lucas, assistant chief of the PHS's Venereal Disease branch, concluded, "Nothing learned will prevent, find, or cure a single case of infectious syphilis or bring us closer to our basic mission of controlling venereal disease in the United States."[54] The study did, however, generate publications, scientific tools, and scientific stature for the PHS researchers.

PHS researchers lacked scientific as well as ethical integrity: Early in the experiment, Raymond Vondelehr had triumphantly announced that the clinical assessments provided proof of a divergent "white" and "black" syphilis: Black syphilitics, he said, clearly suffered primarily cardiovascular complications, whereas whites suffered neurological devastation. But a ten-member blue-ribbon panel of the American Heart Association disagreed. In 1933, they condemned the data as inaccurately interpreted: The racial dimorphism existed only in the PHS researchers' minds. Yet the experiment in racial comparison was continued, as if this had never been determined.

Some claim that the Tuskegee Syphilis Study was not a racist study because it simply mirrored a "parallel" study of Norwegian whites by Dr. E. Bruusgaard. In 1929, Bruusgaard reviewed the charts of two thousand Oslo-area syphilis patients who for various reasons had not received medications between 1891 and 1910. However, equating the Tuskegee study with the Oslo study is inaccurate, because the latter was a retrospective analysis of Norwegian treatment data *that already had been collected,* not an experiment in malign neglect designed deliberately to withhold treatment from the unwitting. Even if the PHS had used a parallel design, it would be absurd to compare the racial dynamics driving black-white health consumption in segregated Alabama to that of whites in a more racially homogeneous social-welfare state such as Norway.

Apologists for the study often make the error of assuming that because there were no national laws governing human medical experimentation in the 1930s, there were no ethical strictures upon what a physician could and could not do with his patients. But in the era of the Tuskegee Syphilis Study, physicians *were* constrained by hospital regulations and AMA codes to share diagnoses and to request permission for experimentation and usually for treatment—the ethical norm of the time. There were also laws that forbade many of the PHS practices at Tuskegee. Among the examples given by historian Susan Lederer is the 1929 observation by lawyer George Weinman that "the unauthorized autopsy of a dead human body is a tort, giving rise to a cause of action for damages."[55] This norm was often violated in the case of African Americans.

Transforming the Legacy

On May 16, 1997, a quarter of a century after the Tuskegee Syphilis Study ended, President William Jefferson Clinton formally apologized for the study in a dignified White House ceremony that allowed the mere eight survivors and their families to join the activists and historians who had championed their cause.

> To the survivors, to the wives and family members, the children and the grandchildren, I say what you know: No power on Earth can give you back the lives lost, the pain suffered, the years of internal torment and anguish. What was done cannot be undone. But we can end the silence. We can stop turning our heads away. We can look at you in the eye and finally say on behalf of the American people, what the United States government did was shameful, and I am sorry. . . . To Macon County, to Tuskegee, to the doctors who have been wrongly associated with the events there, you have our apology, as well. To our African American citizens, I am sorry that your federal government orchestrated a study so clearly racist. That can never be allowed to happen again.

Clamorous applause greeted the President's acknowledgment of the racism and immorality of the study. Under the hot press lights, the survivors shared their remembrances and their hope that such an abuse would never be repeated. "It is time," ninety-four-year-old Herman Shaw declaimed, "to put this horrible nightmare behind us as a nation. . . . We must never allow a tragedy like the Tuskegee Study to happen again."

The apology incorporated a permanent, tangible legacy, as well—the Tuskegee University National Center for Bioethics in Research and Health Care, supported in part by a $200,000 grant President Clinton allocated as part of the apology. It opened May 12, 1998, with the stated goal of training and educating African Americans in bioethics. The center's multiethnic staff has forged scholarly partnerships with mainstream bioethics centers at other universities. Unlike other such centers, however, Tuskegee has also invested heavily in community education.

More than thirty years after its unmasking, the study still horribly fascinates. It may be the study's essentially vacuous nature, because it embodies coolly designed crimes of omission by featureless government martinets who illustrate Hannah Arendt's "banality of evil" to appalling perfection. Or perhaps it is medicine's betrayal by physicians of the Public Health Service, the very government entity charged with protecting our health. Then again, it may have been the carefully orchestrated complicity of so many powerful, privileged physicians utterly bent upon destroying the health of a group of poor, powerless, vulnerable black men.

Or the very longevity of the syphilis study may be what holds us in thrall. Discovering a murderously racist experiment that had been secretly coddled from the interbellum era to the Nixon administration is a bit like finding one of those gruesome prehistoric fish, long thought extinct, in the deep end of your swimming pool. The syphilis study, like those Jurassic holdovers, has forced us to confront a living, breathing monster that we would rather have consigned to history.

Yet the Tuskegee Syphilis Study has not really ended, because it continues to fascinate: The flow of books, plays, poems, songs, and films continues as Americans probe and worry the experiment for lessons. I suspect we are partly motivated by our desire to extract some valuable meaning that will produce good as a counterweight to its evil. Maybe what is important is that blacks and whites are united in their outrage over this medical nightmare and that whites actively attacked this racist viper at the breast of medicine. A white whistle-blower challenged the study, a white journalist forced it onto the national stage, and white and black panel members joined to end it.

But if we had learned what we should have, this book would stop here. The greatest tragedy of the study is that it has failed to serve as a cautionary tale for researchers. Its inception marked the dawn of many other experimental evils against blacks, detailed in the chapters to come.

PART 2
THE USUAL SUBJECTS

CHAPTER 8

THE BLACK STORK

The Eugenic Control of African American Reproduction

*We don't allow dogs to breed. We spay them. We neuter them. We try
to keep them from having unwanted puppies, and yet these women
are literally having litters of children. . . .*
—BARBARA HARRIS, FOUNDER OF CHILDREN REQUIRING

A CARING KOMMUNITY (CRACK), C. 1990

National Socialism is nothing but applied biology.
—RUDOLF HESS, BERLIN, 1934

She might easily have endured the life of quiet desperation dictated by
her birth, then vanished without a ripple. The granddaughter of a slave,
the daughter of sharecroppers, and younger sister to nineteen siblings,
she was intelligent, hardworking, and loved to read, but she was also
dark-skinned, uneducated, and a woman, a recipe for failure in rural
Mississippi. The year was 1961, but it might as well have been 1861. She
helped her family eke a hardscrabble existence on a plantation in Sunflower County by picking three hundred to four hundred pounds of cotton a day for one dollar a hundredweight. They spent their days
exhausted, hungry, and shabbily garbed, but her family never earned
enough to break the cycle of debt and remained trapped in the usurious
latter-day slavery called sharecropping. But she was not angry: A deeply
religious person, she focused her energies on helping others and eagerly
awaited the day she would have her own family.

Her name was Fannie Lou Hamer.

One day in 1961, Hamer entered the hospital to have "a knot on my
stomach"—probably a benign uterine fibroid tumor—removed. She
then returned to her family's shack on the plantation to recuperate. But
in the big house, ominous tidings circulated. The owner's wife, Vera Ali-

cia Marlow, was a cousin of the surgeon who had treated Hamer. Marlow gossiped to the cook that Hamer had lost more than a tumor while unconscious—the surgeon had removed her uterus, rendering Hamer sterile. The cook repeated the news to others, including a woman who happened to be Hamer's cousin, and thus Hamer was one of the last people on the plantation to learn that she would never have a family of her own.

"I went to the doctor who did that to me and I asked him, 'Why? Why had he done that to me?' He didn't have to say nothing—and he didn't. If he was going to give that sort of operation then he should have told me. I would have loved to have had children." But a lawsuit was out of the question, Hamer recalled. "At that time? Me? Getting a white lawyer against a white doctor? I would have been taking my hands and screwing tacks in my casket."[1]

A rage seized her and she complained bitterly about her fate. But she also grew fascinated by political power as a means to redress injustice, and soon she did the unthinkable: She tried to register to vote. But she was rejected at the polling booth, and when she arrived home, the angry owner threw her off the plantation where she had lived for nineteen years.

It didn't matter, because Hamer was no longer a sharecropper. She was now an uncompromising political dynamo who would become one of the most powerful leaders and symbols of the southern civil rights movement. She always spoke of her "Mississippi appendectomy" as the galvanizing force that propelled her into a national leadership role, and she always spoke regretfully of the children she would never have.[2]

She was a lifelong opponent of birth control.

Evolutionary Laggards

The twentieth century saw the dawn of the medical philosophy *eugenics,* derived from the Greek word *eugenes,* meaning "well-born." The word was coined by Francis Galton, a cousin of Charles Darwin. Between 1900 and 1910, geneticists discovered human traits that adhered to a Mendelian pattern of inheritance, one in which the breeding of two carrier parents resulted in a mathematically predictable mixture of well, ill, and carrier offspring. Several metabolic conditions were among these Mendelian discoveries, including sickle-cell anemia, red-green color blindness, and polydactyly (having more than the normal number of fingers or toes).[3] The birth of an affected child from unaffected parents signaled that the parents were carriers.

Armed with this knowledge, Galton first formulated the desirability of using selective procreation to refine the human race while conquering social dysfunction. This goal was widely embraced on both scientific and popular levels by the 1930s, not only in the United States, but also abroad, and eugenic yardsticks were applied to not only populations but to individuals.[4] Eugenicists proposed that society use medical information about disease and trait inheritance to end social ills by encouraging the birth of children with good, healthy, and beautiful traits. This was positive eugenics, but the movement also had a negative face: Eugenicists promulgated the weeding out of undesirable societal elements by discouraging or preventing the birth of children with "bad" genetic profiles. The term *well-born* has a double meaning of "born healthy" and "born wealthy," and this is fitting, because eugenic scientists and their disciples constantly confused the concepts of biological hereditary fitness with those of class and race. Highly educated persons of good social class were considered eugenically superior; the poor, the uneducated, criminals, recent immigrants, blacks, and the feebleminded were eugenic misfits. Eugenicists invoked the term *racial hygiene* as frequently as they did the word *eugenics,* and even a cursory glance at the charts, photographs, and diagrams used to popularize eugenic ideals reveals that the unfit were "swarthy" "black" and ugly by Anglo-Saxon standards, with flattened noses, wiry black hair, and prognathous profiles.[5]

African Americans were roundly disparaged by eugenic theory as scientists continued to seek and find wide physiologic evidence of black inferiority. In a refinement of earlier scientific racism, eugenics was appropriated to label black women as sexually indiscriminate and as bad mothers who were constrained by biology to give birth to defective children. The demonization of black parents, particularly mothers, as medically and behaviorally unfit has a long history, but twentieth-century eugenicists provided the necessary biological underpinnings to scientifically validate these beliefs. The sexual irrepressibility and the bad mothering were biologically located in the hereditary apparatus, they contended. Thus eugenics undergirded medicosocial movements that placed the sexual behavior and reproduction of blacks under strict scrutiny and disproportionately forced them into sterility, both temporary and permanent. Scientists also vigorously researched black fertility, compiling data on black birth rates and using women of color predominantly to test many reproductive technologies and strategies, from involuntary sterilization to Norplant to "the shot."

In 1915, Dr. Harry J. Haiselden heralded the first wave of U.S. eugenics when he gained fame and wealth by exploiting the evil legacy of the black mother. Haiselden was as famous in his time as Dr. Jack Kevorkian was in our own, and for an eerily similar reason: Both hastened the death of those they perceived as "unfit for life," and both chose their victims from the poles of life. Kevorkian preyed upon the old or ill; Haiselden on sick, "defective" infants. On November 12, 1915, he announced to newspapers that he had allowed the ailing but viable newborn of his patient Anna Bollinger to die in Chicago's German-American Hospital because he would have gone through life as a defective.[6] Between 1915 and 1918, Haiselden killed five other babies, drawing fawning attention from the press each time. Practicing negative eugenics very publicly, Haiselden encouraged parents and other pediatricians to follow his example by killing or allowing the deaths of the "genetically inferior." Parents began openly to recruit doctors to kill their children who were born with birth defects, and doctors came forward with their own proud confessions of infanticide.[7] Like Kevorkian, Haiselden arranged "photo ops" with his dying patients and their mothers.

When he decided to make a film to popularize his eugenic ideals, starring himself, it became a hit, making him a wealthy movie star. That film was *The Black Stork*. It begins with the story of a white, wealthy, well-born slave owner who, in a moment of inebriation, is seduced by his "vile, filthy" black servant.[8] The resulting child supplies a genetic taint to his family that haunts his progeny, making them unfit to marry. One scene showcases a panoply of defective children, and the very first image is that of a black child.[9]

In titling the film, Haiselden was mindful of both the negative and the racial connotations of the word *black*. Martin Pernick, Ph.D., the premier expert on Haiselden and his work, points out that Haiselden repeatedly equated *black* with ugliness and undesirability.[10] The fact that her white master—but not she—must be addled by drink before they have sexual congress speaks to the black woman's innate shamelessness. At the film's end, the tainted descendant of the union is subjected to euthanasia, with the approval of a berobed Jesus, who stands over the cradle. This ham-handed bit of eugenic propaganda buoyed popular sentiment toward eugenics.

Soon, life began to imitate Haiselden's art.

German doctors became obsessed with regaining an imaginary Nordic purity even before the 1933 rise of Hitler and National Socialism. But U.S. national eugenics policies had employed unconscionable medical violations against those they considered unfit, including blacks, since 1910. The lions of American and German eugenics were united not only by a shared vision of racial purity but also by the International Society for Racial Hygiene. Chief among its American members was mathematician and biologist Charles Davenport, Ph.D., who established the Station for Experiment Evolution (SEE) and, in 1910, the privately funded and seminal Eugenics Record Office (ERO) at Cold Spring Harbor on Long Island, New York, which joined with the SEE in 1920 under the aegis of the Carnegie Institution.

Davenport was fascinated by biometrics, the quantitative study of evolution. Under him, the ERO conducted research on human heredity by means of numerically mapping human traits, collecting large amounts of eugenic data from scientists and physicians who shared their patients' family and medical histories. The ERO also informed popular and legal opinion concerning eugenics, as when Davenport's deputy, Harry Hamilton Laughlin, provided the extensive statistical research that proved essential to the National Origins Act of 1924. It barred immigrants from Southern and Eastern European countries as "dysgenic." The ERO was so indispensable to the prestige of eugenic science that when Carnegie withdrew its funding support on December 31, 1939, its closing marked the official end of the eugenics era.[11] Laughlin, who was also head of the SEE, worried in print that no two races had ever maintained their purity while living in as close proximity as U.S. blacks and whites did. In 1910, he published a research study of the skin colors that resulted from black-white matings.[12]

Predictably warm relations reigned between American eugenicists and the Germans, who shared Laughlin's abhorrence of black-white mating. In 1933, Davenport's *Eugenical News* praised the German race-hygiene movement and published abstracts of articles from German eugenics journals such as *Archiv für Rassen- und Gesellschaftsbiologie.* Laughlin shared detailed information about eugenic sterilization in the United States with Eugen Fischer, director of Berlin's Kaiser Wilhelm Institut für Anthropologie, Menschliche Erblehre und Eugenik (Institute for Anthropology, Human Genetics and Eugenics).[13] In gratitude, Heidelberg University awarded Laughlin an honorary doctor of medicine degree in 1936.

Although their cruel acts of genocide were primarily directed against Jews and white Europeans, National Socialists also considered any admixture with people of African descent intolerable. For example, the *"Rheinlandbastarde"* were the offspring, born during the 1920s, of German women and French Somalian soldiers who were stationed in the Rhineland during its post–World War I occupation.[14] The Reichsbauernführer Richard-Walther Darre declared, "As a Rhinelander, I demand: sterilization for all mulattoes with whom we were saddled by the black shame on the Rhine."[15] German Hereditary Health Courts judged the reproductive fitness of poor and ill Gentiles on a case-by-case basis, but for blacks and Afro-Germans, visual or verbal evidence of African ancestry was enough to justify immediate secret sterilization in on-site clinics under Special Commission No. 3, which was devised by Eugen Fischer in 1937. For example, Frankfurt health office records for June 19, 1937, note:

> The German citizen Josef Feck, born on 26 September 1920 and residing in Mainz is a descendant of the former colonial occupation troops (North Africa) and distinctly displays the corresponding anthropological characteristics. For that reason he is to be sterilized. His mother consents to the sterilization.[16]

Upon demand, Afro-German men had to produce health documents certifying that they had been sterilized, and although the sterilization of at least 385 children is well documented, an entire generation of Afro-Germans was robbed of its fertility.[17]

However, Nazi eugenicists frequently observed that their laws to bar Jewish-Aryan mating were more liberal than were American laws to separate people of African descent from the white genetic pool. Germans held that a person who was one-quarter Jewish was a legal Aryan and thus fit to marry a German, but parallel marriages and matings between whites and blacks were illegal in much of the United States and, in effect, punishable by death—lynching. The "one-drop" laws of many southern states counted anyone who had even one thirty-second African heritage as black. Other laws, such as the 1924 Virginia Racial Integrity Act, denominated anyone with any "Negro blood" at all as black.[18] Editors of German medical journals learned a great deal about eugenic proscription by studying American medical journals, whose charts precisely detailed which racial mixtures were tolerable in marriages to whites, who was "white" enough to vote, and so on. In fact, a cordial rivalry characterized the relationship between German and American eugenicists: "The Germans are beating us at our own game," Virginian eugenicist Dr. Joseph S. Dejarnette sighed in thinly veiled admiration during a 1934 speech in which he urged the Virginia legislature to expand its sterilization laws.[19]

However, eugenics initiatives, like much of the unethical racial experimentation in the United States, suffered from more than moral flaws: They were simply illogical. There are several reasons why any experiments in improving health and purifying racial stock by removing certain "tainted" individuals from populations will fail to root out the unwanted genes, but scientists had known of at least one since 1917. Before the advent of genetic screening tests, one had only classic Mendelian genetics to rely upon, and one could determine whether a person was a carrier of a genetic taint only by the health of his children—too late for eugenic measures to prevent breeding. English geneticist P. C. Punnett had determined by 1917 that eugenic steps to prevent the reproduction of people exhibiting disease symptoms would fail to detect so many carriers that they would be rendered useless.[20] This knowledge made eugenic strategies and goals scientifically invalid as well as morally repugnant.

The Negro Project

Margaret Sanger, born to a Corning, New York, socialist in 1883, was the most famous American populizer of eugenics, although she is usually lauded as a powerful birth-control pioneer and as a feminist. All these labels fit. Her abundant writings, speeches, and myriad projects reveal a complex, passionate woman whose mission changed over time from women's rights advocacy to eugenics. Sanger shaped American reproductive policy by toppling the "Comstock laws" against contraceptive distribution, by catalyzing the development of the birth-control pill, and by founding the organization that became Planned Parenthood, the nation's twelfth-largest charitable organization. But she did so in alliance with eugenicists, and through initiatives such as the Negro Project, Sanger exploited black stereotypes in order to reduce the fertility of African Americans.

Sanger was a cautious speaker, so it is important to examine not only what she said but what she did. In her 1922 eugenics tome, *The Pivot of Civilisation*, she claimed, "Eugenics is chiefly valuable in its negative aspects. . . . On its so-called positive or constructive side, it fails to awaken any permanent interest." In this book, Sanger popularized her research into the eugenic value of various types of Americans by offering up a slew of case histories. She published a dysgenic family case history to describe the eugenic problems black families presented:

> The parents of a feeble-minded girl, twenty years of age, who was committed to the Kansas State Industrial Farm on a vagrancy charge, lived in a thickly populated Negro district which was reported by the police to be the headquarters for the criminal element of the surrounding State.

Sanger tells us at great length and in detail that all of the girl's family died early or went on to lead lives of hyperfecundity, prostitution, violent crime, or all three. The "Negro district" itself, we are told, is the "headquarters for the criminal element," so clearly we are meant to take the black girl's dysfunctional family as representative.[21]

While Sanger's early campaigns were aimed primarily at Eastern Europeans, she turned her attention to blacks in 1929. That year, Lothrop Stoddard wrote his book *The Rising Tide of Color Against White World Supremacy* while serving on the board of directors of Sanger's American Birth Control League (ABCL), and Sanger's lover, Havelock Ellis, reviewed it favorably in her journal *Birth Control Review*.[22] That year, she also discarded labels such as "good or bad breeding stock" in favor of "class" or "income level." As she began researching birth patterns in Harlem, where 224,760 of New York City's 330,000 African Americans lived,[23] Sanger entitled the June 1932 *Birth Control Review* "The Negro

Number," and she recruited black leaders to contribute articles in support of the eugenic cause. The National Association for the Advancement of Colored People's founder, W. E. B. Du Bois wrote (and Sanger often quoted), "The mass of ignorant Negroes still breed carelessly and disastrously, so that the increase among Negroes, even more than the increase among whites, is from that portion of the population least intelligent and fit, and least able to rear their children properly."[24]

Charles S. Johnson, Fisk University's first black president, wrote that "eugenic discrimination" was necessary for blacks, and a dozen black writers agreed in print. In January 1939, Sanger's American Birth Control League merged with the Clinical Research Bureau to form the Birth Control Federation of America (BCFA). Later that year, Sanger devised the Negro Project, which "was established for the benefit of the colored people," specifically black women who were being denied access to city health services. These first experimental "family planning centers" sought to find the best way of reducing the black population by promoting eugenic principles and were also founded in black areas such as Macon County, Alabama, site of the notorious PHS syphilis study. Du Bois also suggested approaching black churches, declaring them open to "intelligent propaganda of any sort," and added that her organization and "other agencies ought to get their speakers before church congregations and their arguments in the Negro newspapers."

Sanger took Du Bois's advice, writing, "The most successful educational approach to the Negro is through a religious appeal. . . . We do not want the word to get out that we want to exterminate the Negro population, and the minister is the man who can straighten out that idea if it occurs to any of their more rebellious members." She recruited the support of such luminaries as Adam Clayton Powell, Jr., of the Abyssinian Baptist Church and, later, the Rev. Martin Luther King, Jr. Sanger also wanted a black doctor and social worker to staff the clinic in order to gain black patients' trust. She assured the doubtful BCFA that the black physician's authority would be limited and he, like the clinic board members, would be chosen for tractability. "His work, in my opinion, should be entirely with the Negro profession and the nurses, hospital, social workers, as well as the County's white doctors. His success will depend upon his personality and his training by us." When the black Harlem clinic personnel eventually protested their lack of autonomy, the BCFA withdrew support and the clinic closed. But Sanger's experiment of addressing black social ills with the application of negative eugenics via black birth-control clinics was so successful that it persists today.

Sanger left another important legacy: She supported the development of the birth-control pill. Waves of social and political transformation roiled the 1960s and 1970s, but some of the most lasting revolutions were triggered by a single medical event: the development of the Pill. It placed cheap, easy contraception within every woman's grasp for the first time, with an ideal "laboratory" rate of 98 percent effectiveness. The women's movement was galvanized by the sudden ability to reliably uncouple sex from procreation. So was the sexual revolution.

The birth-control pill was developed during an era in which abortion was still illegal, but laws prohibiting contraceptive use also remained in effect until the 1960s and the distribution of information about contraception was not legalized until 1971. Legal spermicidal creams and jellies were expensive, hard to obtain, and unreliable. So were the back-alley abortions from which thousands of women died horribly.

The Pill was made available to poor black women free or cheaply from government-sponsored Planned Parenthood clinics in central urban areas, facilities that were the direct progeny of Sanger's Negro Project clinics. Clinics had many other contraceptive technologies in their arsenals, including condoms and diaphragms, "barrier" methods that physically blocked access of semen to the uterine neck, backed up by spermicidal jellies and creams. Clinics also fitted more African American women than white women with intrauterine devices, or IUDs.

But a history of forcible sterilization fed suspicions that the federally financed birth-control clinics in their neighborhoods were attempts to discover the best way to limit or even to erase the black presence in America.[25] Florida NAACP director Marvin Davies argued that blacks needed to produce as many babies as possible until blacks constituted 30 to 35 percent of Americans. In 1962, the National Urban League rescinded its support of contraception, and so did many local NAACP chapters.[26] Twenty-eight percent of the blacks surveyed in the late 1960s agreed that "encouraging blacks to use birth control is comparable to trying to eliminate this group from society."[27] These genocidal fears were dismissed as paranoia, but prominent white physicians had long advocated a reduction in black births as a means of pinching off the race. In 1903, for example, politically influential physician Charles S. Bacon, M.D. advocated that "the Black Belt will be defined by the government as a negro reservation similar to Indian reservations . . . the plan that has worked so well in its treatment of the Indian question until it has practically eliminated the question with the race."[28]

The 1967 Black Power Conference in Newark, New Jersey, passed a resolution that equated birth control with "black genocide," and that year, a crowd of blacks chanted "Genocide!" as they burned down a Cleveland, Ohio, contraceptive clinic.

Those who cried "genocide" found support in a United Nations resolution. On December 9, 1948, in reaction to the Nazi-engineered European Holocaust, the United Nations Convention on the Prevention and Punishment of the Crime of Genocide unanimously passed a genocide provision proscribing any attempt to destroy a racial or religious group by killing or harming its members. Resolution 260 (III) A of the United Nations General Assembly of 1948 states in part:

> Genocide means any of the following acts committed with intent to destroy, in whole or in part, a national, ethnical, racial or religious group, as such: . . . (a) Killing members of the group; (b) *Causing serious bodily or mental harm to members of the group* [emphasis added]; (c) Deliberately inflicting on the group conditions of life calculated to bring about its physical destruction in whole or in part . . .

The document also prohibited "(d) *Imposing measures intended to prevent births within the group*" [emphasis added], and "(e) Forcibly transferring children of the group to another group."[29]

Many blacks argue that the birth-control movement per se constitutes genocide under Article D because its negative eugenic stance has consistently targeted blacks. By 1972, the *American Journal of Public Health* verified that the lode of genocidal fears had widened. Forty percent of surveyed blacks now believed birth-control clinics were a ploy to eradicate blacks and these respondents expressed a deep distrust of sterilization programs, abortion clinics, and any birth-control programs run by whites.

However, a strong gender divide prevailed: Men were much more likely to denounce birth control as genocide than women, especially young, less well educated, poor, and northern men. In contrast, most black women embraced birth control and more women than men countenanced abortion. In 1970, social activist Donald Bogue found that 80 percent of the black women he surveyed in Chicago approved of birth control and 75 percent were using it.[30] Unlike Fannie Lou Hamer, many black women of the post-Pill generation had career options, thanks to the racial integration of schools and workplaces. Women were eager to leave unskilled labor behind and to enter the professional sphere, so they wished to delay the responsibilities of motherhood until they were ready.[31]

But many black women who desired and used birth control did so despite a strong distrust of the whites who distributed contraception in their communities. In 1972, black social worker Urelia Brown voiced this ambiguity: "Negroes don't want children they can't take care of, but we are afraid to trust you when your offered help has so often turned out to be exploitation."[32] Black Chicago activist Lonny Myers confessed her discomfort with the fact that some birth-control funding came from those "racists" who simply "wished to decrease the number of blacks in the city," but she noted that "any cause has strange bedfellows." Blacks also drew a distinction between physician-controlled methods and those they could control themselves: 87 percent of surveyed blacks said they approved of public contraceptive clinics, while 47 percent rejected sterilization.

Considering these social complexities, is the term *genocide* an accurate description of the birth-control initiatives directed at African Americans? The proliferation of birth-control clinics that were clearly aimed at an African American population falls neatly within the U.N. definitions—they were intended to selectively reduce births within the group. Also, these clinics were numerous and well funded at a time when health advocates failed to address more pressing African American health issues, such as abysmal nutrition, poor control of infectious disease, high infant mortality, low life expectancy, poor quality health care, scarce mental health care, and even a lack of access to hospitals and physicians. This medical myopia cripples any argument that birth-control clinics were erected with the health of African Americans in mind.

But although the proliferation of birth-control clinics was unethical, the general rise of reproductive clinics in black neighborhoods did not constitute genocide because, whatever the intent of the whites who introduced them, such measures were widely embraced by black women. They welcomed contraceptive choice, however warily they eyed those who offered it.

But, as we will soon see, some contraceptive initiatives did richly earn the "genocide" label.

After the first giddy honeymoon, women and their doctors realized that the Pill's high levels of hormones were harmful. It was dangerous for women who smoked and it inflated hypertension and stroke risks—serious flaws for African Americans, who are especially vulnerable to both conditions. Moreover, forgotten and late pills lowered the contraceptive's real-world effectiveness rate to only 70–80 percent. The same vulnerability haunted most other popular birth-control methods, except one: the intrauterine device, or IUD, a favorite with the birth-control clinics that served inner-city women. The IUD had many forms but was essentially a small, thin, and oddly shaped wire coil that a doctor inserted into the uterus, where it prevented pregnancy until the physician removed it.

The IUD proved disastrous for African Americans. Initially, researchers were not sure how it worked, but after several years, they speculated that it continually irritated the uterine lining, creating an inhospitable environment that prevented the implantation of a fertilized egg. This discovery enraged many black women, because it seemed like murdering an unborn child. Also, black women are particularly vulnerable to uterine conditions such as fibroids, endometriosis, and cancer, making constant irritation of the uterus seem ill-advised. Finally, the IUD was unmasked as a killer: It became associated with deadly infections that hampered or destroyed users' fertility. Later, scientists determined that the braided string descending from the wire of the Dalkon Shield IUD provided a breeding ground for dangerous bacteria. Most IUDs were taken off the market by the 1980s. Because Dalkon Shields were primarily dispensed in inner-city clinics, some activists charged that black women had been targeted to test a form of birth control known to cause sterility.[33] However, this is unlikely: Scientists clearly hoped that the devices would work well, not fail.

But researchers did introduce racial bias by overwhelmingly apportioning the *potential* health risks of experimental birth-control technologies to women of color, including black American women. The Pill, Nor-plant, and the Depo-Provera shot were first tested in Mexico, Africa, Brazil, Puerto Rico, and India. Once approved, they were administered to large numbers of girls and women in U.S. venues that are disproportionately and, usually, overwhelmingly African American and Hispanic. These include urban Planned Parenthood clinics, school-based clinics, and urban health clinics that serve Medicaid patients. Many serious effects emerge for the first time during this postapproval stage, when very large numbers of women begin taking a drug. Thus, the immediately postapproval use of contraceptive methods in large numbers of closely monitored poor women of color constituted a final testing arm, so that they were unwittingly participating in a research study. At this stage, serious health complications emerged with methods such as the IUD, Nor-plant, and the shot before they ever gained popularity with middle- or upper-class white women who are cared for by private physicians. In patterns too consistent to be accidental, reproductive drug testing makes poor women of color, at home and abroad, bear the brunt of any health risks that emerge.

The "Mississippi Appendectomy"

The Pill may have been flawed and the IUD deadly, but these methods were at least quasi-voluntary and their effects were usually temporary. The most damaging threat to African American reproductive freedom has been invasive and permanent: compulsory surgical sterilization. When the infamous German eugenic sterilization initiative began in January 1934, seventeen U.S. states were already performing sterilizations routinely, and that year, between two thousand and four thousand Americans were sterilized. Indiana passed legislation requiring the sterilization of the mentally unfit in 1907. By 1911, six states had passed laws providing for compulsory sterilization of the "mentally unfit." In 1935, twenty-seven states had such laws for the feebleminded, those on welfare, or those with genetic defects. Forced sterilization was encouraged by the infamous 1927 *Buck v. Bell* decision, wherein Justice Oliver Wendell Holmes ordered the sterilization of the allegedly imbecilic poor white girl Carrie Buck, intoning, "Three generations of imbeciles are enough."[34] By the 1930s, compulsory sterilization had become a global enterprise, and by 1941, sterilization had been forced upon 70,000 to 100,000 Americans, 9,931 of them in California alone.[35]

African Americans have always been staggeringly overrepresented in the ranks of the sterilized. When the North Carolina Eugenic Commission sterilized 8,000 mentally retarded persons throughout the 1930s, 5,000 were black.[36] By 1983, when blacks constituted only 12 percent of the population, 43 percent of the women sterilized in federally funded family planning programs were African Americans.[37]

This has been achieved under the auspices of a government fed by the myth of the lazy, hyperfertile welfare mother. Say "welfare mother" and most people think of an unemployed black woman, yet most women on welfare are not black. A 1990 survey revealed that 78 percent of whites think blacks prefer welfare to employment. But most black women are employed full-time and hold at least one job, and women on welfare are likely to be employed part-time at low-wage jobs with few if any benefits. However, a black woman *is* more likely to receive AFDC (Aid to Dependent Children, the form of public assistance given to people with minor children) than is a white woman. Black women constitute 6 percent of the population but represent one-third of those on AFDC. And in some poor urban areas such as Baltimore, which is 86 percent black, the majority of people on welfare are also black.

Forced sterilization and welfare have been linked for nearly half a century. Mississippi state legislator David H. Glass instituted a bold experiment when he sought legal means to force sterilization upon welfare mothers in 1958. By 1960, his "act to discourage immorality of unmarried females by providing for sterilization of the unwed mothers" passed in the House by a vote of seventy-two to thirty-seven but died in the Senate as the black activist Student Nonviolent Coordinating Committee (SNCC) protested and distributed a pamphlet entitled "Genocide in Mississippi."[38]

But most sterilizations of poor black women have been performed outside the law and in violation of medical mores. In June 1973, the abuse of two young sisters in Montgomery, Alabama, exposed the decades of stolen African American fertility. Twelve-year-old Mary Alice Relf and her sister Minnie, fourteen, lived on relief with their parents, who had left their meager living as field hands in an unsuccessful search for work in the city. A Montgomery Community Action Agency nurse took the girls to the hospital for a federally funded contraceptive shot and obtained the "X" of each illiterate parent on the consent form. But their parents later learned that the girls had been surgically sterilized, and they asked Atlanta's Southern Poverty Law Center for help. When SPLC filed a class-action lawsuit to end the use of federal funds for involuntary sterilization, its lawyers discovered that 100,000 to 150,000 women had been sterilized using federal funds and that half these women were black.[39] Today, one-third of all adult Mississippi women and 57 percent of all Mississippi women sixty-five and older say they have undergone a hysterectomy.

Sometimes the physician removed the woman's uterus on some pretext after coercing or tricking her into assent for unnecessary sterilization. The women were also sterilized while unconscious, as Fannie Lou Hamer was. In the South, rendering black women infertile without their knowledge during other surgery was so common that the procedure was called a "Mississippi appendectomy."

Involuntary hysterectomies were also commonly practiced in the North. A 1973 study by Bernard Rosenfeld of Los Angeles County Hospital discovered that "doctors . . . are cavalierly subjecting women, most of them poor and black, to surgical sterilization without explaining either the potential hazards or alternate methods of birth control. In most major teaching hospitals of New York it was the unwritten policy to do elective hysterectomies on poor black and Puerto Rican women with minimal indications to train residents."[40] In 1972, medical students at Boston City Hospital (BCH) protested the policy of performing unnecessary hysterectomies on black women in order to allow residents to practice. The students also complained that experimental procedures, the coercion of patient signatures, and falsifying medical records were common practices among black patients.[41] So did students at Columbia University.[42] The chairman of the BCH OB-GYN program did not deny the charges, but blamed "one bad apple."[43]

Across the nation, black women who trusted obstetricians to deliver their children were being surreptitiously sterilized, and this revelation poisoned relationships between them and their doctors. To accomplish the sterilizations, practitioners lied to patients, forged consent forms, or falsified medical records to reflect an "appendectomy" or "gallbladder removal," so it is now impossible to know the exact number of African American women who were sterilized without their knowledge. Nor is there any record of how many such hysterectomies, if any, were medically justified. Some women, like Fannie Lou Hamer, were never told by their doctors that they had been sterilized, and others never found out. One of the few methodical surveys conducted revealed that at least 60 percent of the black women in Hamer's native Sunflower County (Mississippi) unwittingly suffered postpartum hysterectomies.

By 1980, sterilization had become the most common form of birth control, and it still is, edging out condom use by 1 percent.[44] But African American women remain far more likely than whites to undergo a hysterectomy, although researchers have known for over a decade that they are at higher risk of the procedure's complications and are more likely to die from the surgery.[45] According to the National Center for Health Statistics (NCHS), 41 percent of black women who use contraception were sterilized, compared with only 27 percent of white women.[46]

Within a century, reproductive coercion had taken a 180-degree turn for black women. During slavery, black women had been forced to procreate, but now they were being forced into sterility. The consistent factor was white control.[47]

Women were also forced into sterility by governmental welfare programs, upon which unskilled black women workers relied to supplement their meager wages. While a social worker in upstate New York during the 1980s, I learned from old case files that during the 1960s and 1970s, social workers conducted frequent late-night raids on the homes of aid recipients. If a man was discovered, the family's aid could be cut off unless the woman agreed to sterilization, guaranteeing there would be no additional children for the state to support.

Black women are still more likely than white women to be pressured or misled into sterilization, which tripled between 1970 and 1980, in part because hysterectomies are offered as the only curative option for ailments that can be treated more conservatively, such as fibroids and endometriosis.[48]

By 1978, doctors also began administering the drug Depo-Provera— but only in research studies and almost exclusively to poor women of color.[49] Depo-Provera is the Upjohn Company's brand name for medroxyprogesterone acetate, which is also called DMPA. In 1978, the drug had just been FDA-approved for use as a cancer therapy. In 1973, after the government discovered that beagles on which the drug had been tested developed breast cancer, it had refused to fund further testing of the drug as a contraceptive. Cancer medications carry significant risks, which are acceptable when one is fighting a deadly illness but not when a healthy woman is simply trying to avoid pregnancy. However, licensed physicians may administer legal medications for any use they deem appropriate, and American doctors found it appropriate to administer Depo-Provera as an experimental contraceptive to healthy Native American and black patients. In 1978, the FDA criticized an Emory University study of Depo-Provera as having needlessly imperiled the lives of 4,700 women, all black, and in 1992 an FDA board warned, "Never has a drug whose target population is entirely healthy people been shown to be so pervasively carcinogenic in animals as has Depo-Provera."[50]

Listening to Norplant

Depo-Provera seemed discredited as a contraceptive, but in December 1990, the Food and Drug Administration approved another physician-controlled contraceptive, levonorgestrel (the Norplant Contraceptive System) for use as a long-term contraceptive. Norplant consists of six small rods that a physician surgically implants into a woman's upper arm, using special tools and a local anesthetic. The rods slowly dispense the contraceptive progestin levonorgestrel, a form of the female hormone progesterone, for five years, after which the surgeon replaces the rods.

Norplant suppresses ovulation, thickens the cervical mucus to bar the entry of sperm, prevents the development of a hospitable uterine environment, and may also discourage ovulation by suppressing the hormone lutenin. It is extraordinarily efficient, with an annual failure rate of only 0.3–0.6 percent. With perfect condom use, one out of every fifty women will become pregnant each year, and so will one out of every one hundred women who use the Pill assiduously, but only one out of every five hundred women using Norplant will become pregnant.

A 1995 *Journal of the American Medical Association* article attributed Norplant's effectiveness to the fact that it is controlled by the doctor, citing "the steady serum levels of levonorgestrel achieved and the fact that *user compliance is necessarily 100% as long as the capsules are in place* [emphasis added]."

Norplant was developed by the Population Council, a New York foundation that researches and tests contraceptives on poor women of color abroad. It has subsequently been used by more than a million U.S. women, nearly all poor: Planned Parenthood notes that 90 percent of Norplant implantations are paid through Medicaid in forty-three states. A higher proportion of African American women than white women receive these implants, chiefly in public and low-income clinics.[51] Why? Frederick Osborn, a Population Council founder, wrote, "Birth control and abortion are turning out to be major eugenic steps. But if they had been advanced for eugenic reasons . . . [that] would have retarded or stopped their acceptance."

From the first, Norplant was selectively marketed not only to poor black women but also to thousands of young black girls. The fifty thousand Norplant kits implanted in 1991–1992 included some for black teenagers between thirteen to nineteen years old in the overwhelmingly African American Baltimore public high schools. This was justified by pointing to teenage pregnancy rates. But this "solution" to the teenage pregnancy problem was based on racist mythology rather than fact. In 1992, 73 percent of fifteen-year-old girls and 50 percent of seventeen-year old girls were virgins and more white teenaged girls than black girls became pregnant. Although epidemiologists did not immediately recognize it, the American teenage pregnancy rate had already begun falling and the pregnancy rate of black girls displayed, and continues to display, the *sharpest decline of any ethnic group.*[52]

However, Baltimore is atypical in that it is mostly black and has a teen pregnancy rate that was three times the national average, and 10 percent of its girls aged fifteen to seventeen are already mothers. These demographics made the city a useful setting for a national experiment with a racial agenda. The Laurence G. Paquin Middle School clinic became the first site for Norplant implantation; 345 of its 350 girls were black. Thus policy makers focused upon the fertility of black girls, and Norplant was deployed via school-based health clinics, the first one hundred of which opened at black or minority schools.[53]

The Population Council has argued that the contraceptive's safety has been proven by fifteen years of data from 55,000 women in 170 clinical trials.[54] But in 1992, Norplant had never been tested in such young girls; researchers were monitoring their health and reactions for the Population Council. In other words, Norplant implantation in these girls

constituted a large-scale national experiment, and this research component placed pressure upon the school's clinic staff to achieve as near a 100
percent participation rate as possible.[55] They, in turn, pressured all the
girls to undergo implantation, typically citing confidentiality to bypass
their parents.[56] As one aggrieved African American parent put it, "My
daughter can be implanted with Norplant or have an abortion without
my input or knowledge via the school-based clinic, but my suburban co-
workers field calls from [school] nurses who must get their permission
to give their daughters an aspirin."[57]

It is not surprising that the conservative *National Review* praised the
Baltimore experiment, declaring, "better a prophylactic than an abor-
tion," as if these were the only two options for black girls. But so did the
New York Times and the *Philadelphia Inquirer*. The latter suggested in an
infamous December 12, 1990, editorial that black women be paid to have
Norplant implanted in order to "reduce the underclass."

Can Contraception Reduce the Underclass?

Two stories from yesterday's newspaper:
- The U.S. Food and Drug Administration approves a contraceptive that can keep a woman from getting pregnant for five
  years.
- A research organization reports that nearly half the nation's
  children are living in poverty—and that the younger the child,
  the more likely he or she is to be living with a single mother
  on welfare. "Growing numbers of them will not succeed," the
  study's author says.

As we read those two stories, we asked ourselves: Dare we
mention them in the same breath? To do so might be considered
deplorably insensitive, perhaps raising the specter of eugenics. But
it would be worse to avoid drawing the logical conclusion that
foolproof contraception could be invaluable in breaking the cycle
of inner city poverty—one of America's greatest challenges.

Without proof, the editorial went on to link teen pregnancy and
black poverty in a causal relationship, averring, "The main reason more
black children are living in poverty is that people having the most chil-

dren are the ones least capable of supporting them." More black children *are* living in poverty, but the black teen pregnancy rate is falling, not rising, so it cannot be the key impetus behind a surge in black poverty. In fact, poverty *precedes* pregnancy: The teen mothers are already poor, and children who are poor are at higher risk for precocious pregnancy.

Most media analyses did not speak so directly of Norplant as key to stemming black reproduction; instead, coded terminology such as "inner-city" "underclass," "welfare mother," and "urban poor" was widely understood to denote black women.

Young girls become pregnant because of a complex set of psychological pressures and risk factors that a pill, a shot, or an implanted capsule cannot address alone. Girls at risk tend to be poor, academically struggling, and naïve about sex and reproduction. They are usually preyed upon and even raped by older men.[58] Yet the *Inquirer* reduced the wrenching quandary of teen pregnancy to a matter of Norplant, for which it suggested "welfare mothers"—black women—receive cash bribes. In 1991, Norplant fan David Duke, the Louisiana legislator and former KKK Grand Wizard, introduced legislation whereby women on welfare who agreed to Norplant implantation would be paid one hundred dollars annually, and other lawmakers have followed suit.[59] Offering birth control to poor women is a laudable goal, but such schemes unduly entice them.[60]

The media and lawmakers' debates all stressed that Norplant is a safe contraceptive. But is it? According to a 1995 report in the *Journal of Family Practice,* 95 percent of women in a large-scale trial of Norplant had at least one side effect—80 percent suffered menstrual changes; 32 percent experienced weight gain, 24 percent headaches, 16 percent mood changes, and 15 percent acne. Norplant is contraindicated for women with diabetes, hypertension, cardiovascular disease, a tendency toward blood clots, and acute liver dysfunction, all of which African American women develop and die from at higher rates than do white women. Norplant is also contraindicated in women with breast cancer, a disease that kills African American women at rates up to 20 percent higher than white women.[61] The mood swings and weight gain resulting from Norplant pose serious risks for African American women, who already suffer from the nation's highest rates of life-threatening obesity and major depression. In fact, the contraceptive's efficiency drops from 99 percent to 92 percent in women who weigh more than 155 pounds, because its dosage is calibrated for smaller women. Beyond the viewing of a video-tape, physicians typically were not trained in Norplant insertion and re-moval, which is more often complicated by thick, overgrown keloid scars in black women.[62] "We learned some lessons from Norplant," said Dr. Trent MacKay, a reproductive health specialist at the National Institutes of Health in 2002; "as it turned out, at least in some cases, removal was a difficult process.[63]

Such effects drove one in three women implanted with Norplant to seek its removal within the first year; three years later, half had sought its removal. But women who decided that Norplant and its myriad health hazards were not for them often found themselves tethered to the con-traceptive, because although Medicaid eagerly proffered the cost of in-serting Norplant, it was less forthcoming with the five-hundred-dollar removal fee.[64] Norplant was the subject of a recall in 2000 and it was taken off the market in July 2002.[65] By the latter half of the 1990s, another physician-mediated long-term contraceptive had appeared to replace Norplant in low-cost clinics and African American schools—the Depo-Provera injection, despite its checkered past as a FDA-condemned car-cinogen.

In 1991, twenty-seven-year-old Darlene Johnson's judge made her an offer she could not refuse. The California mother of four had "spanked" her six-year-old daughter with a belt and an electric cord for smoking a cigarette, and her four-year-old got the same punishment when Johnson caught her inserting a wire hanger into an electrical outlet. Now Johnson was frightened: She had pled guilty to three counts of felony child abuse, was facing prison time, and was eight months pregnant. Enter Judge Howard Broadman, who offered her a choice of seven years' jail time or one year in jail and three years' probation—*if* she agreed to Norplant in-sertion. Johnson asked whether it was safe, and Broadman assured her that it was and could easily be removed if she experienced difficulty. Johnson agreed, but when she discovered that Norplant is contraindi-cated in women like herself who suffer from diabetes and hypertension, she changed her mind. Although the ACLU and even the district attor-ney joined her lawyers in urging Broadman to release her from the agree-ment, he would not.[66] Ultimately, Johnson was jailed for violating her probation by using drugs. This rendered her case moot, but not the window it opened into the coercive use of contraception and sterilization by the legal system.

During the fifty years since eugenics's heyday, the American courts have upheld procreation as a legally sacred civil right. In a 1942 decision, for example, the Supreme Court rejected an Oklahoma law allowing the sterilization of people who were convicted of multiple felonies involving "moral turpitude."[67] Yet black women's fertility and their right to refuse medication is treated differently. Many Darlene Johnsons exist, nearly all of them black like her. Black women who abuse drugs are ten times more likely than white women to be subjected to court-ordered long-term contraceptives or sterilization.

Forced contraceptive use in response to allegations of child abuse is punishment, not therapy, because it does not protect the existing children, as counseling would. It delays, not prevents, births for the duration of the Norplant "sentence." In any event, preventing a child's birth is a draconian method of protecting it from abuse.

In 1994, the Center for Reproductive Law and Policy in New York City accused the Medical University of South Carolina in Charleston of illegal drug testing and illegal human experimentation.[68] According to a complaint filed with the National Institutes of Health, the hospital tested poor black women—who had voluntarily gone to the hospital to seek prenatal care—for drugs without their consent, then reported those who tested positive to the police. Between 1989 and 1994, approximately forty of these women were arrested, some of whom gave birth while shackled to their hospital beds. U.S. Department of Health and Human Services civil rights director Dennis Hayashi mounted a civil rights suit because all except one of the prosecuted women were black. The sole white arrestee, as her nurse noted in her medical record, "lived with her boyfriend who is a Negro." The hospital also conducted illegal research with these women.

This selective arrest and prosecution of black women fits an insidious national pattern, according to Zita Lazzarini, J.D., M.P.H., director of the Medical Humanities, Health Law, and Ethics program at the University of Connecticut School of Medicine. Eighty-six percent of women prosecuted and jailed for drug abuse while pregnant were black. A 1993 study of women whose offspring had been exposed to cocaine prenatally found that black and Latino women were 72 percent more likely than white women to have their children removed by Child Protective Services. Public clinics in urban settings test and report more vigorously than do private clinics, and this helps drive the racial disparity. However, contrary to media representations, black and white women abuse drugs at the same rate, so one would expect equal drug-abuse rates among pregnant black and white women. And this is the case. Several studies, including a 1990 *New England Journal of Medicine* report, found no significant racial difference in drug use between pregnant black women (14.1 percent) and pregnant white women (15.4 percent), but these studies indicated that black women were ten times more likely to be reported to law-enforcement officials.[69]

The Myth of the "Crack Baby"

In September 1985, *The New England Journal of Medicine* published research by Dr. Ira Chasnoff, an associate professor of pediatrics and psychiatry at the University of Illinois, that described his findings that babies born to cocaine-using mothers remained smaller, sicker, moodier, and less social than other infants. His investigation, however, was tentative and profoundly flawed: It had no control group and he had studied the children of a mere twenty-three women, far too few to infer anything about prenatal cocaine exposure in general. Chasnoff himself was careful to note these methodological shortcomings as he urged larger, more meaningful studies of prenatal drug exposure.

Instead, his research was swallowed whole, then regurgitated in a racialized form by newspaper, magazine, and even medical accounts that focused sharply on babies harmed by the smokable form of cocaine, crack. African Americans and whites use cocaine at similar rates, but blacks are twice as likely as whites to use it in crack form. However, 80 percent of drug users are white, and in raw numbers, twice as many whites as blacks use crack cocaine. This means that white crack users should be twice as easy to find, but most peoples' image of the crack user is informed by media accounts that had focused nearly exclusively on African American users since the early 1980s. Now, Americans associate crack with blacks, and crack users' infants, dubbed "crack babies," are always portrayed as black. During eighteen years as a news and science editor at metropolitan dailies and national magazines, I have never seen a published photograph of a white crack baby.

The putative harms done to crack babies were first popularized in graphic detail in 1989 by *Washington Post* columnist Charles Krauthammer, who warned, "The inner-city crack epidemic is now giving birth to the newest horror: a bio-underclass, a generation of physically damaged cocaine babies whose biological inferiority is stamped at birth." These infants, he claimed, constitute a "race of (sub) human drones, [whose] future is closed to them from day one. Theirs will be a life of certain suffering, of probable deviance, of permanent inferiority. . . . The dead babies may be the lucky ones."[70] By "inner-city," Krauthammer meant, of course, "black." Douglas Besharov of the American Enterprise Institute, who coined the phrase "bio-underclass," did not shy from the racial label: "This is not stuff that Head Start can fix. This is permanent brain damage. Whether it is 5 percent or 15 percent of the black community, it is there."

Krauthammer's column triggered a cascade of national headlines describing these infants as born addicted to crack and neurologically damaged to the point where they constituted a permanent army of inferiority—miniature Golems who could never be human. *USA Today* bewailed "Crack Babies Born to Life of Suffering." In its piece "Crack's Toll Among Babies: A Joyless View, Even of Toys," the *New York Times* detailed how "maternity wards around the country ring with the high-pitched 'cat cries' of neurologically impaired crack babies."[71]

Americans were told that these children were so easily overstimulated that they had to be secluded in darkened hospital rooms for weeks after birth while hospitals researched the best way to treat these "boarder babies." Pediatricians such as UCLA's Judy Howard, M.D., regularly validated this perspective for journalists, as when she told *Newsweek* that the brain function that "makes us human beings, capable of discussion or reflection," had been "wiped out" in these children.

News accounts warned that as they grew larger and stronger, these children would become fearsome adversaries in the classroom and on the playground. In September 1989, two months after Krauthammer's column, a *Washington Post* article warned of "A Time Bomb in Cocaine Babies"; the next year, the *St. Louis Post-Dispatch* declared flatly, "Disaster in Making: Crack Babies Start to Grow Up." In 1992, a *San Diego Union-Tribune* headline shuddered DRUG BABIES INVADE SCHOOLS.[72]

None of this had been demonstrated by research and none of this was true. Although exposure to cocaine in the uterus can damage a fetus, a baby cannot be born addicted to cocaine, as children are sometimes born addicted to other narcotic drugs. Neither is there any difference between prenatal exposure to cocaine and to crack cocaine. Moreover, the "diagnosis" of "crack baby" is based upon a woman's positive drug test, not upon the baby's clinical picture, so it makes no distinction between mothers who smoked crack habitually and those who did so rarely. There is no such medical entity as a crack baby.

A 1991 meta-analysis—a retrospective analysis of the many research articles dealing with crack babies—in the journal *Teratology* found serious methodological flaws in this research. The studies in question lacked control groups of nonexposed babies for comparison and they failed to differentiate cocaine's effects from those caused by prenatal exposure to other drugs, including tobacco and alcohol (the latter cause much greater long-term disability than does cocaine). The studies also failed to take into account pertinent environmental factors such as poor nutrition and housing conditions and the dearth of quality prenatal care. For more than seven years, Chicago's National Association for Perinatal Addiction Research studied a group of three hundred children born exposed to crack. Researchers found that their IQ scores were the same as children who were not crack-exposed but who lived in similar environments.[73] As sociologist Ernest Drucker notes, "even cocaine use in high doses during pregnancy is not unequivocally linked to any fetal defect other than low birthweight and small size. The vast majority of infants born to drug-using mothers are as 'healthy' as other infants born in poverty."[74]

Why were such glaring research flaws ignored for so long by experts? For example, *Washington Post* columnist Krauthammer, who raised the journalistic hue and cry, is a graduate of Harvard Medical School, and I wonder that he did not consider these dramatic scientific shortcomings before suggesting that the children in question should not have been born. In 1989, the British medical journal *The Lancet* showed how papers reporting that cocaine harmed babies' behavior were more likely to be accepted for publication than those showing no harm, even when the latter described better-designed studies. In 1992, a *Journal of the American Medical Association* editorial condemned the "rush to judgment" about cocaine's long-term effects on children, calling the evidence "far too slim."[75] But the harm has been done. The imaginary crack baby epidemic remains real in the minds of most Americans, providing yet another exemplar of African American "bad mothering." In 1989, the *Los Angeles Times* wrote of how "Parents Who Can't Say 'No' Are Creating a Generation of Misery"; the *Washington Post* told us "For Pregnant Addict, Crack Comes First"; and a *New York Times* headline showcased an awkward amalgam of sympathy and cost-consciousness: CRACK'S TINIEST, COSTLIEST VICTIMS.[76] The myth of the crack baby also helped to fuel criminal prosecutions against pregnant drug abusers, three-quarters of which have been filed against women of color.[77]

Even private citizens promulgate both long- and short-term sterilization as the only solution. In 1997, a group called CRACK (Children Requiring a Caring Kommunity) papered inner-city billboards with offers of two hundred dollars in cash for cocaine-addicted men and women willing to undergo sterilization or submit to long-term physician-mediated birth control such as Norplant. The organization refuses to share current ethnic data, but figures from its unguarded beginnings reveal that 60 percent of its first 158 recipients were black or Hispanic. As of mid-January 2004, CRACK had chapters in at least sixteen cities and had paid 1,141 clients to surrender their fertility. CRACK, or Project Prevention, as it is now known, specializes in crack abuse, not the prenatal use of more dangerous drugs or alcohol, so its claims to put children's health first are specious. Its slogan suggests the depth of its disdain for addicted black women: "Don't Let a Pregnancy Ruin Your Drug Habit."

The reproductive freedom of African Americans has been assailed by discouraging the birth of "inferior" black progeny and by curtailing the fertility of black mothers. Flawed eugenic judgments continue to shadow the lives of African Americans, from the putative "crack babies" who are now stigmatized teenagers to teen girls who are judged rather than counseled and protected from male predators.

CHAPTER 9

NUCLEAR WINTER

Radiation Experiments on African Americans

*If anybody knows how to do a good job of body snatching, they will
really be serving their country.*

—DR. WILLARD LIBBY, NOBEL PRIZE LAUREATE, ON OPERATION SUNSHINE

On a dewy spring morning in 1945, Robert S. Stone, M.D., a usually
quiet, deliberate professor of radiology, burst into a neighboring office at
the government's Oak Ridge, Tennessee, nuclear facility, shouting, "Karl,
you remember that nigger truck driver that had this accident some time
ago?"

"Yes, I remember." Dr. Karl Z. Morgan, director of the Oak Ridge
Health Physics Division, was nonplussed. Why was a trucker's month-
old accident of any consequence? "Well," gushed Stone, "he was rushed
to the military hospital in Oak Ridge and he had multiple fractures. Almost all of his bones were broken, and we were surprised he was alive
when he got to the hospital; we did not expect him to be alive the next
morning. So this was an opportunity we've been waiting for. We gave
him large doses by injection of plutonium-239."[1]

No witnesses lingered to describe the accident, but on March 24,
1945, trucker Ebb Cade, of Greensboro, North Carolina, was one of four
passengers who suffered severe injuries and was taken to the Manhattan
Engineer District Hospital in Oak Ridge. Doctors said he would not live,
but medical fortune smiled on him—he rallied quickly and within days
was recovering nicely.

Then Cabe's luck ran out.

Unknown to him, the hospital physicians assigned to his care were
under contract to the U.S. Atomic Energy Commission (AEC). They
were also under the supervision of Stone, the AEC assistant health director, who had been searching for a moribund patient to inject with pluto-

nium. On April 10, without his consent, and five days before setting his broken bones, military physician Joseph Howland injected Cade with 4.7 micrograms of plutonium—forty-one times the normal lifetime exposure.[2] The man-made element plutonium is a "fiendishly toxic" radioactive substance, one that Cade's body would harbor forever: the half-life, or time it takes half a dose of plutonium to disappear, is 24,056 years. Col. Stafford Warren, director of the Manhattan Project's Medical Section, described plutonium "as the most dangerous chemical known."[3]

"They gave him a whopping dose of plutonium," recalled Morgan in 1995, when speaking to an Advisory Committee on Human Radiation Experiments (ACHRE) interviewer. Wright Langham, the chemist who devised the human experiment, justified the toxic injection by explaining to Manhattan Project physicians that "the subject was an elderly male whose age and general health was such that there is little or no possibility that the injection can have any effect on the normal course of his life." But Cade was only fifty-three and held down a grueling job hauling long trucks. Except for a cataract, he enjoyed excellent health.

Before they set Cade's broken legs, AEC doctors completed higher-priority tasks. They extracted bone chips and pulled fifteen of his teeth to measure Cade's newly elevated plutonium levels; only then, five days later, did they set his broken bones. Six months later, Cade was still in the hospital, and in a September 1945 letter, Capt. David Goldring, M.D., of Oak Ridge informed Langham that "more bone specimens and extracted teeth will be shipped to you very soon for analysis." But before he could lose more teeth or bone, Cade slipped away. One morning, the nurse opened his door, and he was gone. Morgan recalled, "They were surprised that a black man who had been expected to die got up and walked out of the hospital and disappeared." They were also disappointed: Doctors had hoped to autopsy Cade's body, because the purpose of the injection had not been to treat Cade, but to experimentally calibrate the plutonium's physiological devastation. Langham hoped to pinpoint the dosage at which a radioactive element such as plutonium causes illnesses such as leukemia. To do this, doctors injected or otherwise introduced a specific amount of a known radioactive substance into a body; then they periodically measured the amount of radioactivity that lingered in the subject's blood, tissues, bones, urine, and feces. The AEC also sought to follow up changes in the subject's health status to determine the exact health effects of different radioactive elements.

We know today, for example, that different radioactive elements have affinity for particular parts of the body. Radon gas raises the risk of lung cancer, while radium lodges in the bone, where it triggers cancer. AEC scientists sought to make similar determinations that would help them to regulate soldiers' wartime exposures, and to control the level of exposure in peacetime workers at nuclear-power plants or uranium mines. But it was difficult to follow subjects, and the scientists' own errors also sabotaged many experiments. For example, scientists in Stone's laboratory mistakenly mixed Cade's initial preexposure bone samples with samples taken after his injection, rendering future determinations impossible.

Cade returned home to Greensboro, where he died eight years later of heart disease unrelated to his injection. He is one of many involuntary radiation experiment subjects; as this chapter will demonstrate, many of these subjects, perhaps most, were African American.

Between 1944 and 1994 the AEC supported more than two thousand experimental projects utilizing radiation and human subjects. Overall, blacks were at higher risk than whites of being subjected to these harmful nontherapeutic experiments. Between April 1945, scant months before the bombing of Hiroshima, and July 1947, the scientists of the Manhattan Project followed the construction of the atomic bomb with a chilling second act: medical experimentation on hundreds of unsuspecting Americans. Pioneers of nuclear science, such as J. Robert Oppenheimer, Louis Hempelmann, and Stafford Warren, masterminded scores of radiation experiments from the headquarters they carved out of the shimmering rust-colored earth of the New Mexico desert, in Los Alamos. In one series of experiments, Manhattan Project doctors injected plutonium into between eighteen and twenty men, women, and children.[4] They acted without obtaining the consent of these people, informed or otherwise, and without therapeutic intent. The Manhattan Project scientists shrouded themselves in secrecy, referring to their subjects only in code: Cade's was HP-12; the "HP" stood for "human product." Scientists never publicly referred to the nature of the injections: the word *plutonium* was barred from their vocabularies by a December 1972 memo from Argonne National Laboratory investigator Robert E. Rowland, who reinforced a long-standing verbal taboo: "Outside of CHR we will *never* use the word *plutonium* in regard to these cases."[5] In AEC parlance, plutonium became "product" or "49," an inversion of its atomic number, 94.

Ebb Cade was the first American to be injected with massive doses of plutonium during this small 1940s pilot program under the direction of the AEC and the DOE. As in the syphilis study of Tuskegee, the victims thought their doctors were caring for them. Claims of imminent death were made in order to justify the toxic injections, but most subjects left the hospital alive, and ten lived for many years after the exposures.

Such outrages strike our post-Tuskegee world as positively diabolical. But the medical wunderkinder and politically savvy scientists who designed these experiments thought it necessary and logical to expand the boundaries of scientific medical knowledge into new radioactive frontiers.

We might never have know the details and the identities of the victims had not reporter Eileen Welsome masterfully investigated dozens of such experiments in her 1987 Pulitzer Prize–winning series for the *Albuquerque Journal* and her book *The Plutonium Files*. Through seven years of unreturned phone calls, governmental rebuffs, and derailed Freedom of Information requests, she doggedly pursued victims' identities.

In one such program, soldiers were shipped to the desert for deliberate exposure to the detonation of nuclear bombs. In another, unsuspecting patients in private and public hospitals—from Strong Memorial Hospital in Rochester, New York, to Vanderbilt University Hospital's prenatal clinic in Nashville—were injected with plutonium infused with fluorine or otherwise used as subjects in various experiments to calibrate the physical damage associated with various dosages of radioactive matter. The moribund pregnant women and their fetuses, the poor, the mentally ill, and children in institutions all risked attracting the fatal attention of doctors of the Manhattan Project. Products of this research, including exposure data, death rates and cancer incidence statistics, and even radioactive excreta and body parts, were forwarded to Los Alamos. The percentage of African American subjects in 1945 hovered around 10 percent, but lawyer E. Cooper Brown, who represented plaintiffs in radiation suits, has estimated that "60 percent were people of color, mostly African American."

One such subject, Elmer Allen, was on top of the world when his path intersected with that of government doctors wielding syringes of plutonium. He was happily married to the former Fredna Hadley and the father of two children, Elmerine and William. Allen had escaped the gravity of the preintegration South for a California life that he loved. Leaping from trains into the mild evening air, Allen sauntered home to nearby Richmond as mists rolling between the perfect cobalt skies and the waters of San Francisco Bay provided a postcard background. The halos crowning the lights of the bay imparted a dreamlike atmosphere, within which every ambition must have seemed in reach. For a black man who had grown up bound by the rigidly circumscribed racial mores of the segregated South, where hostility tainted the very air and violent constraint was never far off, the Bay Area offered intoxicating freedom, its colorful streets buzzing with genial people of every hue and nationality. Allen's job as a Pullman porter paid four hundred dollars a month—rich wages for that time—so he could afford to indulge his wife and spoil his children while dreaming of the education and opportunities they would soon enjoy.

Everything changed in an instant on September 3, 1946, when Allen fell from a train in Chicago. He fractured his left leg, a very common occupational injury for a Pullman porter, for whom bouncing from just-stopped trains to platforms was part of the job.[6] But the Pullman Company refused to accept responsibility for the accident, and Allen hobbled from the hospital to his home for a recuperation that was never to be. The Pullman Company terminated him without compensation of any kind, leaving him unemployed and unemployable, with a dwindling bank account and a painfully swollen ulcerated leg that wouldn't heal. A private physician diagnosed chronic inflammation and hemorrhage in his knee but could make no recommendations for a cure. Suddenly, the sunny foothills and swirling mists of the bay composed a mocking backdrop to Allen's growing anxieties. With a painfully halting gait, he dragged himself up and down the steep streets of San Francisco, searching for a doctor who could straighten his leg and deaden the raging pain. A year later, his knee had swollen to three times its normal size, while his bank account shrank to twenty-five dollars. Mounting medical bills and overdue rent drove him in desperation to the place he had avoided for so long—the University of California–San Francisco's (UCSF) free clinic.

There, he was diagnosed with chondrosarcoma, a cancer of the bone. On July 18, 1947, Allen's left leg was injected with plutonium-238, an even more radioactive isotope than the plutonium-239 given the other patients.

He had just become subject CAL-3.[7]

This never should have happened, because in late 1946, between the injections of Cade and Allen, the Judicial Council of the American Medical Association had set new standards for the protection of human subjects:

> In order to conform to the ethics of the American Medical Association, three requirements must be satisfied: (1) the voluntary consent of the person on whom the experiment is to be performed, (2) the danger of each experiment must be previously investigated by animal experimentation, and (3) the experiment must be performed under proper medical protection and management.[8]

Furthermore, the AEC physicians could hardly have pleaded exemption on the grounds of military or governmental expediency, because in April, just a few months before Allen was injected, the AEC had passed its own, more specific, rules governing medical experiments with humans:

> It should be susceptible to proof from official reason that prior to treatment each individual patients [sic] being of an understanding state of mind was clearly informed of the nature of the treatment and its possible effects and expressed his willingness to receive the treatment. In view of your recommendation the Commission does not request that written release be obtained in such cases but it does request that in every case at least two doctors should certify in writing (made part of the official record) to the patient's understanding state of mind to the explanation furnished him and to his willingness to accept the treatment.[9]

These dense, wordy AEC regulations also required an "expectation that it may have therapeutic effect," but after a February 1995 UCSF review of the case file, the hospital admitted that Allen's physicians had expected no therapeutic effect, so the experiment violated that rule, as well.[10] Allen's medical record indicates that he was told something of the procedure he was about to undergo, and two doctors signed a medical chart note to that effect, but the statement did not conform to the AEC's own standards because the physicians neither explained the true purpose of the injection nor sought Allen's permission. Allen's family says that the injection was described as a form of therapy, a last-ditch measure to save the leg,

Allen's daughter, Elmerine Whitfield Bell, adds, "My father was not an educated man. Even had they told my father that he was injected with plutonium, that would be like telling him that he was injected with ice cream. He would not know the difference."

Three days later, Allen's leg was amputated.

Today, Bell feels certain that her father's bone cancer was a deliberate misdiagnosis, made so that researchers could amputate and study his leg. "I don't think there is any record anyplace of anyone living more than eight years with the sort of bone cancer he is supposed to have had." Actually people with chondrosarcoma that is treated appropriately often live a normal life span, so Allen's longevity was not unusual. In Allen's medical chart, UCSF doctors had indicated that patients with this type of tumor "frequently surviv[e] many years beyond diagnosis if there is complete excision of the primary tumor."[11] This provided a compelling therapeutic reason to excise the area around the tumor and, perhaps, to amputate Allen's leg. The doctors characterized his tumor as "malignant but slow growing and late to metastasize. Prognosis therefore moderately good."[12] They were right: Allen lived until age eighty, forty-four years after his diagnosis of bone cancer. But who could not understand his daughter's distrust, which was shared by her close-knit community, after the revelation of her father's exploitation? "The first thing people did when they learned of this was express sympathy: The next question they always asked was 'Was everyone in the experiment black?' "

They were not. By most accounts, eighteen Americans were injected with plutonium. But, according to a July 1947 statement by Robert Stone, "By race there were 15 white and 5 blacks" injected.[13] Thus, in the plutonium experiment, blacks constituted 25 percent of the subjects at a time when they were approximately 10 percent of the population; this means their rate of involvement was two and a half times greater than it should have been, given what proportion of the population they constituted. However, there is no indication that blacks were specifically sought out for plutonium injections, as they were in some other experiments.

The dearest costs of Allen's experimental status were not medical, but social. Although he lived for four decades after his amputation, these were dark ones for Allen. He moved with his family to his wife's hometown of Italy, Texas, but was unable to readjust to life in the South, where his physical disability and psychological pain made it difficult to find steady work. Allen drank excessively for a while and suffered epileptic seizures; worse, he was unable to shake off the conviction that he had been abused by the San Francisco doctors and robbed unnecessarily of his leg. With uncanny accuracy, he insisted that he had been subjected to experiments related to the injection he had been given and insisted that doctors had taken his leg not to save his life but in order to study it. Allen spoke often and bitterly of these convictions, but not even his family members took his suspicions seriously enough to ask why they had arisen. Only Allen's best friend, Joe Speed, believed him. Speed told journalists flatly in 1994, "They guinea-pigged him."

When I called Elmer Allen's widow, Fredna Allen, in 1994, she was gracious but firm. "My emotions won't allow me to discuss this. But you can try talking to my daughter, Elmerine."

"My father's life was not good," Elmerine Whitfield Bell sighs from her home in Italy, where she has taught for decades at the Edison Middle Learning Center in nearby West Dallas. "You know how difficult things are for African American men, especially a man with little education. Think of it: He was lucky enough to land a job paying four hundred dollars a month, plus tips, in the 1940s. He worked there six years, but to suddenly lose a leg and his job and have to move back to the South from California, which he loved, with two small children, to be supported by his wife—just imagine . . ." Bell's voice trails off. Then, more resolutely, she continues, "Despite it all, my parents managed to send two children to college and lived middle-class lives."

But the AEC's deceit extracted a terrible price. "I remember a lot of things, like how my father would insist that the doctors had experimented on him, then amputated his leg to study it. I felt, 'You're mistaken,'" recalls Bell. "My father and I had a personality clash and I never made peace with my father. I never did understand why he was the way he was. I know now why he always insisted something was wrong with him." His family did not believe that Allen's amputation was medically necessary, either, but they saw it merely as an expression of insensitivity toward devalued African American patients, not as an experimental scheme. Moreover, it did not help Allen's credibility when the family doctor, David Williams, M.D., called him a paranoid schizophrenic:

> What I saw was a fellow who had a loss of limb and became an emotional cripple because of it. He probably had paranoid schizo-phrenia all his life. Far as doing things, I thought he was using this possible exposure as a crutch, a reason, rather than doing as well as I would have liked to have seen him do.[14]

Government scientists had also lied to Williams, denying that any plutonium injection had taken place. In 1973, government scientists at Chicago's Argonne National Laboratory's Center for Human Radiobiol-ogy (CHR) told Williams only that they were bringing Allen to the CHR and to the University of Rochester, two thousand miles away in upstate New York, for follow-up, since, as they put it, "he has this unusual malig-nant tumor and has shown such a long survival time." But the three-week journey to Chicago and Rochester, replete with flowers, limousines, a first-class private car on the Texas Chief, and a four-hundred-dollar honorarium, was not a celebratory jaunt to probe the secret of Allen's longevity. Rather, it was scientifically necessary because the scientists had to retrieve Allen's body tissues in order to inventory the lingering ra-dioactivity and to measure any resultant physical damage from the ex-periment. Argonne placed Allen in its whole-body counter to assess his skeletal radiation. Scientists cataloged his X rays and even collected and tested his urine and excreta. They found radiation-induced jaw abnor-malities and similar changes in Allen's other bones. Allen was then swept off to Rochester, where monitoring of his urine and stool found that, al-though his leg had been removed days after the injection, traces of radi-ation still lingered in his tissues.[15]

Allen died in a nursing home in 1991, just a few years after Eileen Welsome's writings publicly validated his lifelong claims of abuse. "This has really turned our lives upside down, my brother and me," says Bell. "But my mother, my mother relives this experiment every day. Every day she thinks of the fifty years she and my father were together, trying to fig-ure out why she was so naïve and couldn't pick up on the fact that this was the government's doing. My mother has been a very moral person all her life—why, we couldn't even *gossip* in her house, growing up! But now, she doesn't feel too good about herself."

More radiation experiments were to come. In some cases, blacks were only sparsely represented; in some, no evidence can be found for their participation at all; in others, they suffered at higher rates than did whites—that is, they were present at rates greater than their representa-tion in the population. In still other radiation experiments, they consti-tuted a large majority of the subjects, and some of these experiments focused specifically or exclusively upon African Americans. The pluto-nium victims were not the last blacks to be transfigured by radiation.[16] But neither were they the first.

The Cleansing Light of Science

The first recorded black victims of radiation experiments lived around the turn of the century, long before the dropping of the atomic bomb. Near the end of 1895, German physicist Wilhelm Conrad Roentgen dis-covered a magical light. He found that passing electricity through special gases at low pressure generated electromagnetic radiation with strange and powerful properties. The rays imparted fluorescence and enabled him to make images that rendered solid objects transparent. Alive to the rays' potential for seeing inside previously opaque objects but flum-moxed by their mysterious nature, Roentgen resorted to calling them "X rays." Doctors found with delight that the X rays could reveal all manner of skin blemishes, cancers, and even previously hidden internal prob-lems. During the same period, physicians successfully experimented with radium for the purpose of healing. Radiation enjoyed a beneficent med-ical image and scientists sought to seduce African Americans as well as whites with its power to heal and to purify. Any doctor who wished to embrace the newest fad in medicine could advertise his radium or X-ray treatments, and most of the doctors who did so treated patients in pri-vate clinics, rather recklessly by our standards. They were initially un-aware of and later insufficiently concerned by the dangers of repeatedly bombarding patients with high radiation doses. Patients were even given bits of radium in glass tubes to carry about with them so that they could treat their own skin blemishes or superficial cancers.

Physicians soon ventured beyond medical therapy to explore profitable cosmetic uses, and as early as 1900, doctors touted radiation to blacks as an escape into whiteness. A long-winded headline in the January 10, 1904, *New York American* announced, BURNING OUT BIRTH-MARKS, BLEMISHES OF THE SKIN AND EVEN TURNING A NEGRO WHITE WITH THE MAGIC RAYS OF RADIUM, THE NEW MYSTERY OF SCIENCE![17] The *New York Telegraph* predicted, "All Coons to Look White: College Professors Have Scheme to Solve Race Problem," while the *Boston Globe* biblically mused, " 'Can the Ethiopian Change His Skin or the Leopard His Spots': Radium Light Turns Negro's Skin White."[18] All invoked the cutting-edge technology of "scientific light" to efface the dark disability of racial difference, and by every account, the black experimental subjects were not only willing but eager. However, the news accounts were sketchy and error-ridden and no accounts seem to have been recorded in scientific journals, nor were any follow-up studies performed to track injuries.

In 1904, an unnamed black man entered the Philadelphia offices of Dr. Thomas E. Eldridge, asking to have a facial birthmark removed. The doctor told reporters that he successfully used a piece of radium in concert with X rays to bleach the blemish. Then inspiration struck: Why not continue bleaching the man's skin until he achieved whiteness? After a month of daily treatments, Eldridge claimed that half the man's skin was whitened and predicted he would be completely white within a month.

Many newspapers joined the *Boston Globe* in citing Jeremiah 13:23— "Can the Ethiopian change his skin or the leopard his spots?" This was a favored biblical passage of scientific racists, who embraced it as a metaphor for the immutability of racial characteristics. Reporters wondered at the scientists' achievement even as they mocked the racial ambitions of the black subjects:

> Since the news of the marvelous operation on his colored patient
> has become public, Dr. Eldridge has been besieged by negroes who
> detest their natural color and wish to be changed to white men.
> Dusky mamas also have been imploring the doctor all day long
> to make their pickaninnies "jes' like white chillun."[19]

Doctors understood that such irradiation was dangerous. Eldridge himself said, ". . . the danger of burning the skin of the patient being very great unless precautions are taken and the rays allowed for only a short time to strike the spot to be teated*[sic]*." A January 10, 1904, news story in the *North American* (Philadelphia) cataloged the dangers of X-ray bleaching. Its headline read X-RAYS DON'T TURN A NEGRO WHITE, SAYS PROFESSOR PANCOAST: IT IS TOO DANGEROUS: SKIN BURNS AND ATTEMPT TO CHANGE COLOR WOULD BE LONG AND PAINFUL. University of Pennsylvania radiologist Dr. Henry K. Pancoast also questioned its durability. "[When] the skin would regenerate white, would it remain white?" In 1908, the *New York Times* article "White Negro in Paris" reported on a black expatriate who, once ensconced in the City of Lights, "arrived at the conclusion that the only beautiful people were those with white skins." The man went to Philadelphia for radium treatment and, once "white enough," he returned to Paris.

> . . . the man, however, had not reckoned with Nature. He began to feel very uncomfortable. And then his skin began to change colors. In some places it is gray and in others the gray is darkening into black. So that, at the present moment, the negro is full of contrition for having tried to desert his race.

Most journalists assumed that subjects were actuated by a belief that blackness was inferior, not by practical concerns such as escaping race prejudice. When the medical costs in burns and illness were invoked, these consequences were presented not as irresponsibility on the part of the physician but as punished hubris. The new technology afforded scientific observers an opportunity to reaffirm the same belief belabored by chapter 3's accounts of "white negroes" in the circus: Race is more than skin deep, and a "white negro" is still a Negro.

Doctors had probably anticipated a brisk business in bleaching the skins of blacks with radiation, but the publication of its side effects squelched blacks' interest. Physicians were more successful with non-Anglo-Saxon European immigrants, to whom they offered radiation as the cure for another badge of ethnic inferiority—dark and coarse excess hair. Physicians charged enormous fees when they opened X-ray hair-removal clinics with names such as "Hirsutic Laboratories" in the 1920s.

Advertisements in lower-middle-class immigrant neighborhoods reassured the ambitious that "Freedom from Unwanted Hair Opens the Gates to Social Enjoyment That Are Forever Closed to Those So Afflicted." Historian Rebecca Herzig has described how for Mediterranean and Eastern European women, radiation was held out as a technology that would ease their entrée into the impeccably "white" identity they desired by removing telltale dark hair from their upper lips, chins, and lower arms. But instead of hairless white skin, they developed radiation burns, cancers, and horrible disfigurement before suffering painful deaths. The resulting lawsuits spawned legal bans that eventually closed the clinics, and by 1970, researchers calculated that 35 percent of all women's cancers were traceable to X-ray hair removal.[20]

These blacks and ethnic women suffered burns, cancers, discoloration, tissue loss, anemia, severe sores, scarring, and hair loss. Such conditions were recognized as radiation side effects that also struck researchers who worked with X rays or unshielded tubes of radioactive substances. Researcher Clarence Madison Dally, who manipulated X rays in Thomas Edison's laboratory, was the first U.S. researcher to die from radiation-induced cancer, in 1904. By 1911, more than fifty cases of X-ray-induced cancer had been reported. The hands of Nobel laureate Marie Curie, the discoverer of radium, were chronically covered with burns well before her death of radiation-induced leukemia in 1934. That year, black radiologist Rudolph Fisher, M.D., a Columbia University researcher and one of the luminaries of the Harlem Renaissance (he wrote *The Conjure-Man Dies*, the first mystery novel published by an African American), also died of intestinal cancer caused by his work. By 1949, at least sixty-five American scientists had perished as a result of their work with X rays; no one recorded how many technicians, janitors, and support staff died.[21]

But some radiation workers served as canaries in the coal mine. After World War II, the disappointing side effects in bleached Negroes and the ugly deaths of the young white "radium girls"—hired in 1913 by factories such as the Radium Luminous Material Company to paint the dials of luminous watches with radium-226 and the radium isotope mesothorium—joined the carnage in the wake of the Hiroshima and Nagasaki bombings and the X-ray epilation patrons to transform the public's image of X rays and radium. Once beneficial and therapeutic, radioáctivity was now seen as a treacherously malevolent force. American distrust of the scientists who wielded radiation for deadly but profitable schemes was projected onto a plethora of popular science-fiction films that portrayed radiation as the scientific catalyst of horrendous aberrations of nature. Scientists were characterized as willing to exploit radiation's unnatural power for twisted curiosity, wealth, or personal glory. Even the popular meaning of the once-neutral word *mutation* to denote a radiation-triggered change in tissue or genetics became malevolent. The white light of science had been sullied by bloody scandal, and when the government decided to test radiation on Americans after 1944, it chose to do so secretly.

"A Little of the Buchenwald Touch"

The United States also chose to seek Nazi expertise. In 1945, the U.S. State Department, army intelligence, and the OSS, the immediate forerunner of the CIA, recruited former Third Reich scientists, granting them immunity, jobs, and new identities in a resettlement program for Nazi scientists. It was named Operation Paperclip, for the mode of identifying potential recruits—a simple paper clip placed on each of their dossiers. In exchange, the State Department asked that the scientists resume their old habits—working on secret nonconsensual research projects, many of which exploited patients—but this time throughout the United States. Many scientists, from rocket pioneer Dr. Wernher von Braun to former Gestapo chief Klaus Barbie, the "Butcher of Lyon," entered the country under the aegis of Operation Paperclip.

Between 1951 and 1956, for example, German physiologist and former Nazi Herbert Gerstner supervised a total body irradiation (TBI) project of 263 cancer patients, at M. D. Anderson Hospital for Cancer Research in Houston, courtesy of Operation Paperclip.[22] Gerstner irradiated the entire bodies of 30 of the hospital's 263 patients, whose ethnicities were not specified. The irradiation destroyed their bone marrow, resulting in fatal anemia and other complications. The patients died rapidly, and the hospital abandoned the experimental approach.

In a 1950 memo to senior AEC staff, Dr. Joseph Hamilton warned that radioactive experimentation on the unwitting was unethical and illegal, a flouting of the recently adopted Nuremberg Code of 1947. Among other tenets, the code required that all human subjects be fully informed of experiments conducted on them, that animal studies be done first, and that no tests be conducted that might harm human subjects. Hamilton warned that the public would be outraged to find American scientists engaged in the very research for which American military lawyers and physicians had condemned the Nazis, "as admittedly this would have a little of the Buchenwald touch."[23]

Via Operation Paperclip, the U.S. government supplied American hospitals and clinics with seven hundred Nazi scientists.[24] Because the scientists conducted so many disparate studies, all in secret, no racial breakdown of the Operation Paperclip subjects is possible.

By 1947, AEC's Col. E. E. Kirkpatrick expanded the radiation programs when he secretly ordered radioactive injections be given unsuspecting patients and institution inmates throughout America.[25] But why, when the dangers of radiation were already widely known? "My father [Elmer Allen] was injected with plutonium a year and eleven months *after* the bombing of Hiroshima and Nagasaki. Why?" demands Elmerine Whitfield Bell. "You had people exposed to high doses of radiation there. Why study here?"

Scientists did learn much from wartime injuries, but many expressed a need for a more precise quantitative understanding, which would allow researchers and military forces to avoid harm while working with radiation.

However, the strongest clamor for the studies came from the military: Government scientists insisted that a detailed knowledge of radiation's dangers was necessary in order to protect soldiers who were thought to face radiation exposure from the Soviets. Robert Stone, for example, cited an underwater atomic detonation as part of Operation Crossroads in 1947, when radiologists could not reach a consensus about the exact radiation doses that would produce illness in the exposed humans. Experimentation was necessary to settle these questions once and for all, and animal experiments were thought inadequate.

As Lawrence Altman's fascinating book *Who Goes First? The Story of Self-Experimentation in Medicine* documents, Western physicians have adhered to a long and noble tradition of following animal studies with limited self-experimentation by researchers. This tradition may not always have been prudent, but by testing substances or procedures on themselves before experimenting with appreciable numbers of human subjects, doctors symbolically conveyed their belief that the measures were not inordinately harmful and also signaled a researcher's willingness to share the risks as well as the glory of discovery. But in the 1940s, radiation researchers declined to experiment on themselves.[26] Wright Langham observed, "We considered doing such experiments at one time, but plutonium is considered to be sufficiently potentially dangerous to discourage our doing absorption experiments upon ourselves."[27] These doctors needed human subjects, and they turned to the clinic out of habit.

But by what ethical rules were the government scientists bound when exposing unwitting patients to dangerous radiation? Robert Stone, the same doctor who crowed about injecting the "nigger truck driver," was a passionate advocate of human experiments and he offered an elegantly written set of ethical guidelines. He suggested that using only the moribund, prisoners serving life sentences, military personnel, and terminally ill cancer patients was morally acceptable.[28] So, in hospitals, schools, and other institutions across the nation, doctors administered exposures to plutonium, X rays, gamma rays, and radium that far exceeded established tolerance limits. Each time, they claimed to be using subjects in Stone's categories. But as we have seen, Stone and others stretched his "morally acceptable" categories, casting Cade, Allen, and other hardy but uninformed subjects as frail or terminally ill for the sake of convenience.

In June 1947, the Medical Board of Review, a blue-ribbon panel of Manhattan Project scientists and university faculty, convened to examine AEC research. It emerged three days later with an official AEC policy that offered extraordinary protections and was given the blessing of the U.S. Advisory Committee on Biology and Medicine. No substance known to be or suspected of being poisonous or harmful could be utilized in research on human subjects unless each one of the following conditions were met:

(A) that a reasonable hope exists that the administration of such a substance will improve the condition of the patient, (B) that the patient gives his complete and informed consent in writing, and (C) that the responsible next of kin give in writing a similarly complete and informed consent, revocable at any time during the course of treatment.

This document represented a quiet revolution in standards. It is the first occurrence of the term *informed consent* in ethical policy, which meant it was now not enough to gain the assent of radiation subjects; they also had to understand clearly what they were being exposed to and whether this application constituted treatment, research, or both. However, there is even more in the AEC policy: The requirement that the next of kin also give consent was truly progressive. It was important because many of the subjects were too desperate, too poorly educated, or too poorly informed to appreciate what their doctors proposed to do to them. Abusive experiments of the postwar era are often excused on the grounds that critics are wielding present-day standards to judge decades-old research, but this 1947 policy demonstrates that such abusive experiments were as morally unacceptable in their time as they are in ours.

Unfortunately, the sweeping protections of the AEC policy were not widely distributed and scientists routinely flouted their own policy. Stone and his colleagues cited military expediency as the justification for involuntary medical experimentation. But with the exception of AEC physician Shields Warren, they did not seem to realize that they were invoking the same justification that Nazi doctors used in conscripting prisoners and concentration-camp victims for horrific experimental exposures.[29] Shields Warren, however, observed in 1950, "It's not long since we got through trying Germans for doing exactly the same thing."[30] In October 1952, the United States Air Force Military Personnel Center (AFMPC) decided to adopt the ten rules of the Nuremberg Code on the advice of Pentagon personnel lawyer Stephen S. Jackson.

In 1953, Secretary of Defense Charles Wilson issued a memo that established the Nuremberg Code as Defense Department (DOD) policy. Wilson now required experimental subjects to sign an informed-consent statement setting out the "the nature, duration, and purpose of the experiment; the method and means by which it is to be conducted; all inconveniences and hazards reasonably to be expected; and effects upon his health or person which may possibly come from his participation in the experiment."

But despite the adoption of the Nuremberg Code, scientists persisted in approximately fifty experimental radiation abuses within hospital corridors from Los Angeles to Rochester, New York. The Manhattan Project and the Atomic Energy Commission spearheaded research, some of which persisted through the 1970s. Between 1963 and 1971, a Dr. Heller irradiated the gonads of 131 prisoners in Oregon, including at least 66 "negro volunteers," with radioactive thymidine.[31] Vanderbilt University physicians administered radioactive cocktails to pregnant women in Nashville. The University of Chicago fed the radioactive elements strontium and cesium to 102 unwitting patients at state schools. One Dickensian institution, the Fernald School in Waltham, Massachusetts, added radioactive oatmeal to the menus of thirty orphans in a program sponsored by the AEC with the support of the Quaker Oats Company.[32] Old videotapes reveal that some of these Fernald boys were African American, but no records with racial identifiers were ever released. When victims died, government scientists obtained their bodies and autopsied them carefully, measuring the levels of radioactivity and biological damage. To enable large numbers of these grim assessments, at least fifteen thousand bodies were exposed and collected for one project alone: Operation Sunshine. Until the mid-1980s and without the knowledge of patients or their next of kin, this program shipped the bodies and body parts of radiation experiment victims to be dissected at headquarters in Los Alamos, New Mexico.

Between 1960 and 1972, University of Cincinnati radiologist Eugene L. Saenger, M.D., directed experimental high-dose TBI on a total of 200 cancer patients, of whom 150 were black.[33]

The TBI method was dangerous, utilizing magnavolt X rays, cobalt-60, or cesium-137 to administer the equivalent of fifteen thousand chest X rays to the entire body. Patients typically received from one hundred to four hundred rads. A rad is a unit of absorbed radiation with a complex definition: 150 rads, a common TBI dosage, is equivalent to four hundred mammograms. Forty-two percent of the subjects given higher doses died within weeks, and some within days.[34] However, a minority of the subjects received partial-body radiation (PBI), which spared some portions of the body.

When he proposed the experiments in hopes of funding and support from the army director of nuclear medicine in 1958, Saenger gave an experimental rationale, explaining, "These studies are designed to obtain new information about the metabolic effects of total body and partial body irradiation, so as to have a better understanding of the acute and sub-acute effects of irradiation in the human."[35] He deemed such information necessary to allow scientists to protect "military personnel who might be irradiated during a war." The army agreed to fund his experiments, but it expressed doubts, because doctors already knew there were radiosensitive cancers, which responded to radiation treatment, and radioresistant cancers, which typically did not. By the 1940s, TBI was found effective against some radiosensitive cancers (which were disseminated widely throughout the body, such as leukemia and lymphoma), but not against the localized, radioresistant cancers that Saenger studied.

However, the subjects in Saenger's experiments, such as the 82 patients in Cincinnati General Hospital, 51 of whom were black, were told only that the TBI was a treatment for their cancers. Among their catastrophic effects, these high doses destroyed the subjects' bone marrow, and because bone marrow produces red blood cells, the TBI proved quickly fatal to one out of every four subjects, who died within about a month, after suffering anemia, vomiting, and falling white blood cell counts, which left them open to a variety of infections. If one also counts patients who received PBI, 85 of the 111 people Saenger irradiated at Cincinnati General were black.[36] TBI experiments were also conducted by doctors at other Cincinnati hospitals, at Sloan-Kettering Memorial Cancer Center in New York, at Texas's Baylor University College of Medicine, at the Naval Hospital in Bethesda, Maryland, and at the AEC hospital in Oak Ridge. Only one of the administering physicians was an African American—Howard Perry, M.D., who vigorously denied that the experiments had any racial component. He died before this book was conceived, so I had no opportunity to interview him. However, his lawyer, Brian Hurley, wrote to Martha Stephens, author of *The Treatment*, that Perry was a compassionate man who had been falsely accused of "targeting other blacks for radiation experiments." Other radiation scientists assailed the description given by Saenger and his deputy Dr. Clarence Lushbaugh of TBI for radioresistant cancers as "therapy," and insisted that his experiments were too dangerous. Karl Morgan, who had considered Saenger a friend and had worked with Lushbaugh at Oak Ridge, said in 1994, "I think the case of Clarence Lushbaugh's treatment of humans as guinea pigs and Eugene Saenger's at the hospital in Cincinnati are some of the most terrible human studies I ever heard of other than those that took place in Germany, and a few in Japan . . . during the war."[37]

Saenger at first insisted to AEC interviewers in 1994 that written informed consent had been unnecessary for his experiments. Later, Cincinnati General produced consent signatures for TBI subjects, but the subjects' survivors questioned them. For example, Gloria Nelson, the granddaughter of subject Amelia Jackson, pointed out that a signed consent form was produced from her grandmother's file, but that Jackson had never learned to read or write.[38]

Dr. Eugene Saenger stated in congressional hearings that "Race I.Q. or socioeconomic standing were not selection factors."[39] Officially, he explained the racial disparity by saying that the experimental population merely reflected the racial component of the hospital populations where they worked. His testimony, however, is contradicted by his research partner, Clarence Lushbaugh, who explained in 1995 that they chose "slum" patients because "these persons don't have any money and they're black and they're poorly washed. These persons were available in the University of Cincinnati to Dr. Saenger. . . . I did review what he was doing, and I thought it was actually well done."[40]

In 1972, Saenger's TBI projects ended when the DOD cut funding for them—after the university had accrued more than $850,000.[41] Saenger no longer referred to his work as investigative; he defended his experiments as cancer treatments and pointed out that such radiation treatments are used today for cancer treatment. They are used in extreme cases, but today's irradiations—including bone-marrow transplants—bear little resemblance to the experiments carried out by Saenger. Today's procedures are therapeutic and reserved for those whose cancer is widely spread and nonresponsive to other methods. Because the irradiation destroys the bone marrow, marrow for transplant is acquired for reinfusion after the procedure. Unfortunately, it is more difficult to match the bone marrow of African Americans, who tend to have a richer complement of antibodies than do most whites. This means that, like Marion Sims's enslaved vesicovaginal fistula patients, the black TBI subjects' experiences eventually enabled cancer treatments from which blacks are less likely to profit than are whites. Moreover, Saenger's patients did not have to die to provide such information: Researchers had known at least since 1956 that TBI destroys the bone marrow, but now they could calibrate the lethal doses more precisely.

Saenger, who was still a professor emeritus at the University of Cincinnati Medical School as this book went to press, did not reply to my telephoned interview requests through the UC press-relations office or to E-mails in which I asked him to discuss his work. But in his public statements, he defends his research as therapeutic and consensual. The venerable American College of Radiology agreed, exonerating Saenger of wrongdoing on the basis of his denials and by ignoring the rules that governed experimentation during his tenure as a DOD researcher. The trajectory of Saenger's medical career did not falter and he never faced criminal charges.

Martha Stephens, a University of Cincinnati English professor, has written *The Treatment*, a comprehensive and unflinching history of the TBI tests. Its chapters describe the long, bitter fight for justice that finally culminated in a five-million-dollar 1999 settlement between thirteen researchers and the subjects' survivors.[42] The agreement also stipulated that the university would erect a permanent memorial naming the victims, and in June 2000, it complied by installing a small, curiously dated plaque labeled DEDICATED TO THE PATIENTS OF THE RADIATION EXPERIMENTATION, 1973–1974 and listing the names of over 170 patients. The plaque was placed on the medical school grounds, behind a Dumpster and nestled between the kitchen and a parking garage.

Saenger's use of mostly black subjects was a matter of convenience and culture, but other radiation experiments offered scientific rationales for deliberately targeting black subjects. Like the scientific racists of a century earlier, investigators wished to demonstrate that blacks would respond differently to radiation's medical dangers. The design of such experiments *required* African American subjects.

Many such experiments were conducted at the Medical College of Virginia (MCV), part of Virginia Commonwealth University. Between 1949 and 1960, the MCV was home to a secret metabolic laboratory, whose principal focus was the army's preparation for massive nuclear casualties. MCV was chosen in part because it was a heavily research-oriented school in the South and the government had a particular interest in black subjects.

For example, one MCV experiment sought to determine whether radiation inflicted different degrees of damage on the skins of black people than on that of whites. In 1947, Everett Idris Evans, at the behest of the surgeon general of the army, set up the nation's first civilian burn unit at MCV, funded by the army. Evans planned to compare the burn injuries radiation caused in whites to those it caused in blacks. Some were charity patients who had been severely burned in accidents and whose use as experimental material constituted "payment" for their care by MCV staff. But MCV researchers deliberately caused third-degree burns to the skins of other patients at Dooley, a charity hospital for black children, and at St. Philip, its sister hospital for black adults. These hospitals eventually yielded one hundred black subjects a year between the ages of six months and ninety years for similar MCV burn experiments. Doctors used radiation emitted at graduated levels to measure the precise amount of energy necessary to induce specific levels of first- to third-degree burns. Investigators also produced the radiation burns on the arms of forty-four whites at different area hospitals and, at least in some cases, scientists acknowledged that these were produced for "investigational purposes." The doctors and radiation physicians used their data to calculate the numbers of people who would die at specific distances from a nuclear bomb like that detonated over Hiroshima (approximately twenty kilotons). Evans's team deduced that blacks suffered more intense burns than whites after the same exposure, and from this, researchers concluded that radiation burns from a nuclear event would injure blacks much more severely than whites.[43] Another experimental group of 460 black and 770 white patients in the Medical College of Virginia was injected with a variety of radioactive substances, including phosphorus-32, without their consent.[44] Blacks made up 37 percent of these experimental subjects, nearly four times their representation in the population.

The AEC also sponsored fifteen other radiation studies on three hundred black patients at New Orleans Charity Hospital; the studies were conducted by Tulane University physicians. The most toxic of these experiments involved dispensing mercury, in yet another study of disparate racial reactions to radiation. Twenty-two black patients were made to swallow radioactive mercury in order to calibrate its symptoms and the length of time the body took to excrete the toxic metal. In another Tulane experiment, doctors surreptitiously placed radioactive mercury into the open sores that remained just after they had removed blisters from a dozen "colored" and three white patients in order to judge the metal's effects on healing times. They amassed no clinically meaningful data.[45]

Despite the MCV findings that blacks were more vulnerable to radiation burn damage, an illogical belief persisted among doctors and radiologic technicians that African Americans could tolerate increased amounts of radiation than could whites without ill effect. Like the belief that blacks better tolerate pain than do whites, this stubborn myth gave license to conduct painful and dangerous experimental radiation practices. In 1968, consumer activist Ralph Nader complained to the *Washington Post* about the nationwide practice of "giving Negroes 25 to 50 percent stronger [X-ray] doses than white patients." G. J. Tarleton, a professor of radiology at the predominantly black Meharry Medical College in Nashville, Tennessee, swiftly dismissed the claim as "a fantastic charge." But California radiologic technicians conducting a 1966 survey revealed that 72 percent of the state's X-ray technicians had opted on their own initiative to administer these higher X-ray exposures to blacks because of their vague beliefs that African Americans were physiologically different: " 'Their bones are harder and denser. . . . Their skin is darker. . . . Their flesh is tougher.' " Physicians from the Public Health Service and the American College of Radiology denied ever issuing such advisories to doctors, but it was technicians, not doctors, who were making the experimental adjustments without citing their actions in the official medical records. Also, despite the denials, physicians *were* being taught to administer higher-than-indicated radiation doses to blacks. For example, the 1963 edition of *X-Ray Technology,* by Charles A. Jacobi and Don Q. Paris, a standard textbook, contained a charted recommendation that the standard radiation doses should be increased for Negro X-ray patients.[46] In 1968 a study commissioned by Bernard Goldman, director of the New York State Bureau of X-Ray, also found that a "significant portion" of technicians had exposed blacks to higher radiation doses than whites, leading the New York State health department to specifically prohibit the practice.

There were many other racially mediated radiation experiments. For example, the AEC irradiated 235 African American newborns in 1953–1954 in various hospitals across the nation, but the released radiation records give very sparse details. However, we know that biophysics professor Dr. Lester Van Middlesworth injected each of six black newborns with 1.5 microcuries of radioactive iodine-131 in a 1940 program at Vanderbilt University in Nashville. Records also reveal that six of the seven infants injected at John Gaston Hospital, a now-defunct public hospital in Memphis, were also black, and their doctors measured their uptake of iodine, which targets the thyroid gland, twenty-four hours later so that they could learn more about how the gland functions in infants.[47] Today, radioactive tracers are used for therapeutic or screening purposes in smaller, safer amounts; no one should avoid such tests, which trade a low radiation risk for significant health benefits. But these were not therapeutic injections and their risks were unjustifiable.

The experimental use of radiation to harm and to stigmatize African Americans is not entirely relegated to the distant past. In 1978, scientists revisited an experiment that had been conducted between 1940 and 1959 at several sites, including New York University Hospital. There, scientists irradiated the scalps of 2,500 children, 625 of them black, to treat their tinea capitis, or ringworm. Without notification to their parents, children were taken from classrooms for the X-ray treatments and their burns and side effects were carefully assessed, raising the question whether the X-ray "treatments" were chiefly experimental rather than therapeutic in nature. Blacks made up 9.8 percent of the U.S. population in 1940, so these children were represented at two and a half times their rate in the population. Between 1910 and 1959, before effective topical medications were developed, 200,000 children around the world received about 175 rads each for treatment of ringworm. But by 1940, when NYU irradiated children, researchers had known for over twenty-five years that this level of radiation was extremely dangerous, and the standard treatment for ringworm was not irradiation, but ultraviolet light or topical chemotherapy. In 1978, the *American Journal of Public Health* published an article in which NYU researchers assessed the psychiatric results this irradiation had had on the developing brains of 177 of the subjects. They administered the Minnesota Multiphasic Personality Inventory (MMPI) to 118 whites and 59 blacks. (NYU had included in the experiment a control group of 1,800 children who had been treated with chemotherapy, 450 of whom, or 25 percent, were black.) Researchers found more psychological symptoms and deviant personality scores among the adult whites who had been treated by irradiation than among those who had been treated with topical medication. But they found that the radiation-treated black subjects had no more psychiatric symptoms than medically treated blacks, and this suggested to them that radiation levels that could cause brain damage in whites did not affect blacks: "[Some researchers] have suggested brain insults at birth have relatively less impact among blacks on the risk of subsequent neuropsychiatric disorders than among whites," the article stated.

This conclusion recalls both the baseless belief that higher doses of radiation were needed in blacks to produce the same effects as in whites and the previously discussed belief that some disorders such as syphilis and tuberculosis affect blacks in a manner that spares their nervous systems and brains. However, investigators admitted to serious flaws in their experimental design: The MMPI is ethnically biased and less sensitive in discerning pathology among African Americans; also, researchers tested fewer than 10 percent of the original subjects, and this small sample size may also have distorted the results.[48]

Black-Body Radiation

"In more cases than not, the victims are African Americans. You're dealing with a majority of people of African American descent. My mother thinks it's a grand-scale plan," insists Elmerine Whitfield Bell. Is she right? For some radiation-research programs, the racial breakdown has been obscured by the engineered atmosphere of deceit and secrecy—even patient names are missing, lost forever with case records. But all extant data indicate that a higher number of African Americans than whites *were* used in many clandestine radiation experiments. As mentioned earlier, subject advocate E. Cooper Brown of the National Committee for Radiation Victims estimated that three of every five radiation victims were people of color.[49] Seventy-five percent of the subjects in the University of Cincinnati irradiation experiments were African American. But the real significance is the fact that African Americans were typically used in significantly greater proportions than the 10 to 12 percent of the population they have constituted.

In 1993, DOE secretary Hazel O'Leary, the first African American to hold that position, displayed refreshing candor as she reacted to graphic press allegations of the government's experimentation on its own citizens. She admitted the agency's guilt and ordered the selective declassification of vital nuclear information. In December 1993, she ordered the opening of all DOE records of the 435 human radiation experiments conducted between 1944 and the 1990s. O'Leary's investigation ushered in a new atmosphere of openness to replace decades of Machiavellian Cold War secretiveness. As she explained, "We've learned that openness helps to bring a corrective to government, and quickly." She ordered 665 cubic feet of original declassified documents and investigation results stored in the National Archives and mounted on DOE Web sites. This is the sort of forthrightness that would have prevented the investigative failures of the Tuskegee ad hoc committee.

On January 15, 1994, President Clinton created the Advisory Committee on Human Radiation Experiments (ACHRE) to investigate fully the genesis of these experiments and to judge them. The committee was also charged with making sure that these abuses could never be repeated. Clinton also issued an apology on October 3, 1995, but few seem to know this: It was drowned out by the din that accompanied the O. J. Simpson verdict, which was announced a few hours later. Clinton's brief remarks did not mention any racial component of the studies.

The revelations of the committee facilitated civil lawsuits brought against the government and universities by hundreds of victims and survivors. Some cases have been successful, such as those mounted by the chiefly black victims of the Cincinnati TBI experiments. Others are still being contested. However, the ACHRE chose to interview the researchers and publish the resultant oral histories instead of charging them with crimes. None of the physicians conducting the radiation experiments were ever placed on trial.

The radiation experiments capture the moment when an important group of physician-scientists ceased to view themselves as healers and benefactors first, with disastrous results for their victims and for American medicine. For African Americans, the full costs in lost health and lost trust are still being reckoned.

Even today, events occasionally remind us that racism and radiation experimentation remain linked at locations such as the Savannah River Site. Locals call it simply the "SRS." Located just outside Aiken, South Carolina, owned by the DOE, and managed by South Carolina's Westinghouse Savannah River Company (WSRC), this high-tech manufacturing facility once produced tritium and plutonium-239 for nuclear weapons. Now that the Cold War has abated, it processes nuclear waste.

Approximately 2,800 of the SRS's 14,000 employees are black, and by

2002, they had filed at least twenty-two lawsuits. These complain that black employees were denied promotions, were subjected to racist graffiti, found nooses hanging in their lockers, and were subjected to higher radiation levels than were whites. "We have disciplined employees, including terminating an employee for incidents involving nooses," WSRC president Robert Pedde confirmed for the *Augusta Chronicle* in 2002. In 1997, the Department of Labor ordered Westinghouse to compensate seven black SRS workers.

But even worse, blacks complain that they are relegated to the high-radiation areas of the plant, dubbed the "coon areas" by whites. James Ruttenber of the University of Colorado School of Medicine assessed employee radiation readings between 1991 and 1998, using their dosimeters (individual radiation counters). His findings corroborate these workers' claims:

> When all annual dose measurements are grouped by race, the doses for blacks are higher than for whites in all dose categories. . . . The annual penetrating doses for blacks are about 1.8 times as high as the doses for whites . . . the analyses support the hypothesis that these differences are due to job-placement practices that put blacks in jobs that have higher radiation exposures than whites.[50]

Yet their requests for transfer to safer areas have been denied. Jimmy Walker, for example, inhaled plutonium at the plant in 1977. This drove his exposure beyond the permitted lifetime dose of fifty rems (a rem is a measure of radiation dose—essentially, a rad that is adjusted for its biological effect). In 2002, after multiple permanent-transfer requests were ignored, his radiation level soared to more than eighty rems, nearly twice the permitted lifetime exposure, and he retired at age forty-eight in poor health.

The exposures also placed Walker at risk of becoming an experimental subject. At a 2002 checkup, a company doctor pressed into Walker's hands a leaflet suggesting he donate his body to a radiation-research project at Washington State University. In return, his family would receive five hundred dollars. "I feel betrayed by the company, by the government," Walker told London's *Independent* newspaper in 2002. "Now they have admitted the radiation causes cancer. All the time they were telling me there was nothing to worry about." By 2002, the DOE had paid out $25 million to black workers in sixty-two settlements, but the company admits no wrongdoing.

African American radiation victims are neither silent nor passive. Elmer Allen's daughter, Elmerine Whitfield Bell, is an activist who challenges abusive experimentation and refuses to let the memory of her father and the other radiation victims fade from memory with the headlines. "What I really want to come from this," Bell says, "is some type of coalition of victims and survivors of radiation treatments and experiments, so that we can get together and really speak to the issue on a national and on an international basis. I'm determined that as long as I breathe, I will address the issue of radiation and how to eradicate this sort of experimentation from the earth. It will always be used against poor folk. We have to do something."[51]

CHAPTER 10

CAGED SUBJECTS

Research on Black Prisoners

I am disturbed that the World Medical Association is now hedging on its clause about [not] using criminals as experimental material. The American influence has been at work on its suspension. One of the nicest [American] scientists I know was heard to say, "Criminals in our penitentiaries are fine experimental material—and much cheaper than chimpanzees."

—"PERTINAX," BRITISH MEDICAL JOURNAL, JANUARY 1963

On a brightly promising early spring day in 2004, Jesse Williams and I shared brunch in a Philadelphia seafood house splashed with bright jewel-like colors. Against a backdrop of sunny seascapes and murmuring besuited executives, Williams affably recited his résumé, detailing the grim expertise in pain and survival he had accrued during his four decades imprisoned in the Holmesburg Prison system, the stygian scientific kingdom of University of Pennsylvania dermatologist Dr. Albert M. Kligman.

The evening before, Williams, a massive, imposing man with a boxer's build, a bald head, a piercing gaze, and stentorian delivery, had spoken eloquently at a showing of *Acres of Skin*, the documentary based upon Allen Hornblum's incisive book of the same title, an exposé of the decades of Kligman's medical experimentation at Holmesburg.

Williams told the audience of being burned by radiation and sulfuric acid, of immersing his arms in chemicals that had tanned his skin like leather, and of how physicians and technicians had rubbed acid into his scrotum until the skin fell away—all for three dollars a session. Researchers had cut his armpits to study the glands and had laced his back with scars in an attempt to induce the disfiguring ropy overgrowths called keloids. Not only patches of poison oak and ivy but also cadaveric tissue had been implanted in his back, and he had inhaled vapors infused with influenza and other viruses. Patch tests of various harsh chemicals and ointments had left a checkerboard of rectangular scars on his back; detergents whose names he did not know had removed his hair and abraded his scalp. Williams had offered himself up for as many as twelve experiments at once, bringing in from thirty to fifty dollars for each multisession research study. Yet, he said, "We were never told what was going on. We never had witnesses or a receipt for [copy of] anything we signed."

Before the audience, Williams had been practiced and powerful, but I shared a tête-à-tête with a more subdued man, one invested with a gentle but direct manner and who spoke with complete candor about a violent past that included jail stints for robbery and assault. "I've done it all," he admitted quietly. He is now a Christian, and he spoke sadly of the many former inmates who died in broken health and of his concern for another seriously ill subject. Only after being prodded to speak of his own plight did he lament his myriad physical problems, from leg ulcers to mental changes to chronic skin problems, which he ascribed to the testing. "The doctors can't tell me what it is. They don't know what I was tested with." Williams confided his regret of never having achieved the education he desperately wanted and he voiced ambivalence about displaying his scars, physical and mental, for strangers in order to gain support for an inmates' lawsuit. "I feel I'm on display in the zoo sometimes." He sat back and sighed softly. "No one should ever have to go through what we went through. Not again. Not in a civilized country."[1]

When Robert Boyle, the seventeenth-century father of chemistry, mused upon the feasibility of scientific research with humans, he proposed, "Trayal might be made on some genuine human bodies, especially those of Malefactors." From the testing of inoculation practices to the use of cadavers for dissection and display, the medical community has turned to jail inmates first when it sought experimental subjects. Even a 1910 editorial in the black physicians' chief publication, the fledgling *Journal of the National Medical Association,* proposed that prisoners were the most appropriate medical research subjects. The *JNMA* suggested that prisoners might simultaneously expiate their debt to society and protect others, especially African Americans, by substituting for them as unwilling research subjects.[2] Black physicians wished to pursue research while protecting their African American patients, and the use of prisoners was an alternative with which everyone, black and white, could be comfortable.

But why are prisoners such universally desirable subjects for medical research? Boyle was only adhering to the inexorable logic of his profession when he suggested that medical experimentation was most acceptable when practiced upon prisoners. In his time, prisoners were vulnerable, stigmatized, and expendable; they tended to be poor and uneducated; they were likely to belong to despised and powerless minority groups; they had already lost most important civil rights; and their crimes or alleged crimes made them feared and hated. They were barred from assuming any useful role in society, which, in turn, begrudged them even the sparsest expenditures for their room and board—for which some eighteenth-century prisoners were billed. Few had families or much support from the family they had. In Boyle's time, as in our own, prisoners were viewed as dangerous parasites who would not be missed should something happen to them. Boyle's shrewd suggestion has even been shared by prisoners, as some clamor for inclusion in medical investigations for reasons that are examined hereafter.

But in our time, there has been another motivation: Prisoners are ideal subjects for Phase I trials. Federal regulations dictate that modern human medical experiments consist of at least three formal phases. Highly simplified, these are: Phase I, which asks, "How safe is this drug?"; Phase II, which continues evaluating safety while also seeking to determine "How effective is this drug?"; and if the treatment seems safe and effective, the trial proceeds to Phase III, which compares the treatment to the standard treatment, using subjects treated with the investigative therapy and a control group treated with the current standard of care, if one exists. If not, the control group may be given a placebo, an inert sham treatment to enable a comparison with the new therapy.

Phase I trials use healthy volunteers to test the safety of the treatment, looking for side effects and the best mode of administration. Because they are the first human tests, Phase I trials carry a higher risk of problems, such as side effects, than do other trials. For this reason, companies prefer Phase I trials to take place in institutions where subjects can be carefully monitored and are unlikely to be lost to follow-up: If serious problems develop, the researchers want to know. Prisoners fit the bill nicely. Around 1963, Robert Batterman, M.D., an expert in pharmaceutical experimentation, said, "Phase I is very big in prisons. The FDA prefers Phase I to be on an inpatient basis—the only place available for large scale toxicity studies is prison." He also added, "The vast majority of new drugs—more than 90 percent—never get into medical practice. They prove too toxic and fall by the wayside in Phase II."[3]

That Jesse Williams and thousands of his fellow incarcerated research subjects were African American is no accident. African Americans have always been dramatically overrepresented in jails and prisons (at national rates of 40 to 61 percent of all the incarcerated), so any discussion of U.S. inmates is closely bound up with race, and medical experimentation behind bars is no exception.

Some influential white scientists, such as Italian physician Cesare Lombroso, whose theories were discussed in chapter 3, did not distinguish between blacks and criminals. In 1911, Lombroso observed, *"There exists a group of criminals, born for evil, against whom all social cures break as though against a rock* [emphasis added]—a fact which compels us to eliminate them completely, even if by death." This group consisted of men who were inherently, immutably evil because of their deranged physiology. They were also, in his view, more likely to be black than white.

When Lombroso sought to illustrate his theories of "criminal man," he unhesitatingly chose an African society, the Dinka of the Upper Nile, as the perfect example of born savage criminals. The Dinka were no more bellicose than many other societies on other continents, but their dark skin was enough to qualify them for this distinction. Among the physical stigmata that conclusively signaled their criminal nature were dark skin and the concomitant inability to blush. "Inability to blush has always been considered the accompaniment of crime and shamelessness," warned Lombroso. "Blushing is very rare among idiots and savages."[4]

Medical theories of criminality are important because medicine has long claimed a special provenance over criminality. The very frequent reference to a prison as a site of rehabilitation and treatment is the sine qua non of modern penology. Illegal behavior was medicalized in an 1870 statement of the Congress of the American Prison Association:

A Criminal is a man who has suffered under a disease evinced by the perpetration of a crime, and who may reasonably be held to be under the dominion of such disease until his conduct has afforded very strong presumption not only that he is free from its immediate influence but that the chances of its recurrence have become exceedingly remote.[5]

Dr. Karl Menninger, often called the "dean of American psychiatry," was a psychoanalyst, Harvard professor, and scion of the dynasty of psychiatrists who founded the Menninger Clinic in Topeka, Kansas. His lectures and readable books helped bring mental disorders out of the dark closet of shame and secrecy in which they had languished until the mid-twentieth century. He also had a special sympathy for prisoners, but he attributed criminal behavior not to the constitutional evil of Lombroso's conscience-deprived "criminal man" but to a limited psyche, "the spasms and struggles of a sub-marginal human being trying to make it in our complex society with inadequate equipment. . . ."

African American behavior has long been pathologized in a similar manner. In fact, the imaginary black diseases dreamed up by the American school of ethology are psychiatric disorders with a strong forensic bias. As described in chapter 1, they ascribed illegal behavior as well as pathological behavior to blacks, and the "medicine" Dr. Samuel A. Cartwright prescribed was punishment by whips or hard labor.

Twentieth-century corrections personnel perpetuated this medical pathologizing of behavior by making references to borderline personality disorders, antisocial personalities, and sociopaths within their walls who had never been so diagnosed by a medical professional. San Quentin prison psychiatrist Dr. Harvey Powelson, for example, discussed how in the 1950s, staff recklessly made diagnoses of inmates from Rorschach tests, a then-popular diagnostic tool that involved interpreting responses to "ink-blot" patterns. "My sense of the situation is that Adult Authority used the tests for rationalizations for what they'd already decided based upon their own intuition."

Dark Days at Holmesburg Prison

In 1998, Allen Hornblum published *Acres of Skin,* which documents the abusive experimentation conducted at Philadelphia's Holmesburg Prison complex by Dr. Albert M. Kligman between the 1950s and 1970s. "Most of this research was practiced upon African American men," says

Hornblum. "Not only that, but they were used for the worst, most dangerous experiments." Kligman, a dermatologist, was initially invited to Holmesburg Prison in 1951 to treat an outbreak of athlete's foot. But his initial reaction to Holmesburg was far from therapeutic and gave Hornblum's book its title: "All I saw before me were acres of skin. It was like a farmer seeing a fertile field for the first time." Soon Kligman was inducing foot fungus, not treating it, because he saw the opportunity to conduct lucrative experiments upon thousands of captive bodies for at least thirty-three major pharmaceutical and cosmetic companies, such as Johnson & Johnson, Merck, Helena Rubenstein, and DuPont. During World War II, prisoners had been commonly used as research subjects, and after the war, the United States was the only nation in the world continuing to legally use prisoners in clinical trials.[6] Federal, pharmaceutical, and cosmetic companies' money catalyzed a thirty-year boom in research with prisoners.

Throughout the 1950s and 1960s, Kligman gained exclusive experimental use of inmate bodies, testing 153 experimental drugs between 1962 and 1966 alone. Seventy-five percent of Holmesburg's inmate population, including Jesse Williams, were administered cosmetics, powders, and shampoos that caused baldness, extensive scarring, and permanent skin and nail injury.

Fingernails were removed or deformed by punch biopsies, in which a physician employs a special forceps or a biopsy punch to obtain a full-thickness circular sample of skin or nail. The subjects' backs were so covered by flayed, discolored, and scarred skin from various patch tests of chemicals that the distinctive checkerboard or striped skin was a sure tip-off that the man was an ex-con. "If you ever saw guys on the beach you would know where the hell they've been," explained former guard Joseph Dade. Withers Ponton, a lifer in his eighties, complained of a back "all marked up with bad blackheads and scars" after a quarter century of patch tests. "That first test nearly killed me: It was so painful I nearly went through the wall." But he eventually participated in more than fifty tests during a forty-month stint at a county jail, for which he earned several thousand dollars.

When Kligman used prisoners to devise the anti-acne medication Retin-A, it made him a millionaire. Jailed subjects were also inoculated with herpes, vaccinia, and wart viruses and were exposed to *Staphylococ-*

cus and *Monilia*. Their skin was exposed to everything from radioisotopes to temperature extremes. Dow Chemical Company also paid Kligman to test dioxin, a suspected carcinogen, which he applied to the skin of seventy prisoners, mostly black. He also inoculated men with syphilis, gonorrhea, malaria, and amoebic dysentery. Each participant earned anywhere from ten to seven hundred dollars, depending upon the length, danger, and unpleasantness of the research.

But in the fall of 1965, the FDA became alarmed when the *Journal of the American Medical Association (JAMA)* published Kligman's article based on research in which he covered inmates' torsos with the banned substance dimethylsulfoxide (DSMO), an oily industrial solvent. The FDA began scrutinizing his work, and its documents cite "irregularities and falsification of reports," alarm over Kligman's extremely large number of investigations, and concern that he was dabbling in areas far removed from his specialty, dermatology. FDA documents also condemned Kligman's practice of routinely enrolling inmates in multiple studies simultaneously, which multiplied their health risks and clouded the source of any adverse effects. What's more, Kligman's record-keeping discrepancies were rife—he, like many other prison investigators, destroyed or "lost" medical files. This allowed them to claim later, among other things, that African Americans were not disproportionately represented in abusive procedures. On July 19, the FDA removed Kligman from its list of approved researchers and notified sponsors that he no longer was eligible to perform drug testing. But just a month later, the FDA restored his privileges.[7]

The FDA's concern that Kligman was venturing too far afield of dermatology, his area of expertise, was certainly warranted. He began performing chemical-warfare tests for the army and the CIA, using psychotropic agents. Perhaps the most harrowing experimental accounts are those of CIA mind-control experiments in which psychoactive substances, including Schedule II drugs (those with a high abuse risk), were administered to inmates as part of the MK-ULTRA program, a CIA research program conducted from 1953 through the 1970s to produce the perfect "truth drug" for interrogating Soviet intelligence operatives.[8] According to Kligman's own statements, he was operating essentially unregulated and with inmates who participated because they had been told neither the nature of the tests nor the risks they were taking. In 1972, he

enthused, "It was years before the authorities knew that I was conducting various studies on prisoner volunteers. Things were simple then. Informed consent was unheard of. No one asked me what I was doing. It
was a wonderful time."9

The government tests were conducted from three trailers on the
prison grounds. Some inmates gave these tests a wide berth because it
was rumored that they involved LSD and drove men crazy. But others
eventually entered them, drawn by the money, which was much more
than what was paid for skin tests. Half of these subjects reported frightening hallucinations that lasted for days, but prisoners say that they
were never given consent forms or told what drugs they were being
given. Edward Anthony, a black Holmesburg inmate during the mid-
1960s, said that after he suffered rashes from the skin tests, he moved on
to the more lucrative army experiments. "I don't remember much of
what happened after I was given the injection," he said. "But I know
once it wore off, I was a different person than before. I used to be a
mild-mannered person, but now I have drastic mood swings and have
trouble controlling my temper." Jesse Williams gives a similar account of
his time in the trailers. "I used to be into nonconfrontational crimes—
burglary, stealing cars. But after the mind tests, I was a different person,
more confrontational. I would go to bars actively seeking trouble; I
never was like that before."

Some drugs caused temporary paralysis or helplessness, or even
placed the subject into a catatonic state, from which he could neither
communicate nor react to his surroundings. Others caused prolonged
nausea, and still others, such as the drugs Williams and Anthony took,
provoked long-term violent behavior. We still cannot know which drugs
the men were given because they were investigational and identified only
by number. The test results are classified, but the army acknowledges
that it conducted such experiments at Holmesburg. "There was limited
Army involvement with the University of Pennsylvania many years ago,"
admitted Lt. Col. Bill Wheelehan, a Pentagon spokesman. "The Army
does not engage in this type of medical research today."

In a 1973 congressional hearing on human experimentation, the Senate Labor and Public Welfare Committee's health subcommittee heard
testimony from former Holmesburg inmates Leodus Jones and Allan
Lawson, who charged the university was deceptive in the handling of

consent procedures and informing inmates of possible risks. In January 1974, the Philadelphia prison system's board of trustees terminated the program.[10]

Twenty-four years later, when *Acres of Skin* was published, many former subjects realized for the first time that they had rights as experimental subjects and could sue the University of Pennsylvania, Kligman's home institution, despite the indemnification waivers that some had signed. In September 2000, 298 former Holmesburg prisoners filed a class-action lawsuit against the university, Johnson & Johnson, Dow Chemical Company, Dr. Kligman and his company—Ivy Research Labs—and the city of Philadelphia. But the years and the experiments had taken their physical toll. Most subjects are dead, and the survivors, now in their fifties and sixties, suffer from skin and nail problems, breathing difficulties, cancers, and stubborn, sometimes unidentified infections. Seventy former inmates have joined as Community Assistance for Prisoners to pursue legal redress, heartened by the $2.4 million settlement awarded in 2000 to Washington State prison inmates whose testicles had been cut and irradiated between 1963 and 1973. But the Holmesburg suit has been stymied by the statute of limitations.

The University of Pennsylvania insists that its research was ethical because the inmates gave informed consent, signed waivers, and took payment. Senior vice dean Richard Tannen, M.D., of the university medical center, contends that because human research was widely accepted at the time of the Holmesburg experiments, Kligman was not considered to be in violation of any Hippocratic ideals. The hospital offered the men free evaluations and treatment, should its doctors find a causal relationship between the experiments and their current ailments. Jesse Williams responded, "We don't trust them. How can we?" Kligman doesn't respond to interview requests, but he defended his work in a prepared 1997 statement: "To the best of my knowledge, the result of those experiments advanced our knowledge of the pathogenesis of skin disease, and no long-term harm was done to any person who voluntarily participated in the research program."

Holmesburg was no anomaly. In 1952, Chester M. Southam of the Sloan-Kettering Institute injected at least 396 inmates at Ohio State Prison—more than 180 of them black—with live human cancer cells. Southam said he wished to study the process by which healthy bodies neutralized and killed off cancer cells. One of the sponsors for Southam's research was the National Institutes of Health, which also sponsored the PHS syphilis study at Tuskegee. Southam assured inmates that the experiments were perfectly safe because "any cancer that took would spread slowly . . . and could be removed surgically."[11]

Inmates also were used in flawed blood-plasma trials testing "high-volume plasmapheresis"—transfusions utilizing large amounts of plasma—between 1967 and 1969 throughout the state of Alabama. The study was managed by Dr. Austin R. Stough at Kilby, Draper, and McAlester prisons—very sloppily, by all accounts. According to the *New York Times*, there was no informed consent and no accurate records were kept, so no racial breakdowns of his subjects are available. The record keeping and the management of the study were so poor that many men sickened and died not from experimental risks but from simple poor hygiene and from plasma transfusions of the wrong blood type. Sterile technique was all but ignored by the poorly trained technicians, and the laboratory, where blood and fluids pooled on the floors and stained every available surface, was filthy. As a result, 28 percent of the subjects developed hepatitis, in contrast to only 1 percent of inmates who were not subjects. Dr. Stough was expelled several times from hospitals and prisons after his subjects sickened and died from a variety of diseases, but not before he netted roughly two million dollars in profits.

In other prisons across the nation, hundreds of black and white inmates were subjected to flash burns (burns caused by excessive skin or corneal exposure to heat radiation, rather than the direct application of heated tools). Burns were specifically inflicted upon African Americans at sites such as the cornea of the eyes (where they sometimes led to permanent vision problems), forearms, and backs because scientists wished to learn how thermal radiation affected darker skins as opposed to white skin. Some of these experiments duplicated the experiments conducted by the Medical College of Virginia, which were described in chapter 9.

Often under the guise of treatment, psychiatric experimentation with imprisoned African Americans has spanned the poles of barbarity and sophisticated personality destruction. In the 1950s, Tulane University psychiatrist Dr. Robert Heath selected black prisoners specifically for use in psychosurgery experiments. These involved implanting electrodes into inmates' brains to repeatedly stimulate their pleasure centers. Heath also conducted CIA-funded drug experiments, which included LSD and a drug called bulbocapnine. In high doses, bulbocapnine produces "catatonia and stupor," a statuelike state, which Heath and his associate Harry Bailey, M.D., thought would be useful for controlling violent prisoners. According to one memo, the CIA sought information as to whether the drug could cause "loss of speech, loss of sensitivity to pain, loss of memory, loss of will power and an increase in toxicity in persons *with a weak type of central nervous system.*" They tested the drug exclusively on African American prisoners, whom Bailey routinely referred to as "niggers," at the Louisiana State Penitentiary.

Engineered Invisbility?

Despite the extensive history of using black bodies as research subjects, despite the consistently high African American population in prisons, despite the popularity of research studies with a racial emphasis, and despite the penchant for using blacks in the most dangerous or distasteful experiments, jailed African American research subjects remained largely invisible in the medical and popular literature until the 1960s. In his book *Undue Risk,* Jonathan Moreno writes that African Americans were usually excluded from earlier prison studies.[12]

> Ironically, prison research in the United States, including the testicular irradiation research [conducted by Dr. Carl G. Heller and his colleagues during the 1960s], was generally confined to white men, because participating in prison research was considered a privilege, it was denied to minorities—at least until the civil rights movement succeeded in equalizing social opportunities for African Americans, including research opportunities.[13]

Even the Report of the Advisory Committee on Human Radiation Experiments (ACHRE), discussed in chapter 9, agreed, noting:

> In 1975, the National Commission carefully examined the racial composition of the research subjects at a prison with a major drug testing program. The Commission found that African Americans made up only 31% of the subject population, while this racial "minority" comprised 68% of the general prison population.[14]

The ACHRE's broad suggestion that blacks were underrepresented in prison medical experimentation is fatally weakened by the fact that the commission looked at only one (unnamed) prison experiment at one point in time, and thus was not representative. But even the straw man the ACHRE set up demonstrates the disproportionate use of African Americans in prison research. Black Americans in 1975 constituted only about 11 percent of the U.S. population, so that the 31 percent utilized in this prison's experiment meant that African Americans were subjected to research at a rate just under *three times higher* than their presence in the nation's population.

The ACHRE looked at this high black experimentation rate only in comparison to the even higher black incarceration rate. This is myopic, because it looks only at the artificial universe of prisons, rather than at the entire community of African Americans. This is an essentially *communitarian* fallacy, which means that the analyses have ignored the most cohesive affected community: the community of African Americans, not the community of prison inmates.

Moreover, although scientists' early prison-research records were notoriously sloppy and frequently "lost," extant records do make specific references to black prison subjects. Also, those researchers who had a dearth of black subjects, such as Heller, complained of their frustrations in gaining a more diverse subject population, suggesting that they considered the inclusion of African American prisoners in research the norm.

However, various prison studies had different racial compositions and a few recorded experiments were designed as all-white, just as some used only blacks or mostly blacks. Chapter 6, has already described how Joseph Goldberger, M.D., chose to induce pellagra only in white prison inmates to dramatize that pellagra was not a "black disease," but would strike malnourished whites, as well.

Other medical experiments were reserved for African Americans, and these were often the most risky and painful, explains Hornblum. At the Holmesburg Prison complex, where decisions about who participated in particular experiments were often left to inmate-assistants, he explains, "it is possible that the racism in American culture was reflected in the inmates' decisions about who participated in a given test."[15]

For example, only "healthy colored male" volunteers were permitted to enroll in a protocol for one 1957 Philadelphia experiment "to promote the inoculation of human skin with ... herpes simplex and herpes zoster,"[16] which were painful, incurable viral infections. However, another Holmesburg experiment, which targeted young white volunteers, required only that they lower an arm into a detergent, sodium laurel sulfate (found in many shampoos), for an hour daily over fifty-five consecutive days.[17]

Prison researchers often veiled the racial composition of their research population for the same reason that Marion Sims once hid the racial composition of his vesicovaginal fistula patients: concern that scientists would appear to exploit powerless black patients. For example, when researchers wrote journal articles about the approximately fifteen thousand Maryland inmates of state juvenile institutions subjected to genetic tests for XYY syndrome, 85 percent of whom were black, they focused upon the mostly white minority subset of this research program to hide this true racial composition of the experiment, as will be detailed in chapter 11.[18]

Perhaps the belief that black prisoners were exempt from early experimentation can best be understood as emanating from such carefully maintained invisibility. Stripped of their freedom, their civil rights, and their family and community connections, black prison subjects were almost as legally invisible as the slaves in antebellum experiments. Their invisibility was perpetuated in no small measure by the news media, which gave most Americans their only window into prison research.

Until the 1970s, the early news coverage of prison research was almost universally laudatory. Researchers and prison administrators welcomed journalists' determination to celebrate the heroism of criminals who submitted themselves to medical experimentation. *New York Times* profiles of incarcerated volunteers are all of white men, such as Sing Sing lifer Louis Boy. In 1949, the *Times* sympathetically chronicled the risky and medically unsubstantiated experiment to which Boy submitted in an attempt to save the life of an eight-year-old cancer-ridden girl. Boy lay on a gurney next to the dying girl while their circulatory systems were joined by rubber tubing so that his body could act as a filter for her "poisoned blood." The girl died, but Boy survived, and news articles strongly suggested that his selfless act had helped to expiate his crimes. The press attention generated intense human interest, culminating in Boy's Christmastime pardon.[19] In Illinois, Statesville inmate Nathan Leopold, half of

the infamous Leopold and Loeb thrill-killing duo, had been the nefarious architect of the highly publicized "Crime of the Century"—the
coolly executed 1924 kidnapping and murder of fourteen-year-old
Bobby Franks, whom they dispassionately bludgeoned to death and discarded in a marsh on Chicago's South Side. But profiles in the *New York
Times* and other newspapers detailed his key role in recruiting other inmates to join malaria experiments and in signing inmates up for potentially sight-saving corneal donations. In his memoir, *Life Plus 99 Years,*
Leopold boasted of his prison-research roles, and this coverage helped to
transform his "thrill killer" image and boosted his successful parole bid
in 1958.[20]

But this hagiographic approach to inmate subjects had the curious
effect of effacing the participation of black prisoners in medical research
from the period between the world wars until the mid-1970s. News accounts do not refer to black participation, and the images gracing these
paeans to social redemption are of white inmates lying on gurneys. In
Life magazine's profile of Dr. Kligman's laboratories and *New York Times*
photos of inmates queued up to give blood or tissue, no discernibly black
bodies appear. Black volunteers may have been ignored because physicians were nearly always white males who, when approached for the
name of an inmate to profile, proffered a white male for several reasons.
The inmate, like Boy and Leopold, would be treated to a laudatory profile and would reap glory and other advantages, including a possible parole, so doctors cited the names of prisoners whom they thought worthy
of such advantages and whose freedom they could anticipate with com-
fort—essentially, prisoners with whom they could most easily identify.

Mainstream journalists, too, were nearly universally white until the
late 1960s, and they also identified with Leopold's articulateness, intellectual attainments, and socioeconomic level in a manner they could never
have identified with Jesse Williams. White volunteers were also more
likely, like Leopold, to have obtained good educations and thus were
more likely to find an audience for their memoirs, which, not surprisingly, cast them in the most sympathetic light. Among some researchers,
especially in southern prisons, frank racism also precluded black medical
volunteers from reaping positive publicity.[21]

Volunteer Medical Slavery

But were prisoners, black or white, really volunteers? In 1947, the International Military Tribunal in Nuremberg charged Nazi doctors with war crimes, including experimentation upon prisoners of war. The Germans' ably conducted defense hinged upon Dr. Gerhard Rose's contention that U.S. doctors were guilty of exactly the same abuses—regularly subjecting prisoners to dangerous, painful involuntary experiments.

The trials culminated not only in the conviction and execution of many accused physicians but also in the Nuremberg Code, which was devised to govern future medical experimentation.

The U.S. delegation to the Nuremberg trials included Andrew Ivy, M.D., the American Medical Association representative. He offered an idealistic view of American prison research, assuring the public that the highest standards were upheld. Ivy specifically claimed that American prisoners had never been abused or used involuntarily. But he was wrong. In fact, a mere year after Nuremberg, the *Journal of the American Medical Association* praised the Statesville Prison malaria experiments, which violated the Nuremberg proscription against experimentation by using prisoners.[22]

Unfortunately, American researchers have never thought of the code as pertinent to their own research.[23] Yale Law School ethicist Jay Katz, M.D., avers that in the eyes of many American researchers it was "a good code for barbarians but an unnecessary code for ordinary physicians." In *The Nazi Doctors and the Nuremberg Code*,[24] George Annas and Michael Grodin analyze how U.S. investigators rejected Nuremberg and replaced it with naught but hollow assurances that American medical researchers needed no such constraints.[25] The Nuremberg Code is also toothless, carrying no penalties for its breach, and so it is widely ignored.[26]

The vague unsubstantiated claims proposed by Ivy stood in opposition to the judgments of all the pertinent medical organizations, which by the end of World War II had already weighed experimentation with prisoners in their ethical balances and found it wanting. Even a specially appointed research committee of the AMA denounced experimentation with prisoners as a human-rights violation (despite the AMA's praise of the malaria experiments). In 1952, this AMA House of Delegates accordingly issued a resolution entitled "Disapproval of Participation in Scientific Experiments by Inmates of Penal Institutions." Physicians, universities, or jails could not claim to be unaware of this position, because the AMA sent copies of the resolution to governors, state and federal prison officials, and parole boards. Similarly, the Ethical Committee of the World Medical Association, in its 1961 code of ethics on human experimentation, declared, "Persons detained in prisons, penitentiaries, or reformatories—being 'captive groups'—should not be used as subjects of human experiment; nor persons . . . in a position in which they are incapable of exercising the power of free choice."[27]

But none of these prohibitions on medical experimentation with prisoners was ever enforced, so they were blithely ignored by researchers, who were allowed to police themselves. Researchers, wardens, pharmaceutical companies, and universities echoed Ivy's claim that prisoners chose to participate voluntarily, and even clamored for inclusion in experiments.

Were prison subjects, black and white, willing volunteers who freely consented to inoculation with deadly infectious diseases and to testing that removed or damaged their skin, hair, and nails? Did they voluntarily submit to castration for a few dollars and the transplantation of animal tissues or cancer cells, as well as exposure to chemical-warfare agents and untried psychoactive drugs?

Usually, no. The supposedly "free consent" of American prisoners was circumscribed in several ways. In the most extreme cases, some prisoners' right to say no simply did not exist. For example, between January 1967 and April 1968, imprisoned subjects at the California Medical Facility were paralyzed with succinylcholine, also known then as Anectine, a neuromuscular compound that paralyzed muscles so that the prisoner could not move—or breathe. Many likened the terrifying experience to drowning in fetters. When five of the sixty-four selected prisoners refused to participate in the experiment, the institution's Special Treatment Board gave permission on behalf of the recalcitrant men for them to be injected—against their will.

But prison administrations usually exerted subtler pressure, in the form of authority figures and even prisoner advocates, such as social workers, who steered penniless inmates to research studies. Former Holmesburg social worker Priscilla Becroft recalls, "If somebody didn't have money for the commissary and wasn't on the list for a job, the social worker would say you can go to the U of P testing operation." Another social worker admitted harboring doubts about the medical studies to which he referred inmates. "We questioned it among ourselves, but nobody looked into it. The medical personnel walked around in white coats and looked very official and authoritative. . . ."[28]

Parole boards exerted considerable pressure, as well. The well-publicized releases of volunteers such as Louis Boy, Nathan Leopold, and the fifty-nine survivors of the Statesville malaria experiment dangled a tantalizing carrot of freedom before potential subjects. Although volunteers usually did not receive parole, administrators often placed letters of thanks or commendation in volunteers' files, which might have raised their hopes. But parole boards sometimes exerted strong negative pressure as well, according to inmates such as Nick DiSpoldo of the Arizona State Prison, who claimed in a New York Times article that parole boards routinely held a refusal to participate in research against inmates seeking release from his institution.

The prisoners' ability to consent freely was also compromised by a lack of essential information. Informed consent is mandatory for research subjects in all venues, but researchers often did not divulge the true nature of the risks, and often did not even explain the actual nature of the experiments. A New York Times exposé of the multiprison debacle by Dr. Austin Stough, mentioned earlier, reveals that there was no informed consent and that no accurate records were kept. Some researchers who claimed to have consent forms could not produce them. Jesse Williams, veteran of scores of experiments, has repeatedly insisted, "I was never given a consent form. I never saw a consent form." Consent forms made sporadic appearances in prison research, but the average black prisoner was poorly educated or even illiterate, so even when presented with a consent form, he was unlikely to be able to read or understand it. Former black inmate Edward Anthony, for example, insists that he had no idea what researchers meant by terms such as *toxicity* or *efficacy*.[29] Consent forms often were so vague, misleading, and replete with technical data and scientific language that the physicians themselves could not understand them. Although consent forms made only sporadic appearances, legal releases were de rigueur. "Lots of men were burned or scarred and wanted to sue, but they had signed releases and waivers and thought that they couldn't," recalls white former Philadelphia inmate Al Zabala.[30]

Investigators went to remarkable lengths to deceive inmates about the harms inherent in the tests. Jesse Williams spoke of participating in what had been described to him as a "footwear experiment," in which he had to wear boots taped to his feet nonstop for a week. This actually was an experimental attempt to induce a hard-to-eradicate foot fungus. When white inmate Jay Biose worked as a laboratory assistant, doctors suggested that to allay inmates' fear about the tests' safety, Biose affix cotton balls and dummy patches to his own back and arms. In order to heighten the deception, the researchers even paid Biose as if he were a participant.[31]

Prisoners at Holmesburg were often reassured that the shampoos or lotions that were tested on them were perfectly safe and could cause only minor irritation. Thirty to fifty years later, the men remain bald, scarred, or suffer skin and internal organ damage.

But what of other volunteers, those who were neither physically forced nor strongly guided by the prison administration? When they participated, did they offer themselves up voluntarily? The answer hinges upon the meaning of *voluntary*. Copious evidence exists that coercion was a key element of the supposed consent given by most African American prisoners. Today's clinical medical ethicists tend to define *coercion* in medical research very narrowly and without much precision, so many would argue that the inmates may have been induced but were not coerced. However, such critics fail to take into account the coercive features of the prison's special environment. The hell of prison life made the research laboratory, feared and abhorred by African Americans on the outside, an irresistible haven, even a life-support unit, for the African American prisoner.

Except for a few memoirs by famous inmates such as Leopold, the description of inmates' motives for volunteering emanated from researchers and prison administrators. They agreed that the inmates were motivated by money, with which they could purchase items such as cigarettes, radios, and the meager delicacies of the commissary. Researchers also sometimes noted for the press that prisoners enjoyed the special amenities of the prison ward, such as more frequent showers, better meals, and calmer, more secure surroundings. The news media unquestioningly echoed these supposed motivations, subtly sabotaging images of inmate heroism.

But researchers and prison administrators were hardly disinterested observers, and they did not tell everything they knew about prisoners' true motives. Being admitted to the research unit allowed the inmate to avoid the legion of institutional predators. A stint in the lab offered a respite from the ever-present threat of gang rape, shakedowns, racial strife from prison gangs, and deadly assaults for a thousand petty slights. Taking meals in the laboratory unit allowed the subject to escape the mess hall, the dreaded site of frequent melees and stabbings.

The inmates did speak with relish of the better meals and calmer atmosphere of the research laboratory, and freely acknowledged their need for money. There is no question that men participated for the three hundred to four hundred dollars a month or up to fifteen hundred dollars per experiment they could earn, because the few dollars a week the unskilled could earn in the prison laundry or kitchen offered no competition. But a cultural dissonance separated the hostile, violent chaos of the inmate's world and the benign, orderly environment of the university researcher or journalist. Money had a very different meaning for inmates than it had for outsiders. Inmates sought not only commissary baubles and delicacies to brighten life but, more important, the price of freedom—or, at least, of safety.

Poverty, not criminal behavior, is the most common feature of the imprisoned. Jails are full of people, both guilty and innocent, who are there only because they are too poor to make bail. By the 1970s, most prisoners in Holmesburg, for example, were legally innocent men awaiting trial.[32] Between the 1940s and 1970s, bail bondsmen typically would spring an inmate for a down payment of 10 percent of his bail, so that a man jailed in lieu of a five-hundred-dollar bond could buy his freedom within weeks with the fifty dollars he earned from a single medical experiment.

Several inmates also mention a motivation about which the news media kept silent: The human landscape of prison is largely devoid of affection, and incarcerated men described time in the research laboratory as a respite for the psyche, a place where one could go for a while to be addressed and touched with kindness, dignity, and concern.

Researchers such as Kligman knew this, and he imparted the knowledge to medical protégés during lectures:

> Many of the prisoners for the first time in their lives find themselves in the role of important human beings. We say to them

"You're important: we need you." Once this is established these
guys will knock their brains out to please you. If the experiment
does not pan out, they get depressed. They become emotionally involved with the projects. The capacity to respond to love is greater
than most people realize. I feel almost like a scoundrel—like
Machiavelli—because of what I can do to them.[33]

Solomon McBride, Dr. Kligman's chief scientific assistant, was
African American. Although he had no formal education in pharmacology, *Acres of Skin* describes how he managed the Holmesburg testing
program on a daily basis for twenty years, once again illustrating how
some blacks participated in experimental injuries to black subjects.
However, McBride described the studies as "noninvasive procedures"
and claimed "nobody was injured in those tests." When confronted about
the lifelong injuries to inmates, he denied knowledge of such practices:

"I wasn't aware of that," said McBride. "I don't think it ever happened." When asked about the use of radioactive isotopes, he is
quick to respond. "No that wasn't done. I don't think the prison
would permit it." Informed that documents from the Atomic Energy Commission verify the use of isotopes at Holmesburg, he ad-
mits, "I heard about it, but I don't know anything about it. . . . I
was opposed to things that were not kosher. If I saw something
wrong I'd tell 'em to stop. . . . I told the residents not to do stuff
that was dangerous. If they hurt those black brothers . . . I wouldn't
let them do it."[34]

Despite McBride's denials, Holmesburg prisoners suffered psychiatric damage and physical injuries that crippled them for life. Many inmates believe that research physicians had sown the seeds of deadly
cancers during their time in the laboratory, but this claim cannot be
proven because inmates do not know to what they were exposed.
    Inmates also volunteered for experiments because the laboratory
was often the inmate's sole point of entry to medical care, which was
sketchy. On evenings and weekends, medical staff were often simply
unavailable and guards or even trusted inmates performed triage on a
"sick-call" model, assessing who was ill, who was malingering, and who
was sick enough to justify the inconvenience of arranging transport to

distant medical care. Continuous medical care such as quality cancer chemotherapy and regular diabetes maintenance, apart from blood-glucose drugs, were simply unavailable.

Prisons Purge Research

By the 1970s, research in prisons began to disappear, succumbing to scandals that unmasked the racially unbalanced, abusive, dangerous, and scientifically sloppy nature of experimentation with prisoners. The exploitation of large numbers of black male prisoners caused public-relations problems for researchers and institutions in the wake of the increasingly violent and bitter civil rights battles and the revelations of the syphilis study at Tuskegee.

The thalidomide scandal, in which thousands of deformed children were born to European women who took the poorly tested drug, was another important catalyst in tainting the American perception of medical research.[35] Furthermore, Harvard researcher Henry K. Beecher, M.D., had published an article in *The New England Journal of Medicine* that criticized twenty-two cases of exploitative experimentation; an early version of the article had detailed fifty abusive cases.[36] The journal was able to induce Dr. Beecher not to identify the physicians, but the pharmaceutical industry feared that next time, a researcher of Beecher's stature might name names. The very next year, British physician Maurice Pappworth did so.

The formerly fawning news media delivered the coup de grâce by thrusting researcher after researcher into the harsh light of public exposure. On July 29, 1969, the *New York Times* published a page-one article that exposed Dr. Austin Stough's ethically and scientifically sloppy drug-testing program, which had crippled and killed unknown numbers of men throughout the state prisons of Alabama. Unlike the earlier articles, which had praised the experiments, this account suggested that most of his victims were black. In the early 1970s, the *Washington Star* exposed the use of approximately fifteen thousand black boys in Maryland juvenile institutions in XYY experiments. (These are further described in chapter 11.)[37] The malaria experiments that had been lauded as daring a few decades earlier were roundly condemned in the mid-70s as deadly.[38]

Some of the bitterest prison battles were physical as well as verbal, causing the almost universally white investigators to fear for their safety. Dr. Sigmund Weitzman described being slammed against a wall by six-foot-four-inch, 250-pound Roy "Tiger" Williams, a black inmate at Holmesburg who had lost his hair after testing a shampoo formulation. "I was scared to death. He threatened to kill me." Physicians grew frightened of working with the increasingly distrustful inmates and felt intimidated by the growing influence of the Black Muslims, who cast a jaundiced eye on prison experimentation. Burt Cahn, M.D., who worked at Holmesburg Prison from 1959 to 1965, says he left in part because he feared for his personal safety. "I became concerned about the growth of the Muslim movement."[39] The deaths of twenty-nine inmates and eleven white authority figures in the 1971 Attica prison riot also sent a chill through prison medical research programs.

Such programs suffered legal repercussions, as well. Attica inmates won damages for suffering ill treatment and assaults.[40] In 1979, nine Oregon prison subjects shared $2,215 in damages. When a lawsuit by one medical experimentation victim at Holmesburg Prison resulted in a monetary settlement (whose terms are confidential), other pharmaceutical company researchers realized that they, too, could become targets of successful inmate legal action.[41] Charles Miller, a prison-research administrator for pharmaceutical giant Eli Lilly, lamented, "The reason we closed the doggone thing down was that we were getting too much hassle and heat from the press. It just didn't seem worth it."

A January 1973 *Atlantic Monthly* cover story by investigative journalist Jessica Mitford proved even more powerful. She explained that prison medical research consisted of exploitation of the lowest, most vulnerable classes by members of the most privileged. This article became a chapter (entitled "Cheaper Than Chimpanzees") in her 1973 book, *Kind and Usual Punishment,* a dissection of the U.S. prison system.

Soon afterward, Senator Edward Kennedy held hearings that led to the National Commission for the Protection of Biomedical and Behavioral Research (CPBBR), which investigated medical experimentation on prisoners. It considered banning such research outright, as most other Western industrialized countries had done decades earlier. Despite headlines such as GOVERNMENT TO BAN MEDICAL RESEARCH ON FEDERAL INMATES, it decided against this in 1976, partly because not only pharmaceutical companies but also many prisoners opposed a ban.[42] Inmates wished to have the opportunity to participate for several reasons: They could make real money no other way, they sometimes could obtain health care no other way, they missed the safety and amenities of the research laboratory, and they wanted to feel they were contributing to society. In 1979, State Prison of Southern Michigan inmates even filed suit to prevent the FDA from excluding them from research studies.

Instead of banning prison research outright, the CPBBR proposed a detailed accreditation scheme that Secretary of Health, Education, and Welfare Joseph Califano, in consultation with the American Correctional Association, rejected as impractical.

In 1978, HEW produced stringent human-experimentation regulations, which remain in effect today.[43] So did the CPBBR's 1979 report, known as the Belmont Report, which placed the onus on researchers for ensuring that research with prisoners provides informed consent and is therapeutic under what is called the "Common Rule." The Common Rule sets strict limits on nontherapeutic research and research done with prisoners and requires the review of proposed studies by institutional review boards. No study in a prison can present more than a "minimal" risk to the inmate.

In sum, there remain four types of permissible prison research: that on the cause and effect of incarceration and crime; the study of prisons or of incarcerated persons; investigations of conditions that affect prisoners en masse; and therapeutic studies. Although these reforms were necessary and laudable, they are imperfect, especially because the language is vague: What, for example, constitutes "minimal risk"? Even the definition of "therapeutic research" has come into question. Still, research at most prisons, including Holmesburg, ceased by 1976 as a result of public outrage and lawsuits.

Research Renaissance

Most people don't realize that prison medical research, which all but died out in the 1970s, is enjoying a quiet renaissance. Since the late 1980s, investigators in Arkansas, Maryland, South Carolina, Texas, Florida, Connecticut, and Rhode Island have been conducting and proposing research in prisons.

Even more crucial to understand than the past exploitation of

African Americans in prisons is the future medical use and possible abuse of African Americans, because they are the single fastest-growing group in prison populations.[44] Today, research with prisoners means research with blacks, because in 2004 African Americans constituted 44 to 46 percent of all prisoners, which is almost four times their proportion of the general population; clearly, prison experimental abuse is likely to affect African Americans disproportionately.[45] Thanks in large part to mandatory sentencing for drug infractions, women are not spared: Black women make up the fastest-growing population in American prisons.[46] The HIV pandemic and the more recently recognized hepatitis C epidemic have attracted federal dollars and the support of pharmaceutical companies. This has renewed the interest in prisoners as subjects, because 17 percent of the incarcerated have HIV, six times the rate on the outside. Because most HIV-positive people in the United States—and in U.S. prisons—are black, the question of HIV research in prisons is a question of blacks being used in such research.

For hepatitis C virus (HCV), the statistics are even more dire: Inmates have the highest HCV infection rate in the country. Two percent of all Americans but 20 percent of inmates are HCV-infected.[47] For imprisoned black men, the HCV infection rate is much higher, as high as 60 percent. But prison research today is not restricted to these ailments, because inmates suffering from disorders ranging from asthma to cancer have attracted the attention of U.S. researchers, who are conducting ten thousand biomedical research programs. Most of these researchers are funded by the Department of Health and Human Services (HHS), which, for example, supports the Yale School of Medicine with $178.7 million and the University of Miami Medical Center with $191 million.

In 1999, Brown University researchers even mounted a lawsuit to gain access to prisons for HIV research. They cited the high rates of HIV and other infectious diseases in prisons and the need of inmates for cutting-edge treatments, casting their desire to do research as a plea for therapy.[48] They are correct in pointing out that too little attention has been paid to prisoners' health. As early as 1962, physicians complained of a dearth of medical care and therapeutic research aimed at prisoners' ills.[49]

But why, if securing badly needed AIDS, TB, and hepatitis C therapy is the goal, do proposed prison medical programs focus upon the theoretical benefits of research rather than on the known demonstrated benefits of the best available therapy? Few jailed men receive the standard of care for AIDS and HCV, such as protease inhibitors, HAART therapy, or interferon for hepatitis C. Prisons have even failed to take simple public-health measures to reduce the high incidence of anal rape and blood-borne contamination and to restore infectious-disease control to prisons, which would also seem to be a cornerstone of any HIV, HCV, or TB eradication policy.[50]

Brown University researchers have conflated HIV treatment and experimentation, leading one to question whether the real concern is for prisoners' health or whether researchers wish to resume the lucrative jailhouse research of yesterday. The pharmaceutical industry requires research with humans, and the nation's 45,000 researchers are hungrily eyeing the two million Americans behind bars. Today, arguments over the ethical codes have been replaced by utilitarian rationales focusing upon the medical benefits to society and invoking the vague "right" of prisoners to experimentation.

But is prison research, which will take place disproportionately with African Americans, really likely to focus upon therapy and to benefit prisoners?[51] Or will experimental treatments again expose prisoners to dangerous illegal medical risks, despite the federal regulations? Perhaps the best indication of researchers' actual intentions is a glance at some current protocols for research initiatives in American prisons. Researchers are currently conducting studies that involve inducing labor in pregnant inmates, testing different methods of obtaining biopsies, conducting a clinical trial of an experimental HIV vaccine, testing delivery of a potent new cancer chemotherapy agent directly into the liver, and artifically inducing hyperthermia to treat lung cancer. A *St. Petersburg Times* report offered direct evidence that some of the "therapeutic" HIV approaches with HIV-positive inmates may not be centered on the inmates' need for therapy, because participating inmates complained that they felt coerced to participate in such studies and agreed to do so only in order "to escape poor medical care, abusive conditions and lack of access to up-to-date HIV drugs at other Florida prisons."

One particularly troubling study among those mentioned above is Dr. Joseph Zwishenberger's radical new approach to lung cancer, which is to heat the subjects' blood to a temperature where the errant cancer cells theoretically would not thrive. To test his theory, he sedates inmates and connects them to a machine called the BioLogic HT System, which removes blood via venous and cervical tubes. The blood is heated, then returned to the inmate's body, which is kept at a very dangerous elevated temperature of 108.5 degrees. Any adult taken to a hospital with a temperature of 105 degrees would be considered an emergency case and cooling strategies would immediately be undertaken, but in Zwishenberger's protocol, inmates' 108.5 temperatures are sustained for two hours. Subjects sign a consent form that lists death, seizures, congestive heart failure, burns, heart attack, and limb loss as possible complications. Even if the subjects are in a late stage of lung cancer, where the cure rates are infinitesimal, this doesn't excuse such a risky procedure. Although putatively therapeutic, this research surely poses greater than "minimal risk." The consent form includes a waiver that states in part, "I understand that I cannot receive financial remuneration for any injuries resulting from my participation in this project." However, the law specifically prohibits language in an informed-consent document that appears to waive a subject's rights or to release an investigator from liability for negligence or assault.

In July 2000, the Office of Human Research Protections (OHRP) suspended three hundred studies by the University of Texas Medical Branch (UTMB) in Galveston, including Zwishenberger's, after the researchers flouted federal regulations. One hundred and ninety-five of these studies, mostly HIV and AIDS trials, were conducted in Texas prisons, according to the *Austin American-Statesman.* In a September 14, 2000, letter, the OHRP listed numerous UTMB research projects conducted outside of the permissible categories for prison research and cited "scant evidence" that Galveston's institutional review board had adhered to federal law.

The OHRP had approved more than four hundred federally funded studies with prisoners since 2000, but when it froze the UTMB's research projects, a chill once again crept over prison research. However, now that the inmate population has leapt from 200,000 in the 1970s to 2 million, researchers once again seek entrance to prisons, wishing to undertake a wider range of medical studies.

The Institute of Medicine, which provides the federal government guidance on biomedical issues, has appointed the Committee on Ethical

Considerations for Protection of Prisoners Involved in Research to study the issue. It is headed by the brilliant public-health law scholar Lawrence O. Gostin, J.D., professor and director of the Center for Law and the Public's Health at Johns Hopkins and Georgetown universities. The committee will determine whether it is possible to ensure true informed consent in prisons, and whether research on prisoners should be confined to the therapeutic realm. As this book went to press in late 2006, Gostin's group was still weighing the relaxation of the regulations that have muted medical research in prisons since the 1970s, and decisions may result in dramatic modification of prison research policy as early as 2007. If the doors are flung wide to investigators, will they admit in therapy or exploitation?

How can we best protect sick prisoners, many of whom are black, from abusive research without completely banning prison research? As early as 1999, Anne S. De Groot, M.D., suggested that the best way to give prisoners with AIDS access to cutting-edge clinical studies while protecting them from abuse is to ensure that research is done only in prisons that already provide high-quality medical care. This way, prisoners can participate in research without feeling forced into trials.[52]

However, this chapter has demonstrated that the laws enacted to protect prisoners' rights and health consistently have failed to do so. There are no guarantees that today's promises of humane therapeutic research, which often conflates research and care, will protect inmates more effectively. Until American medicine achieves a better record of providing care while avoiding abuse, an utter ban on prison research may be the only protection. However, prisoners are not the only group of African Americans who live with the threat of being involuntarily subjected to research in the name of therapy. The next chapter chronicles the plight of black children who are forced into service as experimental subjects.

CHAPTER 11

THE CHILDREN'S CRUSADE

Research Targets Young African Americans

What's done to children, they will do to society.
—KARL A. MENNINGER, M.D

Like many other parents struggling to bring up children in Brooklyn's Bedford-Stuyvesant area, Charisse Johnson and her husband felt besieged. Neighborhood children ran a gauntlet of ne'er-do-wells and drug dealers on their way to school, and bullets wounded even the innocent who ventured out after dusk. Gang members hounded young children. Her greatest fear was losing her sons to the streets. Already, her sixteen-year-old was being held in a detention center in upstate New York. Was he on a slippery slope to adult incarceration? She felt he must avoid this at all costs.

Shortly afterward, in 1992, representatives from Columbia University appeared at Johnson's door, explaining that they wanted her other son, six-year-old Isaac, to go to its hospital for a series of simple interviews and tests, culminating in a onetime overnight stay involving a single dose of harmless medication. The worker explained that Columbia University was offering a safe free test for Isaac in order to discover whether he might have any medical problems. They would pay her approximately one hundred dollars, and they had something for Isaac, as well—a gift certificate for Toys "R" Us—*if* he agreed to participate.

Johnson hesitated briefly, but eventually she signed.[1] She explained why during a congressional hearing:

> At first I did not understand how and from what source they obtained my name and knew I had a six-year-old son. I later came to the conclusion that this information came to them because of my

16-year-old son's involvement with the juvenile justice system.
Needless to say, I decided to cooperate with the experimenters.
I felt at the time that if they could find me and knew I had a six
year old son they had enough power to affect the wellbeing of my
sixteen year old son who was being held in a detention facility.

American medicine has not spared black children its very worst
abuses in the name of scientific research. This chapter will discuss some
of the many experiments that recruited black children primarily or exclusively, that stigmatized black children, and whose agendas were
specifically racial. These have harmed not only children but also the image of all African Americans.

Over a decade ago, Isaac became ensnared in such a research initiative tailored specifically for children of color. Between 1992 and 1997,
New York City's New York State Psychiatric Institute (NYSPI) and Columbia University's Lowenstein Center for the Study and Prevention of
Childhood Disruptive Behavior Disorders conducted several research
studies that sought to establish a link between genetics and violence.
They performed experiments upon at least 126 boys, most of whom were
between the ages of six and ten, utilizing the drug fenfluramine. Columbia described the population of boys who were given the drug as 44 percent black and 56 percent Hispanic, but this is misleading: Hispanic is an
ethnic category, encompassing people of white, black, and mixed race,
and "all the 'Hispanic' boys lived in the Washington Heights area and
were black Dominicans," observed Rudy M. Brown, Charisse Johnson's
lawyer. The boys were all black, and this was by design: The experimental protocol specifies that eligible participants must be "African American or Hispanic" and specifically excludes whites from participation.[2] In
1998, I asked psychiatrist Timothy Walsh, M.D., who headed the institutional review board (IRB) that approved the study, why. He explained
that the protocol simply reflected the ethnic component of Columbia
Medical Center's nearby catchment area, from which it drew its subjects.
But this is untrue: Not only are there numerous white enclaves in Washington Heights but some of the black boys, including Isaac Johnson,
were drawn from as far away as Brooklyn.

The boys had something in common besides their dark skins: As
Charisse Johnson suspected, they had been selected because their older

brothers had had contact with the probation system. Although it is illegal to breach the confidentiality of juvenile court records in this manner, a Department of Probation internal memo dated August 30, 1991, states: "We are participating in a Research project being conducted by Professor Gail Wasserman of Columbia University, regarding younger brothers of male offenders in an effort to identify early predictors of antisocial behavior."[3] The probation department identified them to researchers.[4]

Researchers sought to investigate whether violent behavior might run in families and to identify a biological basis for such behavior. The researchers claimed that the drug fenfluramine could suggest a genetic basis for aggressive or violent behavior in boys because it is a precursor of the neurotransmitter serotonin. Abnormal serotonin levels are implicated in many psychological states.

Administering fenfluramine once or for a very short period normally causes one's serotonin levels to increase, which in turn increases the amount of the hormone prolactin in the blood. The researchers measured the blood prolactin to indirectly assess how much serotonin levels rose. But if prolactin levels increased too dramatically in response, this suggested to Columbia researchers a biological brain dysfunction that may signal a tendency toward aggression. On the strength of this tenuous connection, the investigators claimed that by monitoring how precipitously the boys' prolactin levels increased after an infusion of fenfluramine, they could measure the boys' propensity for aggressive behavior.[5] Why not simply measure the boys' serotonin levels? This might not reveal pathology, because the blood serotonin concentration might not reflect brain levels. Prolactin, however, is produced only in the central nervous system.

But Wasserman and her colleagues claimed that another risk factor fed the boys' purported violent propensities: bad parenting. Black boys were fated to be the violent products of "parental psychopathology" or "adverse rearing environments." Why? According to the researchers, because of their poverty and their ethnicity. To bolster this deterministic claim, researchers interviewed parents to establish their worthiness—or lack thereof. But the interviewers were hardly "blind," or objective: they knew that the researchers sought evidence of pathological child rearing and of aggressive or violent propensities. As Charisse Johnson recalled, "[on] the campus of Columbia University, we were subjected to a series of intimate, degrading questions, tests and interviews.[6] The experimenters also took advantage of my fears for the well-being of my sixteen-year-old son to intrude on the privacy of my home."

After such interviews, psychological assessments, and physical screenings, the researchers winnowed the original 126 study candidates to 66 boys, including Isaac, in several related fenfluramine studies. They did this by carefully selecting only those boys who were perfectly healthy, both physically and mentally, and did not display signs of questionable behavior. Thirty-four of the boys in Isaac's group were given fenfluramine.

If the drug fenfluramine sounds familiar, it is because it constituted half of the notoriously cardiotoxic Fen-Phen weight-loss combination introduced to the U.S. market in 1973, associated with heart-valve damage and deaths among dieters in the 1990s.[7] By the time the FDA banned it in 1997, concern was also circulating among physicians about the brain damage that low doses of fenfluramine induced in experimental animals.[8] Medical reports of these injuries circulated well before the FDA ban and during Columbia's studies.[9]

American researchers have focused intense scrutiny into the genetics of violence among black boys. To their families and communities, the "index cases" (who first bring a family to the researchers' attention)—including Isaac's older brother—might have been misbehaving, acting out, or testing boundaries by breaking minor laws against fighting and shoplifting. However, to Walsh and his colleagues, they were mentally ill. University psychiatrists had diagnosed these boys with such psychiatric ailments as conduct disorder, oppositional defiant disorder, and attention-deficit hyperactivity disorder, diagnoses that describe children's disagreeable behaviors and that are often assigned to children who break the law. Such a psychiatric diagnosis, whether it describes an actual mental illness or not, can consign a child to a limbo between the law and psychiatric medicine, making him vulnerable to stigmatization by both. In fact, one legal observer, Leonard Glantz, remarked, "Indeed, it appears the only 'diagnosis' these children had was the one conferred on them by the investigators."[10] Such a diagnosis also moves a child from the free world of the normal into the civil rights desert of the mentally ill.

The press raised a hue and cry when it discovered the nature of the experiment but failed to recognize it as part of a pattern: This was just one of many psychiatric experiments in a movement to expand diagnoses of mental illness from one family member to others by positing a putative genetic root of the illness, often on very thin evidence. At institutions such as the Harvard School of Public Health, the brothers and sisters of schizophrenics have been closely scrutinized and labeled with mental illness in initiatives that aim to "expand the phenotype" (the physical or mental manifestations of a genetic condition) of schizophrenia. Because the focus is upon identifying, not treating the putative disorders, such experiments are powerfully stigmatizing.

In the cases of Isaac and others, scientists wished to discover whether these boys shared their brothers' purported violent tendencies and the so-called mean gene. To accomplish this, the researchers did much more than simply give the boys a dose of fenfluramine. More than a dozen of the boys were withdrawn from all their medications for a month, including medications for such life-threatening chronic conditions as asthma. For four days, they ate a special low-monoamine diet (basically a low-protein diet), because monoamines affect serotonin levels. The boys were hospitalized the night before, and once they were out of sight of their parents, food was withheld for the duration of the experiment; the next morning, water was withheld, as well. At 8:30 A.M., physicians inserted a catheter and gave each boy fenfluramine hydrochloride by mouth.

Fenfluramine had never been given to children under twelve before this experiment began. Ninety percent of adults given a single dose experience side effects ranging from anxiety, fatigue, headache, light-headedness, difficulty concentrating, visual impairment, diarrhea, nausea, irritability, to a feeling of being "high." Up to 30 percent of adults who take fenfluramine develop heart-valve damage, and it can trigger a life-threatening form of high blood pressure called pulmonary hypertension.[11] One boy complained of a severe headache and others complained of light-headedness, but they were not released.

Beginning at 10:00 A.M., blood was drawn hourly from the boys' catheters and tested to determine fluctuations in serotonin.[12]

The researchers' claim that serotonin levels reveal aggressive tendencies is based upon questionable science. Walsh characterized the causal association of serotonin levels and aggression as "widely accepted," which is incorrect: The correlation has been heavily criticized. In a 1996 *Journal of Neurogenetics* article, Dr. E. Balaban illuminated the specious nature of the research behind the genetics of aggressiveness when he conducted a devastating meta-analysis of thirty-nine scientific studies.

It revealed that no relationship between serotonin and violence was sustained anywhere in the body of research.

> The results confirm an association between low 5-HIAA [a serotonin metabolite] levels and psychiatric disorders, but fail to support any specific relationship between low 5-HIAA levels and impulsive aggression or criminality. It is premature and misleading to speak of "mean genes" (Hen 1996) or a specific neurochemistry of aggressive behavior.[13]

The fictive nature of this cherished correlation proved merely the first layer of logical and design error. Leaving aside for a moment the egregious *social* fallout of selecting only black and Hispanic boys, this racial selection also created a serious *scientific* error. When only one ethnicity is considered in an experiment to elicit general information about a heterogeneous population, an unacknowledged set of socioeconomic variables are introduced. The boys were not only darker but poorer, and they also lived in less healthy physical environments than do most white boys. This distortion is magnified when the majority group is excluded. Most American boys are white, so excluding white boys is a very serious scientific misstep. Furthermore, the study design described no control group, a staple of such research. Finally, the researchers gave no coherent explanation of how they proposed to dissect any serotonergic effects of genetics from those caused by supposedly "adverse rearing."

The experimental results should have dealt a death blow to this sloppily conceived and executed research, because the boys who were ostensibly predisposed to aggression and violence by their adverse rearing and biological propensities actually exhibited normal or *elevated* serotonin levels in response to the brief fenfluramine challenge.[14] However, Wasserman's group responded by reversing themselves: until the mid-1990s, they stated that low serotonin levels are a marker for violent propensities in children, and after their 1997 study, they wrote that elevated levels signal violent propensities.

These scientific errors were legion, but it is difficult to know where to begin in listing the ethical outrages of this study, and it is very hard to believe that it was conducted fairly recently by of one of the nation's most prestigious universities. The experiment is rife with instances of undue inducement, from baiting children with $25 toy certificates to luring their parents with $100, no insignificant sum on the streets of Washington Heights and Bedford-Stuyvesant.[15]

Such racial selection could stigmatize not only the participants but all black and Hispanic boys as "born criminals." The element of stigmatization is key in understanding certain racial disparities in research with children, because such research is not an egregious exception for black children; rather, it is the norm. In 2003, the journal *Pediatrics* published an analysis by University of Chicago researchers of 192 research studies in major U.S. pediatric journals between July 1999 and June 2000. The authors found that "when compared with research participation of child subjects, generally, black children were overrepresented and Hispanic children were underrepresented in clinical trials, and both were underrepresented in therapeutic research. Black and Hispanic children were overrepresented in potentially stigmatizing research." From 52 to 54 percent of the children in nontherapeutic studies were white; this number was far lower than their 69–73 percent representation in the population. In contrast, 26–32 percent of child subjects of nontherapeutic studies are black, twice to almost three times their (13 percent) presence in the population.[16]

An element of intimidation, if not coercion, was introduced by the use of juvenile justice system officers to identify subjects to the medical researchers. Middle-class white Americans may appreciate police and probation officers as guardians who "serve and protect," but inner-city blacks often have hostile relationships with police. These important abuses raise the question of whether it is morally right to use healthy children in a study that is nontherapeutic, dangerous, and stigmatizing. The Department of Health and Human Services (DHHS) would seem to prohibit this. Its Code of Federal Regulations (CFR), title 45, part 46, governs the protection of human experimental subjects and specifically prohibits experiments on healthy children that convey more than "minimal risk."[17] "I would contend that fasting, hospitalization, low monoamine diet, fenfluramine challenge, serial blood sampling, and exhaustive psychological and educational testing, is clearly more than minimal risk," observed Ernest D. Prentice, Ph.D., associate dean for research at the University of Nebraska. "That protocol was not approvable under the regulations."[18] When the Hearing Committee on Governmental Reform and Oversight convened to examine the FDA role in the fenfluramine research, Dr. Walsh, chair of the NYSPI IRB, defended the study by invoking "the recent deadly shootings at schools across our country." John Oldham, NYSPI executive director, shared these concerns. "With the disasters in Littleton and elsewhere, it has become abundantly clear that studies of aggressive behavior in children are imperative."[19] However, the shootings in question had been carried out by white boys, who were clearly troubled and violent, but who were specifically excluded from these studies in favor of children of color. Why were such studies not conducted in suburban or rural, mostly white school systems?

Despite the violation of confidentiality, the undue inducement, the medically risky nontherapeutic research on healthy children that clearly violated federal guidelines, and the racially discriminatory recruitment, the Office for Protection from Research Risks (OPRR) investigation exonerated the research institutions. This sent a clear message that no penalties would be ascribed to dangerous research if it were conducted on black children, declared lawyer and children's advocate Cliff Zucker. "In cities like New York where the poor are disproportionately minorities, OPRR's decision has a discriminatory impact on children of color. These children will be subject to experiments that may not be conducted on middle-class or Caucasian children."

A 2004 study revealed that the fenfluramine experiments may have damaged more than these children's physical health and legal rights. A relatively low single dose of the drug has been implicated in brain damage in humans as well as in animals. Fenfluramine may actually trigger such behavior changes as increased aggression.[20] Sadly, this is not news to Charisse Johnson and Isaac.

Two weeks after he was given the drug he started having sharp painful headaches. Then as the headaches became more unbearable, he started having anxiety attacks and hyperventilating. He would start gasping for breath as if he couldn't breathe, as with someone who was having an asthma attack. . . . He started having horrible nightmares. He would wake up in the night screaming, thinking that someone was in his room. To this day my son continues to suffer the severe consequences of the reckless disregard for him as a human being by those experimenters. To them, he was just another guinea pig.

Johnson has filed a lawsuit for the violation of Isaac's rights. And the other boys? Daniel S. Pine, M.D., the study's principal investigator, told New York's *Amsterdam News* in 1998 that "families overwhelmingly reported that the research experience was a positive one." But no family members have come forward in response to legal and media requests, so we cannot know whether their children suffered serious side effects from the drug. Johnson's lawyer, Rudy Brown, believes that the other families are intimidated by the OPRR decision and the juvenile justice system, too afraid of what might happen to the older brothers of the subjects should they speak out. And, despite Johnson's insight and courage, justice has proven elusive for her, as well. Her civil suit for sixty million dollars against the city, the researchers, the NYSPI, and Columbia-Presbyterian Hospital alleged breach of confidentiality and civil rights violations. But it languished for three years in the teeming files of Judge George B. Daniels of federal district court in Manhattan. Daniels, who is black, was profiled by the *New York Times* in December 2004 as the "unchallenged king of delayed decisions," with 289 civil-case motions pending for longer than six months—more than any other judge in the nation. By the time Brown was able to force a decision through the appellate court in November 2003, Isaac was seventeen, and Columbia was released as a defendant. As this book went to press, Johnson's case was scheduled for late 2006.

The fenfluramine experiments are not without precedent. Thirty years earlier, the National Institutes of Mental Health's Center for Crime and Delinquency awarded a three-year $300,000 grant to Digamber Borgaonkar, Ph.D. Under the aegis of Johns Hopkins University,[21] he undertook a large study to investigate whether adolescent boys, many of whom were wards of Maryland's juvenile justice system, gave indications of a genetic anomaly, XYY.[22]

The XYY syndrome was first discovered in 1961 when Dr. A. Sandberg described a six-foot white male who exhibited no mental or physical abnormalities but who had an unusual chromosomal complement, called an aneuploidy. This condition affected not the workaday somatic chromosomes but the sex chromosomes that determine maleness and femaleness. A normal male inherits one X chromosome from his mother and one Y chromosome from his father (women inherit two X's, one from each parent), but this man's karyotype, or chromosome chart, showed that he had one X and two Y's, an accident of reproduction.[23] The man looked normal except for his height, a little extra abdominal girth, and troubled skin. Most XYY males look so normal that they tend to be detected by accident while doctors are looking for something else. The mere presence of a genetic variation such as XYY does not necessarily result in any appreciable difference in physiology or behavior, but visceral reactions about the presence of two Y chromosomes led scientists to postulate that such men "must" be supermales possessed of unusual degrees of aggressiveness. For example, in 1973, Dr. L. F. Jarvik opined in the pages of the *Journal of the American Medical Association* that "the Y chromosome is the male determining chromosome, therefore it should come out as no surprise that an extra Y chromosome can produce an individual with heightened masculinity, evinced by characteristics such as unusual tallness, increased fertility . . . and powerful aggressive tendencies."[24]

A wealth of other differences were quickly ascribed to XYY as well, including low intelligence, abdominal fat, large teeth, and acne. But by the mid-1970s, only tallness, adult acne, and abdominal fat persisted as demonstrated XYY traits.

The belief that XYY males, with their extra Y chromosome, were aggressive, even violent, and more likely to become criminals than genetically normal males was bolstered by a finding that XYY males were also found in mental penal institutions at a higher rate than other men.[25] The XYY males were not imprisoned for violent crimes or found more frequently in *regular* prisons than were the typical XY males.

Borgaonkar sought to discover the prevalence of XYY males in the U.S. population and to determine whether the XYY genetic anomaly might be responsible for aggressiveness and violent behavior. To do this, he selected 6,000 boys, approximately 85 percent of whom were black, and most of whom were housed in Maryland state institutions for abandoned or delinquent children. He also selected 500 more affluent boys in Edgemeade, a Maryland private psychiatric treatment center, 80 percent of whom were white.[26]

For "normal" controls, the investigators selected 7,500 East Baltimore boys who were enrolled in a free child-care program at Johns Hopkins University. These boys lived in a housing project for low-income families that was 95 percent black.[27]

Like the fenfluramine victims, these boys were subjected to stigmatizing testing, psychological assessments, and blood draws in a three-year experiment that could brand them as latent criminals for life. Parents were told that the blood samples were taken to test for anemia and other medical problems, but it was actually drawn to screen for boys with the extra Y chromosome that made them XYY males instead of normal XY males.

As with the fenfluramine study, the justice system played an active role in study recruitment. A *Washington Daily News* article observed, "Maryland juvenile court probation officers will probably be used to persuade resisting parents to sign a permission [slip] for them to take a blood sample."[28]

No evidence had been offered of genetic assortment of XYY by race, yet racially distinct populations of boys were selected. Approximately 85 percent were African American at a time when African Americans constituted only 10.8 percent of the population. This means that had an association been proven between XYY males and violence, it would have emerged from the data as an association between black boys with XYY and violence. What's more, Borgaonkar often culled his subjects from incarcerated populations and no evidence of consent, written or verbal, was found for most of the enrolled boys.

The XYY study suffered from the same glaring logical flaws as the fenfluramine study.[29] Similar XYY dragnets were instituted using black infants in New York City and in Boston, supported by Harvard University.[30] But in Boston, ethically responsible researchers were able to derail the study before it began. One of the most effective and vocal critics was pioneering Harvard University geneticist Jonathan Beckwith, who declared, "The whole premise of the study was based on terribly faulty science."[31]

It seems strange that accomplished scientists at several major universities would embrace science that was so deeply flawed. However, if one looks beyond the narrowly stated purpose of the studies to the real utility of any data that might result from them, a logical reason emerges for this apparent design error, because a darker logic lurks behind the studies' selection of black males. The studies fit the period's pattern of intense focus on violence in black populations. Between 1960 and 1972, fed by the baby boom, U.S. crime rates soared exponentially. After 1967, the relatively peaceful civil rights movement gave way to spurts of urban violence—race riots—which escalated after the 1968 slaying of the Rev. Martin Luther King, Jr. Some researchers reacted by medicalizing this violence.

Beginning in the 1970s, the Centers for Disease Control (CDC) reported that annual homicide rates for young African-American males were from five to eight times greater than those for young white males. These data have led to conclusions that violence is a peculiarly African American problem; but such conclusions tend to ignore how racism and poverty confound the relationship between violence and race. They also ignore the fact that violence is an American problem, not an African American one. The United States is the industrialized world's most violent society; Scotland is a distant second, with a murder rate that is only one-fourth of the U.S. rate.

The trend toward the medicalization of violence in blacks fed the popularity of genetic violence studies of black boys, but nature failed to cooperate with the politics. Borgaonkar's research and subsequent studies determined that XYY, the supposed marker for violence, is a "white" marker, not a "black" one, in that it is found more commonly in white men than in blacks. If the extra chromosome were indeed the "violence gene," white men would be from 1.5 to 3 times as likely to harbor a propensity for violence.[32] But it is not. No scientific basis for any propensity to violence or criminality in XYY males was found, and the theory, which was always thin and circumstantial, was discredited. However, the XYY theory of hypermale criminality still thrives in popular culture because the news media, which had widely trumpeted the "criminal gene" controversy, largely failed to publicize the findings that exonerated XYY. As a result, people still think of XYY men as harboring a "criminal gene." Journalists muse on the chromosomal status of the serial killer du jour and such murderers as Richard Speck and Arthur Shawcross have often raised a supposed XYY anomaly as a defense in murder trials, sometimes successfully.[33] Novels and films celebrate hypermales, such as those in the film *Alien 3*, whose prison planet is populated by "double Y-chromo" felons so violent that they require off-world incarceration.

Racially discriminating recruitment strategies in the search for the criminal gene helped to solidify a precedent of using captive or coerced populations of African American children, a sparsely examined subtext of American experimental design.

We cannot excuse the XYY experiments by suggesting that no rules forbade such experiments. By 1970, HEW regulations required informed consent be obtained before any federally funded project used humans as research subjects. Johns Hopkins University's policy also required it. In

1961, the relevant rule read, in part, "Persons retained in prisons, penitentiaries or reformatories—being captive groups—should not be used [as] subjects of experimentation, nor persons incapable of giving consent because of age, mental capacity or of being in a position where they are incapable of exercising the power of free choice." The boys in the XYY study fell into most of these protected groups.

Although they were separated by nearly thirty years, the fenfluramine and XYY experiments had much in common. Both sought biological determinants of violence and both chose to look no further than very young black boys with no history of mental illness or of violent or criminal behavior. A minority of white boys with psychiatric problems were victimized in Baltimore, as well. Both studies were nontherapeutic, invasive experiments that could brand boys, via poorly constructed experimental protocols, as potential criminals for life. The fact that these experiments were approved by investigational review boards is especially chilling evidence that IRBs have not afforded the desired protections.

The 1970s XYY experiment and the fenfluramine experiments of the 1990s were simply nodes in a continuous series of abusive experimentation that reflected the social realities of segregation and discrimination. Scientists loaded the statistical dice in the simplest manner—by testing blacks exclusively—to locate the supposed biological propensity toward violence in the hereditary apparatus of blacks[34] "But," as the late naturalist Stephen Jay Gould mused, "why should the violent behavior of some desperate and discouraged people point to a specific disorder of their brain while the corruption and violence of some congressmen and presidents provokes no similar theory?"

Perhaps the answer lies not in the scientific philosophy but in the social effects of such research. Locating black violence in the genetic complement of black boys nourishes excuses to abandon social therapeutic approaches. What good is better education, better nutrition, safe, clean housing, social and psychological support, and a more nurturing home and school environment to a born monster? But this hereditarianism fallacy is specious.[35] An inborn racial propensity to violence has often been postulated but has never been demonstrated, despite a bewildering variety of attempts. Even if such a tendency were discovered, it would in no way negate the mitigating value of social, psychological, and educational interventions, certainly not without trying them first.

Murder of the Black Mind

But another medical trend fueled by the "born criminal" image posed a much more immediate danger to boys: crude, often experimental brain surgeries, backed by a quite coarse understanding of brain function, to excise the alleged seat of violence. Between 1936 and 1960, an estimated fifty thousand lobotomies severed neuronal connections between the frontal lobes and the midbrain of mental patients, both adults and children. Psychiatrists and neurosurgeons who practiced these "blind-cut" lobotomies simply inserted crude tools such as the icepickalon and blindly swept them back and forth within the brain, cutting all the connecting nerves, sight unseen, at one fell swoop. Nothing could be more violent than this clumsy and nightmarish destruction of brain tissue. These acts of unbelievable surgical hostility, which obliterated a child's very seat of thought, ability, and personality— nothing less than a murder of the mind—were forced upon black boys as young as five.[36]

From the 1960s through the early 1970s, disenchantment with the widespread use of tranquilizers fostered interest in brain surgery as an alternative to "quiet" patients.[37] University of Mississippi neurosurgeon Orlando J. Andy, M.D., capitalized on this trend, performing many types of brain ablations, including thalamotomies (destruction of the thalamus, which controls emotions and analyzes sensations),[38] on African American children as young as six who, he decided, were "aggressive" and "hyperactive." Witness his published approach to the behavior of a child he refers to as "J.M.":

> J.M., a boy of 9, had seizures and behavioral disorder (hyperactive, aggressive, combative, explosive, destructive, sadistic).
> Bilateral thalamotomy was done, left (January 12, 1962) right (January 20, 1962). Right thalamotomy was repeated on September 16, 1962. The patient's behavior was markedly improved and enabled him to return to special education school. After one year, symptoms of hyperirritability, aggressiveness, negativism, and combativeness slowly reappeared. A fornicotomy [removal of a fornix, a small paired brain structure that connects areas of the brain that are key to emotions] was performed on January 15, 1965.

Impaired memory for recent events developed and the patient became much more irritable, negativistic and combative [emphasis added].

Consequently, a simultaneous bilateral thalamotomy was done one month later, on February 16, 1965. The patient has again adjusted to his environments and has displayed marked improvement in behavior and memory.[39]

Andy removed six areas of the boy's brain in five surgeries over three years, areas that were then known to be important to emotions, expression, and cognitive function. He also implanted electrodes in the child's brain in a vague, unspecified experimental venture. The surgeon did not explain how he arrived at his assessment of J.M.'s "behavior disorder" and why he thought the extreme remedy of brain surgery was indicated. Therefore, we do not know whether the child had serious behavior problems or whether he was exhibiting the same annoying behaviors displayed by most nine-year-old boys at some point. Andy is not a psychiatrist and J.M. received no bona fide psychiatric diagnosis. We have no description of the effects or duration of the child's behavior, nor what his parents thought of it. There is no indication that the parents were informed of the surgery or whether their permission was asked.

In short, Andy did not even take the trouble to convince us that J.M. needed medical intervention of any kind, to say nothing of having parts of his brain removed. In pondering these shocking acts, it is important to remember that Andy wrote up this case in medical journals—twice—because he was proud of it as an example of his best work.

According to Andy's own chronology, the fornicotomy appears to have caused memory impairment, combativeness, and other unwelcome behavior changes. Andy's response was to remove more brain tissue, which left the child "adjusted" with "marked improvement in behavior." The boy may have been "adjusted" because he had too little brain function left to irritate anyone. Andy seems to have consigned most of J.M.'s personality to the wastebasket, and he expressed concern only with the purported behavior problems: He never mentioned the seizure disorder after the first line. Andy often boasted of his successes in controlling children with such surgeries, but a subsequent report on J.M.'s progress noted that "intellectually, however, the patient is deteriorating."

These surgeries, performed throughout the South by white neurosurgeons like Andy, are imbued with racist barbarity. The unacceptable behavior of black boys (girls are rarely mentioned in the juvenile psychosurgery literature of the period) triggers neither psychotherapy nor counseling, but a violent medical response. The child's "unacceptable" behavior must also be considered in the context of the very narrow range of acceptable behaviors for black men and boys in the segregated South. When the 1955 lynching case of Emmett Till was reopened in 2004, it reminded us that young black boys could be savagely tortured and murdered on suspicion of whistling at a white woman. What transgressions triggered Andy's characterization of a nine-year-old as so unacceptable that the appropriate response was to cut out portions of his brain repeatedly? The surgeon leaves this to one's reeling imagination. Today, Andy is revered as a neurosurgical pioneer, one whose work was never challenged in his lifetime and who never suffered any disciplinary action. This may have reflected the powerlessness of his institutionalized black subjects in pre-civil-rights-era Mississippi, or it may reflect the white male perspective of segregated Mississippi neurosurgery in the 1960s, or both.

However, Andy did not restrict his lobotomy recommendations to black children. He also observed that "the kind of brain damage that could necessitate such radical surgery might be manifested by participation in the Watts Uprising." Its rioters, he hypothesized, "could have abnormal pathological brains."[40]

He was not alone in this conjecture, as brain destruction was employed not only for misbehaving black boys but to ensure the docility of prisoners and, in the 1960s, as a government-funded cure for urban rioters. Three American physicians proposed that such urban uprisings were caused by men who could be cured by psychosurgery. Dr. Vernon Mark, director of neurosurgery at Boston City Hospital, and his colleagues Drs. Frank Ervin and William Sweet swept aside social factors such as poverty, slum housing, and poor education in a 1967 proposal in the *Journal of the American Medical Association*:

> The obviousness of these causes may have blinded us to the more subtle role of other possible factors, *including brain dysfunction* [emphasis added]. . . . The real lesson of the urban rioting is that, besides the need to study the social fabric that creates the riot at-

mosphere, we need intensive research and clinical studies of the individuals committing the violence . . . to pinpoint, diagnose and treat these people with low violence thresholds before they contribute to further tragedies.[41]

The National Institutes of Mental Health (NIMH) and the Law Enforcement Assistance Administration granted the three surgeons $600,000 for brain research on urban rioters.[42]

Lobotomies have fallen out of favor except for narrowly defined causes. Five thousand lobotomies were performed annually in the late 1940s, but by 1980, fewer than five hundred were performed. Laws severely curtailing the surgeries in California and Michigan had a chilling effect, discouraging the practice. Dr. William B. Scoville of Hartford, Connecticut, for example, performed 750 lobotomies a year at state hospitals in the 1950s, but did only 7 or 8 a year by 1980.[43]

Today, some psychiatrists still practice several types of lobotomies. However, the crude abuse of early lobotomies has been eclipsed by a wide variety of therapeutic brain surgeries, both subtle and bold, that save lives and minds. It would be a terrible mistake to condemn all extensive brain surgeries, even experimental ones, in children: This confuses the lifesaving genius of some modern techniques with the abuses of the past. For example, African American neurosurgeon Dr. Benjamin S. Carson, Sr., the chief of pediatric neurosurgery at Johns Hopkins, has devised innovative surgical techniques that use a sophisticated understanding of the brain, maintain a therapeutic focus, and incorporate informed consent. His successful innovations in separating craniopagus conjoined twins (Siamese twins who are joined only at the skull) and employing hemispherectomies to quell life-threatening epileptic seizures have restored health, not mere docility, to an entire generation of children.

But the obsession of American psychiatry with black boys continued and took center stage in February 1992, when Frederick Goodwin, then chief of the Alcohol, Drug Abuse, and Mental Health Administration of the NIMH, appeared before the National Health Advisory Council to champion the Violence Initiative, a group of urban violence studies.

He did so by comparing inner-city boys—young blacks—to rhesus monkeys in the jungle.

If you look, for example, at male monkeys, especially in the wild, roughly half of them survive to adulthood. The other half die by violence. That is the natural way of it for males, to knock each other off and, in fact, there are some interesting evolutionary implications of that because the same hyperaggressive monkeys who kill each other are also hypersexual, so they copulate more and therefore they reproduce more to offset the fact that half of them are dying. Now, one could say that if some of the loss of social structure in this society, and particularly within the high impact inner city areas, has removed some of the civilizing evolutionary things that we have built up and that maybe it isn't just the careless use of the word when people call certain areas of certain cities jungles, that we may have gone back to what might be more natural, without all of the social controls that we have imposed upon ourselves as a civilization over thousands of years in our own evolution.

Many were deeply and vociferously offended by this characterization of young black men, and the then Secretary of Health and Human Services, Dr. Louis Sullivan, who is African American, criticized his remarks. But despite the many calls for Goodwin's removal, Sullivan appointed him head of the National Institutes of Mental Health, from which influential post Goodwin continued to champion Violence Initiative research, such as the New York City fenfluramine studies, and to influence other U.S. medical-research policy.

What's notable about Goodwin's statement is the implication that these black children poison their environment with their atavistic behaviors, instead of a belief that they fall victim to the dangerous, impoverished, and desolate urban landscape into which they are born. In the relentless quest for black pathology, the influence of unusually harmful and violent environments of many black children has often been given short shrift in deference to genetic studies.[44]

But more incisive medical investigations of violence are appearing, often conducted by African American physicians. For example, in 1991, Harvard School of Public Health professor Deborah Prothrow-Stith, M.D., wrote *Deadly Consequences,* an insightful analysis of youth, race, and American violence. Prothrow-Stith used her training as a physician, health-policy expert, and mathematician to make incisive statistical analyses of the myths surrounding violence in black children, and to propose solutions that entail transforming obviously pathological environments, not to offer thinly supported speculation about genes. When a coalition of public-health academics, police, physicians, and ministers made a concerted attack on Boston's youth violence in 1998, violent crime fell precipitously, and that year the teenage murder rate fell to zero, although, as Prothrow-Stith observed, "we didn't change the gene pool."

What sort of research will future scientists be encouraged to pursue with our tax dollars—racist mythology or investigations of violence as an American problem, not a black one? As Stephen Jay Gould warned in 1982, we have a choice to make: "Shall we concentrate upon unfounded speculation for the violence of some—one that follows the determinist philosophy of blaming the victim—or shall we try to eliminate the oppression that builds ghettoes and saps the spirit of the unemployed in the first place?"[45]

The National Commission for the Protection of Human Subjects of Biomedical and Behavioral Research concluded in 1977 that children were an especially vulnerable population because they could not offer consent. Yet, children today are more likely to become research subjects now that federal policies begun in the mid-1990s have changed the face of the "typical research subject." The National Institutes of Health (NIH) Research Revitalization Act mandated the inclusion of women and minorities in all research in 1994 and added children in 1998. So far, the new FDA and NIH policies have placed stress not on protecting children but on ensuring children's access to research—unfortunately, this too often means researchers' access to children. This is an ominous paradigm shift for black children, who already are overrepresented in nontherapeutic and stigmatizing medical research.[46]

Parental Consent

Informed consent is a special concern for African American children. Children are required to give assent for some experiments, which is simply a verbal agreement, but we have seen that children such as the six-year-old fenfluramine subjects will give assent in exchange for a toy. They simply cannot be expected to make good judgments about their health. Certainly children cannot give informed consent, because they cannot understand the medical procedures, or weigh the risks and benefits of participating in medical research.[47] Therefore, researchers substitute parental consent, which is spoken of as the ne plus ultra of subject protection. But as we saw in the fenfluramine experiments, obtaining parental consent opens a child to experimentation but does not always protect him. The first stumbling block to parental permission is legal: Researchers and legislators assume that parents can give consent for their child to join a research study, but as Leonard Glantz points out, "The legal authority of parents or guardians to 'volunteer' their children to participate as research subjects is unclear."[48]

In the case of nontherapeutic and risk-laden experiments such as the fenfluramine and XYY studies, parental permission is ethically questionable, as well. Although we expect parents to act in the best interests of their sick or well child, recent history teaches us that they often cannot or will not do so.[49] Parents have, for example, agreed to fenfluramine administration and to XYY tests during which their children's blood was drawn by unqualified undergraduate students, exposing the child to the risk of infection.

Such injudicious parental consent is garnered because parents are inadequately educated about research studies. To give just one example, a 2004 study of children with leukemia conducted at six U.S. children's hospitals showed that parents who consent to their sick child's participation in medical research often misunderstand the term *randomization*, which means that children are randomly assigned to receive either the standard treatment or the unproven experimental one being tested. A computer, not their doctor, decides which child will receive which drug, but parents tend not to understand this. Parents who do understand randomization are less likely to give consent.[50]

But even well-informed parents do not always fulfill our expectation that they will act in the best interests of the child. Parents may be at the mercy of conflicting motives, especially if a child's illness is causing stress and disruption for the rest of the family. Also, poor parents may find financial incentives for study participation too tempting to resist, even if those incentives consist only of free care for a sick child in a research program. The psychological stress of caring for a sick or dying child may cause parents to grasp at quixotic research straws, as Baby Fae's parents did. She was born on October 14, 1984, with hypoplastic left-heart syndrome, a fatally undeveloped heart. Leonard L. Bailey, M.D., chief of surgery at Loma Linda University, convinced her young, unmarried, poor white parents to allow him to implant the heart of a baboon in their twelve-day-old infant, although no one had ever survived a cross-species organ transplant. Unsurprisingly, Baby Fae died a few weeks later.

A 1992 study suggests that parental consent to medical research is inauspicious for a child, partly because the parents who volunteer their children for research are less well educated, more likely to have substance-abuse or other mental-health problems, and possess lower self-esteem and less confidence than those who withhold permission. In short, the parents who consent are those least likely to make a good decision about study participation.[51]

Perhaps Baltimore's Kennedy Krieger Institute (KKI) best exemplified the dubious protections of parental consent, which it was careful to elicit when it began its "Repair and Maintenance Study" in the mid-1990s. Researchers approached black families in 108 units of decrepit housing encrusted with crumbling, peeling lead paint. Lead paint is a notorious cause of acute illness and chronic mental retardation in young children, who inhale the lead borne on the air and nibble the peeling paint chips, drawn by the appealing sweet taste of the lead. That same sweet taste led Romans to infuse their wine with lead, courting mental devastation, which some historians believe hastened their civilization's decline. Today, it is poor children in crumbling inner-city housing who suffer most from lead. Fortunately, we know how to protect children by banning the use of lead paint and by offering lead-abatement programs. But the agenda of the KKI scientists did not include removing children from lead exposure, because they planned to use these children to evaluate new, cheaper lead-abatement techniques—of unknown efficacy—in old homes with peeling paint.

Because scientists wished to explore cheaper ways of eliminating the lead threat in the future, they purposely arranged with landlords to have children inhabit lead-tainted housing so that they could monitor changes in the children's lead levels as well as the brain and developmental damage that resulted from different kinds of lead-abatement programs. Scientists offered parents of children in these lead-laden homes incentives such as fifteen-dollar payments to cooperate with the study, without divulging that it placed their children at risk of lead exposure. The literature given the parents implied that the study was protecting their children from lead damage and promised to inform parents of any hazards.

KKI researchers simultaneously encouraged landlords of approximately 125 tainted housing units to rent to families with young children by paying for the lead abatement if the landlords rented to such families. They met with chilling success. When the KKI drew blood from one-year-old Ericka Grimes on April 9, 1993, for example, her reading was nine micrograms per deciliter (μg/dl), which is a "normal" reading, according to CDC guidelines. The KKI identified lead-imbued hot spots in the home but did not tell Ericka's parents. When Ericka was retested on September 15, 1994, her blood-lead reading was 32 μg/dl, which CDC charts label a "highly elevated" reading.

The KKI is affiliated with the prestigious Johns Hopkins University, whose IRB approved the protocol.[52] On August 16, 2001, Maryland's top appellate court ruled against the researchers, drawing a parallel to the Tuskegee syphilis experiment.[53] Judge J. Cathell noted, "It can be argued that the researchers intended that the children be the canaries in the mines." His decision noted:

> The IRB was willing to aid researchers in getting around federal regulations designed to protect children used as subjects in non-therapeutic research. An IRB's primary role is to assure the safety of human research subjects—not help researchers avoid safety or health-related requirements.[54]

This is bad news because the university or corporation IRB is considered the prime body charged with protecting the subjects of medical research. Each IRB is required by law to have at least five members, at least one of whom must be a nonscientist. One member must be nonaffiliated with the university, and the board's composition must reflect the community's diversity. But as the fenfluramine study also suggests, these boards are failing to provide the needed protections.

However, if parents have proven to be hobbled protectors in the research setting, institutional abuses such as the XYY experiments suggest that parents still are more desirable guardians than institutional bureaucrats and are far better protectors than no guardian at all. Unfortunately, a black child is more likely than a white one to have his parent completely removed from the informed-consent equation. Black children are far more likely than whites to be institutionalized, in which case the parents are often unable to consent freely or are not consulted at all. Black children throng juvenile detention centers in at least twice their proportion in the population. Their sheer numbers place them at especial risk of being used for research studies there. Nationally, minority-group members, especially blacks, represent 34 percent of children, but they constitute 67 percent of those committed to public facilities.[55] In New York, blacks make up 41 percent of children, but 87 percent of those placed in public juvenile justice facilities. Today, one in sixty-four white boys are taken into custody before their eighth birthday, compared with one in thirteen African American boys.[56] According to a 1999 national *Juvenile Justice* report, black children are more likely to be incarcerated, not because their behavior is worse, but because of biased handling: Their cases are processed differently from those of whites from the very inception of a problem.[57]

Sociologists argue that these orphaning factors combine with the condemnation of blacks as indifferent parents to ensure that the parental consent of African Americans is held in scant regard. For example, Baltimore's 85 percent black XYY studies sought permission only from some fifteen-year-old subjects themselves.

Perhaps the most infamous example of such parental bypass is the case of *Bonner v. Moran*.[58] In 1941, the aunt of fifteen-year-old John Bonner, "a colored boy residing in Washington city," took him to the charity clinic of Episcopal Hospital, where her daughter Clara, John's cousin, was being treated for extensive burns.

Clara's plastic surgeon, Dr. Robert Moran, said that she needed skin grafts, and the doctor and the aunt appealed to John, a junior high school student, to provide some of his own skin. No one asked permission of John's mother, who was sick at home; in fact, she had no idea that John had been taken to the clinic. This surgical attempt at an experimental skin graft was no small matter. John was hospitalized while the plastic surgeon cut a tube of his flesh from his armpit to his waist, then attached the tube to his cousin's side. But the large area of skin failed to take and John himself needed several blood transfusions and two months' hospitalization. He emerged permanently and extensively scarred.

When John's mother recovered, she sued Moran for battery (the legal consequence of nonconsensual surgery), but the court exonerated him on the grounds that Bonner was a mature minor whose consent was legally binding. However, a federal appellate court reversed the ruling, noting that the surgery had not been for John's benefit: "By his own testimony, it clearly appears that he [the physician] failed to explain, even to the infant, the nature or extent of the proposed first operation." Mrs. Bonner and the hospital eventually reached a settlement for damages.[59]

Infants and very young children are even more vulnerable: Not only can they not resist; they cannot even tell what has been done to them. In a 1925 *Journal of the American Medical Association* article, Dr. M. Hines Roberts made no mention of consulting parents or guardians when he wrote of subjecting 423 hospitalized "Negro newborns" in Atlanta, both sick and normal, to risky, painful spinal taps in order to study how such tests could cause injuries—"trauma produced by the needle at the site of puncture." The taps introduced blood into the spinal fluid of some infants and exposed them all to the risks of infections such as meningitis, as well as motor injury, paralysis, and even death.[60] In a 1956 nutrition study, black infants were covertly deprived of the essential nutrient linoleic acid, "essential" because, as the researchers already knew, the body cannot survive without it.

In the late 1980s, many states, including New York, funded research initiatives that tested newborns for HIV infection without their mothers' knowledge, then withheld the knowledge of their HIV status. Sixty-eight percent of HIV-positive infants were African American.[61] The infants suffered irreparable, unnecessary harm because lifesaving treatment was not instituted; the mothers had no idea that their newborns (and they themselves) were HIV-positive. The mothers were victimized because they remained unaware of their own HIV-positive status and thus could not seek treatment. "It was the Tuskegee experiment all over again," says Nettie Mayersohn, the New York assemblywoman who shepherded legislation that would mandate HIV testing and reporting for newborns in New York State.[62] However, in 2004, news emerged of another New York City study. In this case, HIV-positive children in foster care were given high doses of experimental, risky antiretroviral drugs without their parents' knowledge or permission. This study is discussed in detail in chapter 13.

Even an NIH physician, Dr. Lameh Fananapazir, bypassed parents when he implanted pacemakers in fifty-five black children to test a new treatment. The children had been diagnosed with a benign inherited condition that thickens the heart, and Fananapazir wished to see whether the pacemakers would lessen the thickening. But he never articulated a logical therapeutic motive, and the pacemakers did not improve the children's health, which was not threatened by their condition. Instead, the implantation exposed them to surgical risks of pain, infection, and heart damage. Fananapazir's surgeries puzzled his cardiologist colleagues, one of whom dismissed the study by saying, "There's a lot of witchcraft here."[63]

Another type of research with children, experimental vaccines, has gained national notoriety. Today, highly publicized theories link vaccination to everything from autism to sudden death, and even parents who adhere to the vaccination schedules often do so uneasily. Although vaccine skeptics come in every color, recent revelations have sown a deeper-seated uneasiness among African Americans.

Between 1987 and 1991, U.S. researchers administered as much as five hundred times the approved dosage of the experimental Edmonton-Zagreb (EZ) measles vaccine to African American and Hispanic babies in black neighborhoods of Los Angeles. The parents of these children did not know mammoth overdoses were being administered nor that the vaccine was experimental. They also did not know that the vaccine had earlier been given to two thousand Haitian children in Cité Soleil, the most desperately impoverished area of Port-au-Prince, with disastrous results. EZ-vaccinated children, all poor, began to sicken and die by the hundreds there and throughout countries in the Third World, including Senegal, Mexico, and Guinea-Bissau. Horrified by the disastrously high death rates, World Health Organization officials abandoned their plans to administer 250 million EZ doses throughout developing countries. But after these experimental deaths, the vaccine was administered to black and Hispanic Los Angeles children.[64]

Such outrages have prompted African American groups to condemn vaccination.[65] Dr. Abdul Alim Muhammad, Nation of Islam minister of health, recommended "a moratorium on immunizations for all African-American members of the Muslim faith." However, shunning vaccines is itself dangerous.

The vaccine debate encapsulates more than a scientific disagreement; it also reflects the lingering iatrophobia from the exploitative abuse of African American children. This abuse has had a chilling effect on lifesaving research because parents are withholding their permission from positive as well as abusive research. History has shown them how difficult it is to distinguish between the two.

African American children are still being harmed not only by abusive experimentation but also by the fear of research that follows in its wake. For example, the African American infant mortality rate is twice that of whites and Congress has charged the NIH with much-needed research to investigate the reasons for this carnage. However, two years into the five-year project, the National Institutes of Health canceled the study. It gave no official explanation, although rumors flew that the project director had engaged in ethics violations in wangling support for the study. The surrounding community, hearing reports of research fraud, feared that their children would be harmed if they enrolled.[66]

The real victims of this abortive study are the millions of black infants who will die awaiting research into their mortality while a plethora of studies explore supposed genetic links between violence and black children.

PART 3
RACE, TECHNOLOGY, AND MEDICINE

CHAPTER 12

GENETIC PERDITION

The Rise of Molecular Bias

In the age of the technological fix, this country is heading for genetic and behavioral control of society. Who will exercise the control? Who will make the decisions about which genes are defective and which behavior abnormal? Who will make the decisions about the genetic worth of prospective human beings?

—JONATHAN BECKWITH, 1974

"When I went to prison, the concern and worry literally broke my mother's heart. She suffered a series of heart attacks and strokes and died in 1997. She knew I was innocent, because I had been at home with my parents when the crime occurred. And over the years, things just wore her down. When you are in prison, if you are close to your family, your whole family is in prison."

The burden of guilt is common coin in prison, but Calvin Johnson knows the crushing agony of innocence. The twenty-five-year-old Atlanta resident had a bright future, a close-knit family, many friends, and a wedding date when he was convicted of raping a white woman in 1983. He had never seen his "victim" before, but he was convicted, although pubic hairs recovered from her body did not match his. They did come from an African American man, and that, apparently, was enough. "I still had faith in the justice system. I believed it would be just a matter of time before officials realized that they had made a mistake. I was really kind of naïve: I didn't believe that I would be sentenced or convicted of the crimes."

Although the woman identified photographs of someone else as her assailant and although he did not match key elements of her description (the actual rapist had only a mustache, and Johnson wore a full beard), Johnson was convicted by an all-white jury. For seventeen years, Johnson fought to survive in "the hardest work camp in the state of Georgia. I worked in snake-infested swamp waters up to my knees." He also had to stave off assailants. "When you're in prison for a sex offense, if you're not physically strong, the guys around you, they'll try to pick at you. So I lifted weights and became a pretty good size. People left me alone." Johnson lost his youth, his fiancée, and his naïveté, but, he says, "I always believed that God would save me." Faith in God sustained his spirit, and in 1986, Johnson finally found physical deliverance in DNA, which proved him innocent. He was forty-two years old.

Nearly all human cells contain genes, which, in turn, contain deoxyribonucleic acid, or DNA, the molecule that encodes life itself. DNA's genetic code is composed of building blocks called nucleotides, and this code dictates and directs the development of a fertilized egg through processes of protein manufacture so complex that they remain incompletely understood. DNA is passed from parents to children, and it determines or influences many traits, from your eye color to many disease propensities. There is DNA in nearly all your cells, but there are several types of DNA, and less than 1 percent codes for differing traits such as eye color, height, or disease susceptibility. Unless you are an identical twin or the product of another such multiple birth, your DNA is unique. No one else on the planet has your exact genetic code, although humans share a great many genetic similarities.

Today, "DNA fingerprinting" technology enables scientists to identify distinctive genetic patterns.[1] In Johnson's case, the DNA samples from his body ultimately proved that the pubic hairs and other biological evidence left behind by the rapist were not his. At least three types of DNA fingerprinting are in use, but despite the terminology, none is as accurate an identification method as matching a fingerprint. The most popular method at the time of Johnson's conviction, restriction fragment length polymorphism, or RFLP, analysis, compares the DNA of two or more individuals, which varies by only 0.1 percent. That's one difference in a thousand, useful for establishing paternity—or guilt. A newer form of DNA comparison utilizing single nucleotide polymorphisms (SNP) has rapidly outstripped RFLP.

Anyone who doubts that genetic technology can be an important blessing for African Americans should consider its pivotal role in freeing black men such as Calvin Johnson. Johnson was freed by the Innocence Project, the brainchild of O.J. Dream Team members Barry Scheck and

Peter Neufeld, lawyers at the Cardozo School of Law in New York. So far, DNA evidence has helped them and the fifteen to twenty similar projects they have inspired to exonerate more than 328 inmates,[2] including Kirk Bloodsworth and Earl Washington, Jr., who were sentenced to die in Maryland and Virginia, respectively.[3] "These are mostly African American men convicted of raping white women," says Neufeld. "Only 10 percent of reported sex assaults are allegations of white women attacked by black men. Yet most—54 percent—of all convictions proven to be unjust involve African American men wrongfully convicted of assaulting white women. This is a crime that seems associated with many wrong convictions."

So many men have been freed by DNA testing that laws ensuring prisoners' rights to DNA appeals have been passed in some states, including California, New York, and Illinois. Illinois declared a moratorium on capital punishment after an embarrassing string of investigations uncovered many innocent prisoners in its penal institutions.

However, deployment of DNA technology is no panacea. Relatively few inmates can afford the requisite five thousand dollars, and the backlash triggered by the Illinois embarrassment was swift. Some cities, such as Lansing, Michigan, passed laws restricting the use of DNA evidence in inmate appeals. Then again, some criminals leave no testable materials behind, and according to Barry Scheck, even when biological evidence exists, 70 percent of the time it is allowed to deteriorate, is lost, or is discarded during the decades an innocent person languishes in jail.

Human error sometimes sabotages genetic wisdom, as when courts ignore compelling DNA evidence.[4] Scientists and technicians in genetic laboratories have made errors and have even falsified DNA test results. For example, Chicago Laboratory worker Pamela Fish lied or made errors that bolstered at least one erroneous conviction, according to forensic experts who reviewed her testimony before the release of inmate John Willis.[5]

A study by University of Michigan law professor Samuel R. Gross determined that tens of thousands of innocent people are trapped in jail: "If we reviewed [all] prison sentences with the same level of care that we devote to death sentences, there would have been more than 28,500 non-death-row exonerations in the past 15 years rather than the 255 that have in fact occurred."[6]

Even for freed men such as Johnson, justice remains elusive: How do you compensate a man for consigning him to spend his youth in hell? For the loss of his family, friends, income, and good name? States such as California offer a nonnegotiable settlement of one hundred dollars for each day of unjust imprisonment. But two-thirds of those freed by DNA evidence get nothing.[7] And money means nothing to some, such as Frank Lee Smith, a Fort Lauderdale man exonerated by DNA evidence nearly fifteen years after he was sent to death row and eleven months after he died there of cancer.

Clearly, DNA testing is no substitute for justice. In fact, according to experts such as Neufeld, "the real significance is not that DNA got them out, but that DNA provides a window into the criminal justice system to see what went wrong with the system to let so many innocent people be convicted."

But DNA evidence has powerful uses beyond liberating the innocent.

Shades of Gattaca

The film *Gattaca* held a not-too-distant mirror up to a genetic dystopia in which human decisions—and discretion—are removed from all-encompassing judgments about men's worth. In this film, only one's DNA, recognized and assessed by machines, determines one's fate, leaving character, personality, drive, and intent all sublimated to the tyranny of the gene. The biometric dystopia of *Gattaca* doesn't exist yet, and perhaps it never will. But developments over the past few years evoke an unmistakable glimmer of recognition. The FBI, Secret Service, IRS, Social Security Administration, Census Bureau, and Department of Veterans' Affairs all maintain extensive collections of genetic data. Since May 1998, sex offenders have been required to surrender DNA samples to federal databases, and today every state maintains its own DNA database that contains the DNA profiles of felons—and of others, including people merely suspected of crimes or even of innocent people rounded up in DNA sweeps. The samples of 450,000 convicts are stored with identifiers, such as the person's name, description, criminal record, Social Security number, and image. The government has also sponsored the creation of national databases, such as the FBI's Combined DNA Index System

(CODIS), which stores DNA samples, most without identifying information. CODIS went online in 1998 with samples from 8,000 convicted child molesters, and by 2001, it contained the profiles of 1.5 million felons. In 2002, the U.S. Attorney General ordered the FBI to expand CODIS to 50 million profiles, and by 2004, CODIS stored 2.6 million samples containing the DNA of people convicted of almost any crime. In October 2005, the Senate Judiciary Committee approved a law, which was pending when this book went to print, to force anyone who is merely *detained* by federal authorities to provide DNA, and in August 2006 the database contained more than 3.5 million samples. The FBI predicts that CODIS will accommodate 50 million samples "in the near future."[8]

Some scientists warn that the very DNA evidence and technology that has freed hundreds of African American men like Johnson may soon be wielded by police to criminalize and convict black and Hispanic men. From California to London, DNA data banking has allowed the collection of genetic evidence for convicted felons on the premise that those who have been convicted have sacrificed some of their rights to privacy. But Troy Duster, a professor of sociology at Berkeley and author of *Backdoor to Eugenics,* warned in 2001, "The same technology that will exculpate people today is also being used to put people who have merely been *stopped* by the police into genetic databases." He is correct. In 2000, Miami police seeking a violent criminal described vaguely as "black or Hispanic" stopped 2,300 black and Hispanic men on the street and quickly took a buccal swab from each, swabbing the interior of each man's cheek. The police now had samples of their DNA, accompanied by identifying information—suspect profiles—and each man was free to go, for the time being. The samples were tested against DNA left by the rapist at the scene, but none of these men's DNA matched that of the putative assailant. Therefore, all these men have demonstrated their innocence, but police have stored their genetic data in a database to be tapped when they next seek a perp.

This database of innocent black and Hispanic men constitutes a collective presumption of guilt. When weighing the ethical and scientific unacceptability of this tactic, it is important to realize that (1) the term *DNA fingerprinting* is a misnomer: the genetic profile is not as specific as a fingerprint and cannot provide a unique identifier; (2) the description of a "black" or a "Hispanic" suspect is so vague that it yields a racial dragnet, not a description of a suspect; and (3) some "rare" differences that allow one to differentiate individuals based upon a genetic profile become less rare when one looks only within ethnic or kinship groups.

DNA profiling has been questionably imposed upon white men, too, but with important differences. For example, the ACLU of Massachusetts denounced DNA testing as "a serious intrusion on personal privacy" when police in Truro, Massachusetts, used it in investigating the 2002 killing of white fashion writer Christa Worthington. The ACLU also cited the technology's failures in sites such as Baton Rouge and Virginia when DNA samples were coerced from up to eight hundred area men, most of whom were white (in contrast to the thousands taken from black and Hispanic men). The ACLU also argued that the seven thousand forensic DNA samples tested in sweeps have resulted in only one arrest, making DNA sweeps a very expensive and inefficient way of targeting suspects.[9] This is partly because guilty suspects typically refuse to give a sample, even under considerable pressure; it is the innocent who allow themselves to be cajoled or bullied into a buccal swab.

A DNA sweep targeting all Caucasian men, in which police coerce men into supplying DNA to eliminate themselves as suspects, then store it for use the next time they seek a criminal, would be as ethically repugnant as a similar sweep of black men. However, in Truro the donors were not exclusively white and were not targeted on the basis of skin color, so racial bias was not a factor: Truro police asked "all local men" over eighteen years old to provide samples and recorded their various races. What's more, the police agreed to destroy the Truro samples after collection, unlike sites in Miami and Washington, D.C., where the police sought DNA only from men of color.[10] The Truro sweep was still a privacy violation: Many white men felt pressured to give samples and complained that the demand for a DNA sample violated Fourth Amendment protections against unreasonable search and seizure.

Moreover, a black man was arrested for Worthington's murder in April 2005, under troubling circumstances. According to the *Boston Herald*, this suspect, who had an extensive criminal history of violent crimes against women, had given the police permission to take his DNA in April 2002, but police declined to do so until March 2004. During the three years it took them to take, analyze, and act on his DNA analysis, the DNA dragnet of Truro's eight hundred adult men was completed. Some now complain that their privacy was invaded for no reason by DNA testing because police failed to investigate an obviously promising suspect or even to analyze his DNA sample.

California, too, is forcibly taking DNA samples from people presumed innocent—people who have been arrested but not tried and convicted. Defenders of the practice often say that taking and storing such samples is no more intrusive than the common practice of taking a suspect's fingerprints. It is true that fingerprints are taken of arrested persons without too much protest that the innocent are being stigmatized, but again, DNA markers are not fingerprints: They are less specific and far more invasive. In practice, a fingerprint is not a forensically infallible means of identification, but it verifies a person's identity with enough accuracy to satisfy the legal system. However, one's DNA contains intimate information not only about one's identity but also about one's health, including one's future risks of becoming prematurely senile, or developing Huntington's disease or a hard-to-cure cancer. Besides harboring the markers for four thousand disease risks, DNA also contains information about the health and identity of one's forebears and descendants. With a sample of your DNA, a person can predict certain disease and disorder probabilities for you *and* for your children. George Annas, a law professor and bioethicist at Boston University, has referred to one's DNA profile as a "future coded diary," and with the completion of the Human Genome Project, the code has essentially been broken. Therefore, taking the fingerprints of an arrestee and taking a sample of his DNA are not comparable acts; the latter is far more intrusive and revealing—but far less likely to yield a uniquely definitive identification.

In the United States, laws prevent the federal government from retaining DNA samples of the innocent, but the states are doing just this. In 1994, police took samples from 160 black men in Ann Arbor, Michigan, many of whom complained that they had been coerced by police officers who ignored their alibis and threatened to prosecute them if they refused to submit. San Diego police similarly pressured eight hundred black men in order to catch a serial killer described only as "dark-skinned." Black Ann Arbor residents complained that the police tactics "bordered on harassment and abuse," but the men who were approached in Truro often cited subtler peer pressure and vague fears that police would scrutinize them more heavily if they refused to give a sample.

However, Ann Arbor law-enforcement officials denied that their investigation was discriminatory; they insisted that police were simply targeting individuals who met the description of the perpetrator. The Ann Arbor killer—along with several other men—refused to provide police with a DNA sample and was identified only after he was arrested for an unrelated crime.[11]

In mid-April 2001, Syracuse University's Lubin Center hosted a program on forensic genetic technologies, moderated by television journalist Catherine Crier and with a panel of experts that included NYU sociology professor Troy Duster and Howard Safir, the police commissioner of New York City under Mayor Rudolph Giuliani. Safir's new career as a proponent of high-technology security includes the promulgation of his view that police should soon be allowed to use brave new genetic technologies to stop people on the street, take a buccal swab with a portable device, run the database off a satellite, and use their portable computers to see whether they have a "hit."

Such on-the-spot DNA testing is not yet reality, but several biotechnology firms are endeavoring to perfect portable solutions that can allow cops to stop a person, obtain a quick DNA sample, and check it against a database in minutes. One such firm, located in San Diego, is called Nanogen. It utilizes single nucleotide polymerases (SNPs), small DNA fragments that are sites of genetic difference distinctive enough to identify a suspect. Nanogen can put SNPs on a microchip the size of a stamp, technology that scientists have taken to calling "SNPs on chips."[12] Or by analyzing and comparing small areas of DNA called short tandem repeats, or STRs, a police officer armed with DNA from a buccal swab can very speedily check thirteen STRs within minutes. However, some critics argue that thirteen STRs is too few for reliable identification. Police outfitted with portable computers will be able to access the DNA data banks to screen the profiles of thousands of men. The FBI felons' database has samples from eight thousand unsolved crime scenes and state law enforcement has accrued approximately 620,000 samples from lawbreakers, including those suspected or convicted of minor crimes.

Every state now maintains genetic databases that are matched to genetic samples taken from crime scenes, such as blood traces, in order to facilitate finding the person who has committed the crime.[13] Crier echoed the sentiments of many present when she asked why being in the genetic database would be a problem for an innocent black man. "If he is not guilty, what is the problem for a man in the database? He has nothing to worry about."

But he does. Multiple levels of bias feed the all-black and Hispanic databases, and lawsuits such as the Pamela Fish case cited earlier already have verified that DNA evidence is no more immune to fraudulent or incompetent manipulation than is other evidence. Then, too, there is the issue of collective stigmatization: If only men of color are in the database, only men of color become suspects and only they can be convicted. Databases that exclude white men, the numerical majority group, will miss most criminals. As the *American Criminal Law Review* points out, "Optimal effectiveness, however, would require a universal DNA database that contains DNA fingerprint of *every* citizen, otherwise potential matches would be missed."[14] Although a universal DNA database would be more efficient than one based upon skin color, it is also ethically unacceptable because it would necessitate coercion. The DNA sweeps, from Miami to London to Truro, have met with varying levels of resistance and resentment and so cannot be described as voluntary.

Will the novel DNA fingerprinting technology lead to the imprisonment of more African American men than have been freed because of it? This technology's benevolent face has been seen most often, but it has another, sinister, visage. This dual nature holds true for almost every application of genetic science to African American health and welfare. Historically, every boon appears to have been accompanied by a stigmatizing threat to health or freedom. For American blacks, genetics has always been wielded as a two-edged sword.

Sickle-Cell Misstep

African Americans are no strangers to genetic innovation, but unfortunately, genetic therapy has long been sabotaged by racial myths and bad science. The agenda-driven nature of much genetic research with African Americans has rendered many blacks wary of all genetic science. One of the most infamous examples within recent memory has been the family of troubled genetic initiatives surrounding sickle-cell disease.

Chapter 6 described how in 1910, cardiologists James B. Herrick, M.D., and Ernest E. Irons first identified the "thin, elongated, sickle-shaped" red blood cells of a desperately ill twenty-year-old dental student from Grenada. A year later, a Virginia medical journal published a description of a twenty-five-year-old black woman with similar symptoms. Soon, reports of African Americans with sickle-cell anemia, a constellation of dire conditions ascribed to misshapen "sickled" red blood cells, began to flood medical journals. When people with the disorder are exposed to environmental insults such as low-oxygen environments, their red blood cells deform into a sickled shape and become adhesive, sabotaging the cells' ability to carry sufficient oxygen and causing them to block small blood vessels, including capillaries. These events trigger excruciatingly painful episodes, known as sickle-cell crises. A sickle-cell crisis can generate not merely anemia but also bleeding ulcers, strokes, a heart attack, or the loss of limbs and tissues, depending upon the location of the compromised blood vessels. Thus physicians often prefer the term *sickle-cell disease,* pointing out that most of the sufferers' worst medical crises have little to do with anemia. By 1920, an erroneous belief had become firmly entrenched that sickle-cell disease was a racial condition that struck only African Americans.[15] However, it also affects people from Mediterranean, Middle Eastern, and West African regions, but not those from South African and East Asian regions.[16]

After the supposed postwar conquest of infectious disease via antibiotics and after the discovery of DNA's double-helical structure in 1951, genetics gained primacy as the preeminent mode of understanding and attacking disease. In 1949, sickle-cell anemia became the very first molecular disease to be identified. Scientists learned that sickle-cell anemia was the worst of several sickling-cell disorders and that it struck one in every four hundred African American newborns. They also knew that sickle-cell disease and a slew of closely related blood disorders called hemoglobinopathies struck not only blacks but also persons of other races. For example, one such blood disease, thalassemia, affects people of Mediterranean, Middle Eastern, and African extraction. But sickle-cell anemia's identity as a black disease was so firmly entrenched that blacks with thalassemia are still often misdiagnosed with sickle-cell disease.[17]

Sickle-cell disease is recessive: A person must carry two of the recessive genes for sickle-cell disease to develop the illness. People with only one sickle-cell gene are said to be heterozygotes, or carriers, who are essentially well. But if two heterozygotes for sickle-cell disease marry, their offspring run a one-in-four chance of developing the disease. If a carrier marries a person without the gene, none of their children will develop sickle-cell disease, but their children run a one-in-two chance of becoming carriers themselves. Carriers of sickle-cell disease are sometimes referred to as having the sickle-cell trait, but despite the connotation of illness that the word *trait* carries, they are well. (Because of the potential for confusion, this chapter avoids the term *sickle-cell trait* whenever possible.)[18]

By the late 1960s, workplaces instituted genetic screening, ostensibly to protect vulnerable employees by avoiding their placement in work environments that could trigger illness such as a sickle-cell crisis. The federal government supported initiatives that encouraged widespread genetic screening of sickle-cell disease, and African Americans themselves pushed for many of these initiatives to test for and counsel people at risk for sickle-cell disease, so there is no doubt that many of the projects were well intentioned. However, some were not. And in many cases, good intentions paved the medical road to perdition.

"Sickle-cell screening created huge problems," recalls Vernellia Randall, professor of law at Dayton University. "Airlines, for example, said pilots with the trait couldn't fly."

Why not, if they were healthy? In 1968 and 1969, doctors at Fort Bliss in El Paso, Texas, grew concerned that army basic training was suddenly proving more than usually hazardous—even deadly. Within eleven months, four recruits had collapsed and died suddenly, all of them black. Even more alarming were the autopsy results, which showed the men's red blood cells were now sickle-shaped. The soldiers were black and the high altitude of the boot camp—4,060 feet—suggested that the deaths might have been due to sickle-cell disease crises triggered by the low-oxygen environment characteristic of high altitudes. But *The New England Journal of Medicine* report on the men's deaths noted that the sickled cells didn't necessarily mean that the men had sickle-cell disease, because the misshapen cells could have been a consequence, not the cause, of their deaths. When the National Academy of Sciences studied the deaths, it could neither rule out sickle-cell anemia nor prove that it had killed the men.[19]

But the U.S. Air Force Academy rushed to judgment, promptly issuing a directive barring the admission of all black sickle-cell carriers—

healthy people. Carriers were permanently grounded, were banned from copiloting, and were reduced to ground jobs. It is worth noting that by banning black carriers from admission, the academy was effecting a large-scale restoration of its long-standing, nakedly race-based ban on blacks entering the academy, but now it could offer the rationale of protecting them.[20]

Strangely, scientists as well as laypersons confused well sickle-cell carriers with the homozygotes who had both genes for sickle-cell disease and therefore had the disease. However, this confusion was no accident: It resulted in profits for Ortho Pharmaceutical Company of McNeil Laboratories, the company that sold the so-called sickle-cell screening test, which did not differentiate between the sickle-cell trait and sickle-cell disease. Ortho was promoting and distributing a test it called Sickledex that could not discriminate between sickle-cell carriers and people with sickle-cell disease. That is, Sickledex detected the presence of the gene, but not whether one or two genes existed. In order to market the test, employers, military hospitals, and the government extended to carriers the same advice and restrictions that applied to people genuinely ill with sickle-cell anemia. Otherwise, these agencies would have had to admit that the test was of extremely limited therapeutic value because it could not tell a sick person from a well one.[21]

The National Institutes of Health, hospitals, and private organizations disseminated brochures and booklets equating carrier status with the disease, and millions of well black people were informed that they were ill and genetically tainted. Some were told that they had a life expectancy of twenty years. The very first sentence of the preamble of the National Sickle Cell Anemia Control Act, enacted in 1972 to foster sickle-cell research, screening, counseling, and education, is untrue: "Two million Americans suffer from sickle cell disease." Actually, 2 million people were healthy carriers[22] and fewer than 100,000 Americans suffered from sickle-cell anemia. The erroneous claim coupled with its constantly reinforced perception of sickle-cell disease as a black disorder left Americans with the mistaken impression that a good portion—one in twelve—of African Americans suffered from sickle-cell anemia.[23]

The perception of sickle-cell heterozygosity as a disease state is an eloquent illustration of ethnocentrism, because far from being unhealthy, this carrier status confers the distinct biological advantage of immunity to the deadliest strain of malaria. This helps sickle-cell carriers in malarious areas to survive. At the Eighth International Congress of Genetics in 1949, evolutionary biologist J. B. S. Haldane first proposed that people with one gene for sickle-cell disease were "more resistant to attacks by the sporozoa that cause malaria." In parts of Africa and other countries where malaria-carrying mosquitoes thrive, people who have one gene for sickle-cell anemia and one gene for normal hemoglobin are not only healthier than people with sickle-cell anemia but also healthier than people without the trait—those with normal hemoglobin. Being a heterozygote for sickle-cell anemia protects one from invasion by the deadly *P. falciparum* strain of malaria in several ways. A form of the malaria parasite—the plasmodium—infects the person's red blood cells, but in heterozygotes, the plasmodium causes only the infected red blood cells to sickle by making the cell environment more acidic: this increased acidity, in turn, makes the hemoglobin lose oxygen, which further escalates the sickling of the infected cells. However, the resulting lack of oxygen also depletes the infected cells of potassium, which kills the malaria parasites. Any surviving parasites are picked off by the person's immune system, and the sickled cells are taken out of circulation, destroyed, and eliminated from the body along with the parasites. The uninfected red blood cells do not sickle and the person suffers neither from sickle-cell disease nor from malaria.

In malarious environments, sickle-cell heterozygotes are 15 percent more likely to survive and to reproduce than their neighbors with normal hemoglobin.[24] This is called the "heterozygote advantage" and it helps to explain why the common denominator for groups carrying the sickle-cell gene is not being black, but living in proximity to the malaria-bearing anopheles mosquito. Other genetic diseases that also are thought to confer a heterozygote advantage include cystic fibrosis, the most common genetic disease among people of European descent, which protects against the fatal dehydration of cholera and typhoid, and scientists have suggested that heterozygotes for Tay-Sachs disease, which preferentially strikes Ashkenazi Jews, may enjoy increased protection against tuberculosis.

Today, the United States sees only about one thousand cases of malaria annually, so that the heterozygote advantage is not terribly useful to a North American, except for travelers to malarious areas and as an object lesson in the interplay among genetics, disease, and culture.

African Americans were among those confused by the erroneous medical advice the government was dispensing. Many states mounted compulsory genetic-screening programs, which many blacks welcomed, but which caused others, including genetic experts, to feel stigmatized. For example, James Bowman, M.D., an African American professor of genetics at the University of Chicago, was the lone voice crying out in the genetic wilderness when he was invited to address a 1971 Black Panthers event. There, sickle-cell screening was being conducted by community leaders, who warned that anyone who tested positive could expect to live only twenty years longer. Bowman forcefully objected that the testing was unable to identify the genuinely ill, and that in any case, the clinical picture was far less dire. Despite Bowman's credentials and protests, the black and white organizers persisted in the erroneous testing and counseling.

Seventeen states enacted sickle-cell screening laws, often in response to requests from African Americans. But black Americans did not clamor for workplace screenings, which threatened privacy and raised questions that could create a genetic underclass of workers. In 1971, almost nine hundred diseases were known to be genetic, yet screening tests could identify the carriers of only fifty genetic diseases.[25] However, screening for sickle-cell disease was the genetic test performed most often by employers. By 1975, tens of thousands had been screened for Tay-Sachs and thalassemia, but half a million blacks had been screened for sickle-cell disease. *In the Name of Eugenics,* a social history of genetics by Daniel Kevles, notes, "No one argued seriously for the screening of every possible parent, but some did urge the screening of people from groups at comparatively high risk for particular genetic diseases, notably blacks. . . ."[26]

The National Institutes of Health's policies and publications focused exclusively on African Americans, solidifying sickle-cell anemia in the American psyche as a black disease. Unfortunately, the government policies still confused the disease state with being a carrier. Screenings were performed en masse at a variety of sites in an assembly-line fashion with agenda-driven, inaccurate counseling. When screening revealed that a person carried the trait for sickle-cell disease, that information was dumped upon her; she was informed she was sick, given a brochure that erroneously equated the disease with the trait, then often dismissed without further support or answers except for the one piece of advice that was always dispensed—the inadvisability of marriage between two people with the trait, because they could produce children with sickle-cell anemia. This was often the main informational point of the screening, to identify affected people so that they would know not to have children. Such advice led many African Americans to accuse genetic counselors and counseling programs of genocide, especially after 1973. That was the year amniocentesis allowed prenatal testing of the amniotic fluid, first for life-threatening disorders, then for genetic defects, and later for sickle-cell anemia. This was also the year that *Roe v. Wade* gave American women access to legal abortion on demand.

Genetic counselors, who had dispensed pointed advice along with diagnoses since the 1950s, were supposed merely to provide diagnosis and disease information, but they still practiced virtually unregulated and many recommended abortion on the basis of testing that could not discern the trait from the disease.[27] "For at-risk couples who conceived at that time," recalls Vernellia Randall, "the advice was pregnancy termination. Some viewed these as attempts to limit the fertility of blacks."

Discrimination against sickle-cell carriers has been slow to dissipate, lagging well behind scientific knowledge. The U.S. Air Force Academy's admission bar and grounding of heterozygous pilots, for example, was ended only in 1981, by a lawsuit.[28]

Testing, Testing

Today, unscrupulous employers continue to wield genetic screening, but they now do so surreptitiously, without employees' informed consent. In 2001, the Equal Employment Opportunity Commission charged Burlington Northern Santa Fe Railroad with running genetic tests on workers who filed claims for carpal tunnel syndrome. If tests had shown them to have any genetic predisposition to the condition, the railroad could have argued that it should not be held liable.[29] Some lawsuits spawned by such abuses allege racial bias. Perhaps the most egregious was the case of *Norman-Bloodsaw v. Lawrence Berkeley Laboratory,* a research center that the federal government ran in cooperation with the University of California. In 1998, 172 employees, all but one of them black, sued LBL when they learned that they had secretly been tested for syphilis, pregnancy, and sickle-cell trait without their knowledge that the blood and urine they had supplied during required physical examinations would be tested in this manner. These tests were insulting as well as intrusive, and were illegal under the Americans with Disabilities Act. But what is particularly disquieting is the lack of scientific sophistication the laboratory demonstrated in testing only its black employees for the sickle-cell trait: Scientists should have known that not only blacks were at risk and they should also have known that carrier status imparted no reasonable disability risk. The blatantly racial nature of the screening was suggested when plaintiffs learned that the only white employee to have been tested for venereal disease was a white man married to a black woman. In August 2000, the University of California settled the $2.2 million suit brought by these black employees.

The privacy of these workers was illegally assailed and they could have been unfairly stigmatized. But there is another reason that being tested for genetic issues without one's consent is damaging: The price of genetic knowledge can be intolerably high. The health information contained in one's genes can give clues to prevention and self-care, but such information can also generate futile anxiety and lay one open to layers of medical and financial discrimination. "If you know of a genetic condition and lie about it to your insurance company, they can refuse to cover you," observed Marian G. Secundy, Ph.D., the late director of the National Center for Bioethics in Research and Health Care. "If you learn you are at risk for a disease that cannot be treated, the information can be worse than useless: The knowledge will not enable you to protect yourself, and you will suffer mental anguish over an illness that you may never acquire."

Employers who refuse to hire people when they learn of genetic indicators for a disease may relegate them to an "unemployable" biological underclass. And that's not just a concern for those with known genetic disorders, because everyone's genome harbors a few bad apples—genes that could, but do not necessarily, indicate a health problem. The more people are forced to reveal about their genome, the greater their risk of suffering genetic discrimination. Currently, black people are most likely to be subjected to such testing, in large part because testing for sickle-cell disease is the most common genetic screen used by employers and insurers. A 2000 congressional report predicts that such discrimination may become widespread as employers are pressured to contain health-care costs.

Already, black women, who have a higher-than-normal risk of the

BRCA1 gene, which confers as much as a 70 percent higher risk of breast cancer, fear their insurers and employers may discover their status should they seek genetic testing. "Some women seek gene testing on their own and pay for it out of their own pockets because they don't want their insurance company to know," noted Tene Hamilton, an Alabama genetic counselor.

Might other genetic tests preclude African Americans from desirable jobs in the near future? Consider, for example, that a genetic mutation affecting resistance to chemotherapy occurs more frequently in African and African American populations than in Caucasian or Asian populations.[30] A 1998 research study of African Americans and Hispanics living in Manhattan revealed that they harbor a genetic variant (APOE-epsilon4) that places them at a higher relative risk of developing Alzheimer's disease than whites.[31] African Americans are more likely than whites to be healthy carriers of glucose-6-phosphate dehydrogenase (G6PHD) syndrome,[32] which can cause the loss of red blood cells and affects many medical risks and medication reactions. If this carrier status is detected by tests and is miscategorized as a disease state, will blacks be barred from desirable jobs? Of course, each of these genetic complements appears in other ethnic groups as well, but the rates—and thus the risks—are higher among African Americans.

There is also the widespread misconception that simply having a disease gene means you have the disease. This is not so. Most common adult-onset genetically influenced diseases, such as Type II diabetes, hypertension, and cancer, typically result from several genetic factors, not from a single gene. It often also takes environmental triggers (obesity, nutrient deficiency, exposure to noxious chemicals, for example) to cause the disease to manifest. What's more, genes interact to temper one another's effects. All these factors complicate determining who is at risk, and they also hamper scientists' attempts at gene therapy.

Less Than Global: The Human Genome Project

Used therapeutically, genetics hold out promises of enormous improvements in African American health, but the promises have as yet gone unrealized. For example, research into sickle-cell disorder, the first identified molecular disease, remains underfunded and the disease still awaits an effective treatment, but effective genetic therapies were mounted within just a few years after the gene for cystic fibrosis was discovered in 1989. Whites are at much higher risk than blacks for cystic fibrosis.[33] Therapeutic research sometimes bypasses blacks because finding a gene for an illness and curing an illness are two very different things and decades may separate one from the other. Also, the interests of African Americans too often fall below the radar screen of mainstream genetic research, and much more quality research should be undertaken into blacks' genetic risks. This may seem an ironic concern for a book that has focused upon the experimental abuse of blacks, but it is merely the obverse of the research-abuse coin: As research has become an important avenue of therapy the proportionate inclusion of African American in ethical, therapeutic research has become imperative.

Take the Human Genome Project (HGP), which has been touted as a unifying global enterprise to map all of humanity's genes and has been sold to the public on the strength of its role in finding cures for many illnesses. The U.S. National Institutes of Health and London's Wellcome Trust have completed the vital arms of the project, which began in 1990. The 30,000 genes constituting the genetic makeup of a human being have all been identified and mapped.

However, Dr. Georgia Dunston, a geneticist at Howard University, claimed in the mid-1990s that of the more than sixty families whose genes were analyzed by the project, there were no people of African descent.[34] She lamented that severing the African branch of the family tree is a critical error because African gene pools are the oldest and consequently the most diverse on the planet, due to human life's having evolved in Africa. Dunston asked, "What picture of humankind can emerge without Africa?"

Also, of the 100,000 professional HGP scientists from sixteen separate research universities in six countries, only a few, aside from laboratory assistants, were black.[35] Dr. Bettie J. Graham, program manager for the National Human Genome Research Institute at the National Institutes of Health, told the *Journal of Blacks in Higher Education*, "Unfortunately, African Americans have not been involved in the first phase of the Human Genome Project." However, the relatively small numbers of blacks conducting biomedical research for the project also proved a factor.[36]

Howard University was, however, belatedly invited to contribute data and has since received considerable support, which enabled it to open the National Human Genome Center, with Dunston as its director. Today, the center is pursuing several projects of importance to African American health. Among them is a search for candidate genes of complex diseases that are common in African American populations. These include prostate cancer, breast cancer, asthma, Type II diabetes, hypertension, and HIV/AIDS.

The near homogeneity of the HGP is ironic, because the stirring message of the Human Genome Project data is a ringing denunciation of race. Analyses found so little variation among the genomes of what have been thought of as separate racial groups and so many genetic characteristics in common that race was found to have no basis in biology.

This book uses the term *race* because it is accepted argot, a convenient, commonly used way of designating ethnic groups that are perceived as distinct. We all know what we mean (or think we do) when we denote someone's race as "black" or "white." In our nation, race is inarguably important in discussions of health and disease. However, the Human Genome Project has erased any lingering doubts: Biological race does not exist, because all humans share the same genes. Although the proportions of genes differ, meaning that genetic differences exist, these variations map very poorly onto what we think of as races. This seems to introduce a logical contradiction: If race is not real, how can we speak of race-based therapeutics? The answer is that race *is* real, but it is not biological: It is social. What correlates very closely to most "racial" differences in life expectancy, mortality, disease susceptibility, and survival is the race to which one is perceived as belonging.

This is contrary to conventional wisdom and at first blush seems easily refuted: The racial differences between an Icelander and a Nigerian seem obvious. But so do the differences between a dark-skinned Asian from southern India and a pale North African, yet the former person is classified as Caucasian and the latter as "black." Historically, confusion has been sown by the fact that in the early days of the republic and of African enslavement, the Africans who were imported represented only the polar opposite of pale-skinned Europeans in skin color and hair types. Africa is home to people of every skin color, hair type, stature, or other physical measure, but the rich diversity of Africa and, for that matter, of Europe was not represented in seventeenth-century America. Only the dark-skinned denizens of West Africa and principally pale-skinned Anglo-Saxons populated the colonies. If our forebears had included dark-skinned Finns and Mediterraneans on the one hand and North Africans, East Africans, Egyptians, and Somalians on the other, they would have had a better appreciation for the presence of similar phenotypic traits in all ethnic groups. When one looks at the diverse bounty of all peoples, it is easier to appreciate that most of the various criteria we have for sorting people into races—skin color, eye color, hair texture, body type, blood types, disease susceptibility—map very poorly onto genetic frequencies, albeit with a few dramatic exceptions.

For there are exceptions, and although they are rare, it is important from a medical point of view to recognize them when we see them if we want to devise the best-possible medical treatments. However, many genetic diseases are no respecters of race: As we have seen, sickle-cell disease affects Mediterranean peoples, Africans, and South Asians, among others; the autoimmune disorder sarcoidosis afflicts principally African Americans *and* Scandinavians. Some genetic risk factors for diseases such as heart disease, prostate cancer, and low birth weight are present in African Americans but not in Nigerians and West Indians, suggesting that factors other than African heredity are at work.

Today, the commercial marketing of genetic theories is being undertaken with data from the HGP with African American markets very much in mind. A vital part of this marketing plan involves African American pharmacogenomics, the custom-tailoring of medications to exploit genetic variations. But statistically, only a small percentage of genetic variations—about 0.1 percent, one in a thousand—can be laid to race.

Exploiting that real one genetic difference in a thousand to develop more effective medications for African Americans or for any other group is an exciting, very positive tool, especially if it can focus upon major killers such as cancer, heart disease, stroke, and HIV. However, most genetically distinct diseases and differences between ethnic groups account for only a small fraction of the illness and death in any community.

Heart of Darkness

In the late 1990s, the Pharmaceutical Research and Manufacturers of America (PhRMA) boasted that its members had 99 medications in development that addressed the particular medical needs of African American patients. By 2004, that number had grown to 249 medicines. But these were not drugs tailored specifically to black patients' medical needs; nearly all of these medications treated illnesses that African Americans suffer at higher rates than whites, which encompasses nearly every serious ailment.[37] It is certainly laudable that drug companies are producing medications that address black health needs. However, the implication that these were *tailored* to racial needs is easily recognizable as a marketing ploy.

The case of BiDil, a heart drug approved by the FDA in July 2005, is different. BiDil is an oral combination of two drugs, hydralazine and isosorbide dinitrate, that act as antioxidants, widen blood vessels, and produce nitric oxide, which, BiDil makers say, provides beneficial effects for African American heart failure patients. It was developed for its potential to reduce deaths and serious illness among African Americans diagnosed with congestive heart failure.[38] CHF is a condition in which the heart muscle, which has been weakened or otherwise compromised by injury or disease, fails to maintain circulation properly. The overwhelmed heart triggers a cascade of functional deterioration that culminates in a slow death: It is commonly fatal within a decade of diagnosis. People with congestive heart failure may suffer from constant fatigue, swollen legs, and respiratory problems. Or heart failure may be insidiously asymptomatic. BiDil's patent holders say their medication's mechanism of action addresses a genetic anomaly that makes African Americans particulary susceptible to CHF. This medication is in the vanguard of new commercial marketing of genetic therapies for blacks.

NitroMed, the Cambridge, Massachusetts, biotechnology firm that developed BiDil, claims that it is the first specifically tailored medication to treat congestive heart failure in an estimated 750,000 African American patients. Clearly, BiDil should be embraced and supported if it works to decrease death and disability due to CHF. But its marketing as an exclusively African American genetic medication is just as clearly troubling for both scientific and social reasons.

First, is the medication driven by a true biological dimorphism in black heart patients or is it the product of a fertile market? In an illuminating analysis in the *Yale Journal of Health Policy, Law, and Ethics*, Jonathan Kahn has weighed the medical evidence and found it wanting. His investigation reveals that BiDil began life not as a specialized medication tailored for African American heart patients, but as a heart drug aimed at the general public. Neither its first clinical trials in 1987 nor its patent application in 1988 mentioned racial applications, and only after the FDA Advisory Committee refused to approve BiDil's use for a general population in 1997 did NitroMed reanalyze twenty-year-old data from its first trials, looking for possible special applications that might allow it to approach the FDA with a revised application.[39] The Food and Drug Administration's Modernization Act had recently required inclusion of racial minorities and women in clinical trials, and in 1997 Surgeon General David Satcher drafted the resolution that made resolving racial health disparities a national priority. In 1998, BiDil was reborn as a black medication, rescuing the drug from pharmaceutical oblivion.

But how did NitroMed make a case for BiDil's transformation from a medication for everyone to a genetic drug that addresses specific weaknesses in African Americans, even before clinical trials were conducted? Was it based upon a proven special utility for black patients?

In part, NitroMed achieved this by creating a perception of CHF in blacks as a racially distinctive disease, then supplying the medication that was "necessary" to address this biological dimorphism. First, as Kahn has pointed out, BiDil's makers made a case for CHF as a racial disease claiming that there is a huge difference in the mortality rate between black and white patients with CHF. NitroMed scientists claimed that CHF kills blacks at twice the rate it does whites, and publications from *Science* to *Today in Cardiology,* as well as press releases from the Association of Black Cardiologists, affirmed this disparity.[40]

But the data contradict this claim. It is true that proportionately twice as many blacks as whites died of CHF in 1988, but reducing the rate of heart failure in African Americans has been a medical success story, and by 2003 the gap had nearly closed. Most recent CDC figures indicate that the racial ratio of heart-failure deaths is 1.1 blacks for every 1 white—they are almost identical.[41] Kahn traced the provenance of NitroMed's widely disseminated figures and found that they were based upon very old studies, including National Heart, Lung, and Blood Institute (NHLBI) data collected in 1995. At the time NitroMed was using this data, it was already woefully outdated and no longer accurate. NitroMed's researchers used numbers that were not only old but also inappropriate, because they cited National Health and Nutrition Examination

Survey (NHANES) data from 1988 that described prevalence, the number of people *suffering from* CHF, which is very different from mortality, the number of *deaths from* CHF.[42] One 1987 study does seem at first blush to support the NitroMed figures because it indicated that 1.8 black men died of CHF for every affected white man and that 2.4 black women with CHF died for every afflicted white woman. But in addition to being old superseded figures, these figures describe deaths within a specific age range, from thirty-five to seventy-four. Thus they reveal a serious disparity in the age at death, not in absolute deaths. The same percentage of blacks and whites die of CHF, but 50 percent of blacks who die of CHF are between the ages of thirty-five and seventy-four, while only 30 percent of whites who die of CHF are seventy-four or younger: Most whites who die of CHF do so quite late in life. In short, bad data helped BiDil boosters to portray CHF as a racial disease by exaggerating its death rates in blacks and raising the specious question of why so many more blacks than whites die of the disease.

NitroMed explained that only physiology could explain such a dramatic disparity in the death rate. In doing so, BiDil's promoters discount the well-substantiated research into myriad nongenetic factors that drive CHF death rates. Nongenetic interventions in the form of better access to medical care, more preventive lifestyle changes, and high-tech interventions have already cut the African American CHF death rates from twice that of whites in 1988 to essentially the same as whites in 2003. This fairly quick reduction didn't emanate from genetic techniques or changes and thus strongly suggests that nongenetic factors are most important. So does recent research that suggests heart failure is fed by hypertension and kidney disease. Hypertension in blacks, in turn, has been shown to be driven by stress (including the stress of racism), by diets that are high in fat, possibly by salt sensitivity, by overweight, and by obesity. There is even evidence that hantavirus infection spread by rodents in urban settings can cause kidney disease and hypertension.[43] So can exposures to some poisons in such urban settings. A slew of reports, beginning with those published by *The New England Journal of Medicine* in February 1998, have shown that limited access to high-tech care has also fed blacks' higher mortality from heart disease. But researchers and news articles that discuss the merits of BiDil tend to give the nongenetic factors short shrift. As Kahn points out, Clyde Yancy, a black cardiologist on the steering committee of BiDil's trial, says that the data "do not support socioeconomic factors as important contributors to the excess mortality rate seen in African Americans affected with heart failure."

BiDil patent holder Jay Cohn, M.D., and his colleagues wrote papers positing a genetic mechanism for CHF in blacks: "a pathophysiology found primarily in black patients that may involve nitric oxide insufficiency," which makes the cause of their heart failure different from that of whites. Clyde Yancy agreed, saying, "Heart failure in blacks is likely to be a different disease" and adds "the emerging field of genomic medicine has provided insight into potential mechanisms to explain racial variability in disease expression."

But even if the putative difference in nitric-oxide metabolism were found primarily in African American patients, this would not mean that *all* African American patients in heart failure harbor it, or even most African American patients. Nor would it mean that such an anomaly is restricted to blacks.

Since the publication of Kahn's analysis, NitroMed has quietly revised the numbers in its promotional materials. It no longer claims that African American CHF deaths are double those of whites. But the alarm sounded by its earlier claims already served its purpose: The FDA gave the drug another opportunity in clinical trials, this time to prove that the drug is efficacious against CHF in African Americans

In 2003, NitroMed, with the Association of Black Cardiologists as a highly visible participant and supporter, mounted a clinical trial. NitroMed enrolled 1,050 African Americans for the trial of BiDil as a treatment for heart failure in African American subjects. The trial was called A-HeFT, an acronym for the African American Heart Failure Trials,[44] and it tested BiDil not on its own but in conjunction with fully approved heart medications. In August 2004, the clinical trials to demonstrate BiDil's safety and efficacy were halted because, its makers say, the results were clearly beneficial to blacks suffering from heart failure. The results showed that 6.2 percent of patients given BiDil died; 10.2 of patients who did not receive BiDil died, constituting a 43 percent survival advantage for those taking the medications.

The FDA has approved BiDil's race-based labeling. This means that although a doctor may choose to prescribe it for non–African Americans in an "off-label" use, insurers will not have to cover its cost for them. The study should have included whites in order to provide evidence that the drugs works differently in blacks, but because the patents for use in all races will expire in 2007, there is no economic incentive to test the drug in whites. (NitroMed will hold the patent for the use of BiDil in blacks until 2020.) In an ironic twist, whites are being subjected to racial exclusion by being denied access to testing or use of a heart drug that could benefit them or even save their lives.

NitroMed stock rode the good news from the A-HeFT trials to a 73 percent leap in share price. Because it was tested only with other drugs, BiDil typically will be prescribed for use in concert with other drugs, not instead of them, so that BiDil will not compete in the marketplace with established heart medications. This will help BiDil's sales and this could even explain why BiDil was tested only against a placebo: Had BiDil been tested alone, researchers would have run the risk that the study results could have been different, finding that BiDil provided less protection to black patients than standard medications.

Because heart disease is the number-two killer of blacks—and whites—BiDil should be embraced if it indeed conveys a racial benefit to blacks with CHF. So should any other therapy that accurately targets clinically meaningful disease vulnerabilities in African Americans. But the development of a genetic drug for what has been newly dubbed "a racial disease" also raises long-term issues that temper its immediate benefits.

We soon will see other medications marketed for "genetically distinct" populations of African Americans. The glaucoma medication Travatan is being promoted to African Americans as "the first glaucoma drug to demonstrate greater effectiveness in black patients," although the FDA-required informational insert indicates in fine print that eye color may be a better indicator of its effectiveness than race. Prostate-cancer therapies genetically tailored for African American men are in the pipeline. Recently, 89 percent of breast-cancer tumors from African American women tested positive for a newly found gene, BP1, compared with 57 percent of those from Caucasian women. Can a special medication tailored to the black breast be far behind? It will also be important for African Americans to study and, where applicable, to support such research efforts by joining ethical therapeutic trials that offer the best-possible safety protections. To find these trials, African Americans should discuss them with their personal physicians and consult resources available on-line that offer "how-to" primers on joining clinical trials.

But unsurprisingly, given the subject of this book, I also advise African Americans to look before they leap. Although many black cardiologists and many in the African American news media applaud the BiDil innovation,[45] the specter of neoracial disease based upon questionable genetics should give one pause for many reasons. African Americans must actively support the search for disease risks and therapies, but they must also be conscious of the long-term import of funneling scarce resources into race-based medications unless they provide the best therapeutic approaches.

A genetic fix for a nongenetic disease is unlikely to be the most efficient approach. What's more, racializing CHF allows scientists and policy makers to ignore the environmental factors that are the chief causes of the racial heart-disease disparity. Racial genomics also raises profound social questions. If physicians fall back into the antebellum habit of treating blacks' ailments according to race, will not this condemn many to poorer, stereotyped, less appropriate care? Because race is not a biological reality, medications based upon group biological differences will work only for some African Americans. This will lead to a false sense of security, and will stymie the search for more inclusive, more efficacious, and, in a word, better treatments. We must recognize the powerful stigmatizing potential of genetic approaches to disease, especially when they are touted as the only approach.

From tools that could release or convict to the troubled history of genetic disease fixes that may provide cures or mere stigmatization, genetics offers a cornucopia of medical answers and pitfalls to blacks. The next chapter gives the history of another mixed blessing: research into infectious diseases.

CHAPTER 13

INFECTION AND INEQUITY

Illness as Crime

Unhealthy places and decadent times infect us by their contagion.
—JOSEPH JOUBERT

IIn April 1992, thirty-four-year-old Milton Ellison made the front page of the *New York Times*—after being unshackled. "They had me chained to the bed for three weeks," he told the *Times*. Ellison was not held for assault, rape, or murder. His "crime" was more subtle: He had tuberculosis and had not complied with his doctor's orders to take medication. He was jailed not in a cell at New York City's Rikers Island prison, but in an Orange County, New York, hospital. Health officials had summoned sheriff's deputies, who transported him to the hospital, where his wrist and ankles were shackled to a hospital bed and he was given his medication under the observation of not doctors, but deputies. After his weekslong ordeal, Ellison, who is a schizophrenic, asked, "Why was that necessary? If I were ill, I couldn't go anywhere."

Ellison was not the only patient to be incarcerated. Other major cities, including Boston, San Francisco, Atlanta, and Washington, D.C., have taken the same steps. Public-health expert Georges Benjamin, M.D., who now serves as the editor of the *American Journal of Public Health*, said, "There are rules on the books that allow caregivers to get court orders to force individuals to be hospitalized. You hospitalize them until they are no longer infectious." However, these rules are public-health laws that require a hearing before involuntary commitment, a hearing that Ellison was not given.

A disquieting racial disparity characterizes the patient profiles of those forced to undergo such containment therapy. Between 1988 and

April 1991, the New York City health commissioner ordered thirty-three tuberculosis patients to be held in hospitals against their will until they were no longer infectious. Seventy-nine percent were black.

As we have seen, blacks have long been perceived as particularly vulnerable to some infectious diseases, so perhaps it should not surprise us that when emerging diseases such as AIDS and hepatitis C appeared, these were racialized as well.

What's more, blacks are also frequently presented as vectors of disease, posing a threat of infection to whites. In the 1930s and 1940s, African American public-health advocates following in the footsteps of Booker T. Washington promoted such initiatives as Negro Health Week to provide tuberculosis prevention and care to blacks who rarely gained entrée to quality medical care. But white support of such initiatives was predicated on concerns that the black domestics who cared for their children, cleaned their homes, drove their cars, and prepared their meals might import tuberculosis into white households.

Tuberculosis, often referred to as TB, is an ancient infectious disease that usually attacks the lungs and is often fatal if not treated properly. It was once feared mightily: Just as AIDS displaced cancer in our bestiary of medical horrors, cancer once displaced tuberculosis, after antibiotics seemed to vanquish TB. In the developing world, many deaths from AIDS are still due to the tuberculosis that accompanies it. In the United States, half of incarcerated TB sufferers are not only black but also homeless and many have a history of mental illness, alcohol and drug abuse, or all of the above risk factors.[1]

Until recently we had consigned infectious diseases to the past. This is because fifty years ago, the discovery of antibiotics and the development of vaccines armed scientists with magic bullets against disease-causing microbes such as bacteria and viruses. The Sabin vaccine had tamed polio and antibiotics such as rifampin promised to eradicate tuberculosis. Bubonic plague and bacterial meningitis were being controlled for the first time. The diseases tetanus, diphtheria, and pertussis, once mass murderers, were already memories.

Unfortunately, we then seemed to lose our respect for infective organisms because we had the antibiotic cure handy in a pill or a syringe. The apparent conquest of infectious diseases fostered an ominous hubris as health systems abandoned public-health measures designed to prevent infection. Antibiotics replaced hygiene and basic public-health measures. Hospital wards no longer boasted pathogen-killing ultraviolet lights and special ventilation that constrained the movement of airborne pathogen-laden air. Secure medical wards to quarantine the ill disappeared, as did regular testing in schools and workplaces. Education and "case finding," the regular monitoring of the public to find people with tuberculosis, ended. The result? Over a decade ago, we realized that profligate use of antibiotics and shortsighted public-health measures had combined to turn the common *E. coli* bacteria in hamburger into a killer, to transform the common staphylococcus germ into flesh-eating variants, and to summon even deadlier manifestations of diseases like tuberculosis from their ashes.

Tuberculosis underwent a horrible renaissance because when case finding was abandoned, people with TB went undiagnosed and untreated, at least not attended to in time to save their lives or those they infected. Also, people who should have been taking medication for TB were often noncompliant—that is, they did not take medications at the recommended doses for the necessary length of time. As a result, not all of their TB bacilli were killed, and the surviving TB bacilli were hardier and resistant to some of the drugs that had once vanquished them. "TB is no longer easily cured with the drugs that worked so well fifty years ago," said Roscoe C. Young, M.D., a pulmonary specialist at Meharry Medical School. "Instead of one drug taken for a short time, doctors now must use four drugs in a complicated schedule that can spread over years to treat this deadlier multi drug resistant tuberculosis (MDRTB). We now have highly virulent strains of tuberculosis with the airborne propensity for spreading."

AIDS has also abetted TB cases among African Americans. Two-thirds of people with AIDS die of lung disease, and if they are African American, that lung disease is more likely to be tuberculosis than *Pneumocystis carinii* pneumonia.

Doctors invoke disease resistance to explain why they must reluctantly force treatment upon the drug-resistant such as Ellison. They explain that compared to the earlier, slowly progressing version that took years to contract and develop, today's TB bugs propagate quickly, promiscuously, and with greater lethality. TB patients who repeatedly abandon long, carefully orchestrated regimens of up to four drugs can die, but not before infecting others. Despite this rationale, 27 percent of the infectious persons locked away by New York City do not suffer from drug-resistant strains.

Georges Benjamin, who is African American, emphasizes that locking up patients should be the last resort, and his reluctance to do so is obvious. "There are policies and procedures in place that most public-health officials would try first," he explains. "For example, they try to do directly observed therapy [DOT, in which a nurse or other public-health professional watches a patient to ensure that medications are correctly taken]." But, sadly, funds to support such intermediate measures have dwindled, leaving doctors with fewer options before detaining patients.

Funding may also factor in some decisions to monitor patients closely or to confine them to hospital units, because health institutions earn more for patients undergoing DOT or forced hospital treatment than for voluntary patients, For example, in 1992, Medicaid paid only $38.82 per patient per week for routine doctor visits by the patient, but it paid $95.90 when a worker visited the patient's home for DOT. Hospitals could receive grants of as much as fifty thousand dollars to build DOT programs.[2]

However, the ethical problems of detaining TB patients, who are mostly black men, extend beyond any whiff of financial inducement. Thirty-four percent of the TB cases in the United States affect blacks, who constitute only 12.3 percent of the population—a 300 percent greater TB risk for blacks than for whites. "TB has always been more prevalent in blacks, but not due to genetic susceptibility," explained Margaret Kadree, M.D., chief of infectious disease at Morehouse School of Medicine, "but because of socioeconomic conditions. We have been among the poorest people and often live in urban centers amidst crowded conditions and a lack of access to health care."

One wonders whether, if tuberculosis singled out upper-class whites, less punitive solutions would abound. The history of a persistent TB epidemic at New York's Rikers Island prison may be instructive on that score. In 1982, the Legal Aid Society sued the city's corrections department, demanding that it address inmate illness and deaths resulting from its longtime tuberculosis epidemic. That year, there were 2,268 new TB cases. By late 1991, there were 4,426 cases. In January 1992, a new drug-resistant TB killed twenty-seven inmates.

Then an infected white corrections officer died.

The city responded with alacrity, signing a renovation contract within the month, on February 8 with Mark Corrections, Inc., of Maywood, New Jersey, and building a new high-tech tuberculosis isolation wing, which was speedily erected at a cost of four million dollars.[3]

There is no easy answer to the multidrug-resistant TB threat, but in light of its racially disparate containment approaches, we should give the shackles a rest and fund more medical approaches. Confining medically underserved TB sufferers fails to address impaired health, poor access to care, crowding, and homelessness—the root causes of the tuberculosis upswing. In fact, the fear of being locked up may dissuade people with TB from seeking treatment. There are also "slippery slope" issues. We jail people with TB today. Might we jail people with SARS tomorrow? Alcoholics? Smokers?

Less punitive practices and more medical solutions might include wide-scale vaccination, a step that the government has so far resisted funding, probably because the Bacillus Calmette-Guerin vaccine, the world's most widely used, is imperfect, protecting only four out of five people vaccinated, and triggering a painful reaction called regional lymphadenopathy in a few.[4] Policy makers might also consider a better coordination of public-health systems to give immigrants, the homeless, prisoners, and migrant workers easier access to treatment. Currently, health policy simply abandons or incarcerates the infected as "noncompliant" when they fail to scale the formidable barriers of cost and access between themselves and good medical care.

Drug-resistant tuberculosis proved to be merely a sentinel disease. Within the last few decades, new infectious diseases—or reinvigorated old ones—have materialized as global threats, from the AIDS pandemic to hepatitis C to SARS. An infectious disease represents far more than a physical ailment that is caused by pathogens and the organisms on which they travel—"disease vectors," in medical argot. Infectious diseases also pose a threat to entire populations. Their spread, prevalence, and treatment is closely linked to social factors, including crowding, poverty, inequitable access to medications, incarceration rates, women's rights, and a host of other political and social stressors.

These threats have played out very differently for African Americans than for whites, and a few examples illustrate how biased research and inequitable policies have shaped the uncomfortably close relationship between African Americans and infectious disease.

AIDS

In 2002, HIV infection outstripped the Black Death as the single deadliest pandemic in recorded history.[5] According to the Joint United Nations Programme on HIV/AIDS, 40.3 million people across the globe are infected with HIV, and 3 million died of AIDS in 2005.[6] Sub-Saharan Africa is the most heavily affected region, because it is home to 64 percent of new HIV infections. Closer to home, HIV now constitutes the third leading cause of death for young adult African Americans (those between twenty-five and forty-four years of age). In 2004, the CDC determined that most of the AIDS cases in the United States were diagnosed in African Americans.[7] As this book went to press, AIDS was being diagnosed in black Americans at ten times the rate as in whites; it is twenty-five times more common in black women than in white women and ten times more common in black men than in white men. Nearly all American children infected by HIV, approximately 83 percent, are black or Hispanic, but one reads more about the tragic plight of sub-Saharan African children than about the children in our own backyards. This observation plays into a perception by many African Americans that because AIDS strikes the marginalized, concern and sympathy have been largely replaced by stigmatization, moral judgment, and deadly indifference.

In the 1980s, however, AIDS was first identified in what was then an equally marginalized group—gay white men. They were widely maligned as people with reprehensible lifestyles whose behaviors put them at risk for what was dubbed "the gay plague." When it became clear that intimate relations between gay men and others were facilitating the spread of HIV into populations previously thought immune, such as straight whites, this misplaced moral disdain escalated into accusations that gays were sources of contagion and that their behavior needed to be constrained by public-health laws. The debate was encapsulated in San Francisco journalist Randy Shilts's controversial social history of the pandemic's early days, *And the Band Played On.* Shilts detailed the role of Gaetan Dugas, known as "Patient Zero," who knowingly infected many other men.

But gay men's behavior was not heavily circumscribed, because fierce debates over the human rights and dignity of gays ensued and thus few of the proposed constraints were enacted into law. Bathhouses that facilitated anonymous sex were closed, but the public-health department made no attempt to trace men's sexual contacts, to quarantine those infected men who refused to protect their partners, or to force men to divulge their HIV status. Certainly no one was jailed. In fact, Cuba was almost universally condemned for its claim that it had contained the HIV epidemic by quarantining the infected. Thus the standard public-health tactics of infection control, including contact tracing and selective quarantine, were rejected in the early days of the epidemic, when they might have had the most usefulness in stemming the spread of the pandemic.

However, the focus of the pandemic shifted as black people were infected in large numbers and they became identified with the vectors of the disease. HIV was very early posited to have an origin among people of color, though it was first found among whites.

By the late 1980s, medical journals and news media referred to several classes of the HIV-infected. There was early and frequent reference to "innocent victims of AIDS," which intimated the existence of other, presumably "guilty" victims. The innocent included infected children such as Ryan White and such sympathetic exemplars as Kimberly Bergalis. What they had in common, besides media sympathy, was white skin and virginity. Ryan White was a ten-year-old boy who had been cast out of his school because of his HIV status and whose family had been persecuted by fearful neighbors. This sad tale of cruel discrimination against a sick child was narrated by newspapers and television everywhere and was punctuated by frequent reminders of his "innocent" status. He had not contracted HIV from a sexual encounter or injected drug use; neither had Kimberly Bergalis, another "innocent" victim who had been infected by a dentist implicated in the possibly intentional infections of several other patients—patients we never saw—before his demise from HIV disease. Bergalis was constantly profiled, and her courage, religious faith, and ravaged youth made it impossible not to sympathize with her plight. Her virginity, which certified her status as an innocent victim, was mentioned in a high percentage of the news stories describing her plight.

But the demographics of HIV infections began to change as HIV preyed upon the marginalized, the Africans and, in this country, the poor and black. Early newspaper stories on the shifting demographics were given little prominence; neither were reports that the rural South was emerging as an epicenter of infection. But by 1997, a sea change had taken place and news reports informed us that HIV affected a much larger percentage of blacks than whites, that it had become the chief killer of young African Americans, and that most children with HIV were black and/or Hispanic. First in the minds of many Americans and finally in grim reality, as certified by CDC statistics, AIDS had became a black disease.

Not all the news about AIDS and blacks is bad, although too often, silence greets hopeful news that contradicts AIDS's status as a black disease. For example, although journalists publicize and celebrate hopeful news about white men who have resisted illness despite long-term HIV infections, a resounding media silence followed similar tidings about groups of African women who by 1997 seemed to have achieved what the best laboratories in the world could not: the power to ward off HIV infection. Over six years, 10 percent of a group of the Nairobi prostitutes under study remained uninfected, although each had sex with hundreds of men. The resistant women didn't use condoms or receive medical care any more frequently than their infected counterparts. Scientists aren't sure how their bodies outwitted the virus, but human leukocyte antigens (HLAs), "smart" proteins that recognize foreign invaders, are probably the chief factor.

Many vaccines have been designed by studying people who display puzzling immunities. For example, Edward Jenner first perfected the smallpox vaccine in 1796 after studying milkmaids who became immune after contracting the more benign cowpox. The Nairobi women have the potential to be today's milkmaids, the source of a lifesaving vaccine out of Africa, so one might expect these women to be the focus of media and popular speculation. But popular references to Africans' natural immunities have disappeared, although medical research continues to explore their potential as promising domestic pockets of possible disease resistance.

American attitudes toward people with AIDS have also mutated from protective to punitive. More restrictive laws have evolved into the litmus test for public-health advocates and legislators who wish to be perceived as addressing the pandemic.

TESTING CHILDREN

The term *innocent victims* has largely disappeared from newspaper pages. Not even the infants who were tested for HIV without their mothers' knowledge or the African infants whose mothers lost their prophylactic azidothymidine, or AZT, when U.S. drug trials ended are now specified as "innocent victims."

Children with HIV are increasingly finding that their status is that of involuntary research subjects, not victims. In December 2004, for example, the journal *Nature Medicine*[8] reported that since the early 1990s, HIV-positive orphans have been the subjects of "dozens of national clinical trials run by researchers at Columbia University Medical Center and other [New York City] area hospitals." Mammoth pharmaceutical corporations such as GlaxoSmithKline, the manufacturer of zidovudine, have sponsored the testing of antiretroviral and other pharmaceuticals on scores of HIV-infected orphans housed in New York City's Incarnation Children's Center (ICC). This institution for the HIV-infected is run by Catholic Charities in Washington Heights, a neighborhood where Columbia University conducted fenfluramine violence studies, as detailed in chapter 11. The ICC orphans were born to HIV-positive mothers and their parents either are dead or have been deemed unfit to care for them by the courts.

Within ICC's walls, Columbia University Medical Center physicians manage AIDS drug trials approved by the Pediatric AIDS Clinical Trials Group (PACTG), a network that imposes standards for and evaluates clinical trials for the care of HIV-infected children. These trials were supported by the National Institute of Allergy and Infectious Diseases and the National Institute of Child Health and Human Development, with the approval of New York's Administration for Children's Services (ACS).[9]

Katherine Painter, M.D., the medical director of Incarnation Children's Center, acknowledges that ICC is affiliated with Columbia-Presbyterian and receives HIV-infected children from six New York hospitals—Columbia-Presbyterian, Harlem Hospital, New York Hospital, St. Luke's/Roosevelt, Kings County Hospital in Brooklyn, and SUNY, as well as "from outpatient HIV clinics in the city, in the five boroughs and in Westchester." She also verified that, as was mentioned in chapter

11, the children are subjects in the testing of experimental drugs. "Many of the clinics that refer to us are participating in clinical drug trials," she told the *New York Press* in 2004. "Children participating in a drug trial undergo monitoring, testing, and supply of an experimental drug through their outpatient clinic and we maintain that treatment here."[10]

Thirty-six experiments were conducted at the ICC between 1997 and 2003, and GlaxoSmithKline sponsored four of these. The center's experimental activities are not unique or even unusual for New York, according to the BBC, whose November 2004 television documentary *Guinea Pig Kids* noted that "over 23,000 of the city's children are either in foster care or independent homes run mostly by religious organisations on behalf of the local authorities, and almost 99 percent are black or Hispanic."

Researchers and ICC staff characterize these clinical trials as therapeutic, intended for the benefit of the children; and researchers agree that pediatric drugs require testing in children because children metabolize and react to medications differently than adults do.

However, children's advocates question the therapeutic nature of these experimental drugs, pointing out that they have debilitating, even fatal, side effects, including anemia, muscle wasting, organ failure, fatal destruction of bone marrow (the site of red-blood-cell production), life-threatening liver diseases, cancers, bodily deformations, brain damage, painful and fatal skin conditions, and likely genetic mutations, liver swelling, unsightly fat deposits, and skin necrosis (death and sloughing of the skin).

Some of the candidate AIDS medications are being tested to determine their toxicity. Children as young as four were given cocktails of up to seven potent medications, although physicians are normally reluctant to give young children even approved powerful medications. Little if any benefit accrued to the infants from these risky exposures, because although some were HIV-positive, they were too young to have developed AIDS. One study is of "Stavudine . . . Alone or in Combination with Didanosine," a combination that has killed adult women. An experimental vaccine administered to children as young as twelve months utilizes "live chicken pox virus," even though it can trigger the disease itself. A study titled "HIV Levels in Cerebrospinal Fluid" required that infants undergo a spinal tap, a risky, invasive, and painful procedure.

There was even a study on HIV-negative children that used an experimental HIV vaccine. By law, such a nontherapeutic study on healthy children can convey only minimal risk, but the vaccine's risks are unknown.

Also, some of the experiments did not involve HIV therapeutics: One drug trial tested a herpes medication "for tolerance, safety and pharmacokinetic" information; another investigated reactions to a *doubled* dose of measles vaccine—in six-month-old infants.

For its part, Columbia University released a statement denying that the drugs' side effects were serious enough to warrant discontinuing treatment. However, this should have been the parents' call, not the university's or the ICC's. But guardians and parents who adopted HIV-infected children have found the ICC, ACS, and researchers arrayed against them when they have tried to take children off medications they found to be harmful.

In explaining her take on this struggle, Dr. Painter has said, "We're having an increase in referrals over the last years to deal with medication adherence. There are a fair number of children whose HIV illness may be well controlled but whose families are experiencing difficulty complying with the child's medication regimen." By "referrals," Painter means children who are torn from parents and returned to the various agencies when these parents and guardians balk at dispensing the investigational drugs.

Federal law gives parents the ultimate right to decide when the promise of an experimental treatment exceeds the risks and side effects and gives them the right to withdraw a child from a clinical trial at any point in the experiment.

But most of these children have no parents or their parents have been deemed unfit by the courts to care for them. The children are too young to give legal consent to participate in the HIV studies, and their legal guardian is the city or an allied governmental agency, which is the same entity that has committed to conducting the trial. The New York City Department of Health enrolled the children in drug trials in the early 1990s, and the city's ACS gave permission for the ICC children to be used. The agency receives funds for hosting the trial and needs a minimal number of subjects; therefore, it should not also be the arbiter of the children's participation. It is not disinterested and cannot be objective. Yet the agencies are allowed to enroll the children as research subjects en masse, although federal regulations require individual consent for each child.

In fact, the ICC forces the medications upon children over the objections of foster or adoptive parents. Mona Newberg, a New York City teacher, adopted her great-niece and great-nephew and removed them from the ICC in 2002. She refused to sign papers permitting her children to be used in AIDS experiments but told a journalist in the fall of 2003 that "ACS has signed for me when I didn't want to give Sean [her adopted son] drugs. When I said, 'No,' the ACS caseworker grabbed the form and said, 'I'll sign it. You don't need to.' They're always switching medications—they never ask me if it's okay."[11]

Jacklyn Hoerger is another foster parent, and one with a unique perspective: She is an experienced pediatric nurse who worked at the ICC for years before she fostered two children as a prelude to adopting them. One Saturday morning, ACS came to the door, accused her of child abuse, and seized her children. Her crime? She had withdrawn them from the experimental AIDS medications and insists that they had become happier and healthier. As a medical professional, she is better able than most to ascertain whether the benefit of an experimental drug justifies the harm it is doing the child. But ACS has prevented her from seeing her children.

Painter seems to validate Hoerger's account when she describes the ICC policy toward compliance with the investigational drugs: "What we're asking of our families and patients in terms of adherence is something beyond 100 percent—all of their medicines all the time, whether they have them on hand or not, whether the medication makes them sick, or whether they're sick with a concurrent illness."

Despite Hoerger's status as the children's foster mother and her medical training, the ICC trumps parental consent for these children. Such a scenario evokes the question, Is the state's chief motivation a desire to maximize the children's health or its own desire to complete AIDS research protocols?

The BBC documentary claimed, "If the children refuse the drugs, they're held down and have them force fed. If the children continue to resist, they're taken to Columbia-Presbyterian hospital where a surgeon puts a plastic tube through their abdominal wall into their stomachs. From then on, the drugs are injected directly into their intestines.[12] ICC spokesperson Gerald McKelvey acknowledged that the city sometimes took children from foster parents who had refused to administer the drugs, but he denied to *Nature Medicine* that children were ever forcibly administered medications. "Of course some kids were reluctant, as kids are, to take their medicine," he said. It was not children, however, but recalcitrant parents, some of whom were medical professionals, who were reluctant to administer medications because of the debilitating effects on the children and the fear that they were being exploited as nonconsenting subjects.

For several years U.S. research protocols with African American and Hispanic children, who constitute virtually all the American children living with HIV, have exposed an alarming willingness to jeopardize their health and rights.

A PUBLIC-HEALTH DRAGNET

The legal constraints that had been deemed inappropriately repressive for white gay men in the 1980s and early 1990s have been vigorously applied to African Americans, especially African American men. Increasingly, laws have mandated the testing of whole groups, such as pregnant women and prisoners. At least twenty-nine states punish or incarcerate those who pass the virus on to others, and scores of similar bills are waiting in the wings. "It has bothered me that when more punitive laws have come up, it is black people who are affected," observed the late Dr. Walter Shervington, a New Orleans psychiatrist and former president of the National Medical Association.

The issue of contact tracing best exemplified the shifting mood. There are two types of such tracing. Voluntary notification programs allow the patient with HIV to notify his partners. But in mandatory programs, health department officials notify the patient's sexual contacts that they are at risk and must be tested. Patients are identified by code, which partially preserves confidentiality, or by the person's name, which affords none. New York State, the former infection epicenter, which once championed patient advocacy and privacy protection for AIDS, has legislated a quite restrictive form of mandatory notification. If you test positive for HIV in New York, the doctor must report your name to the state. The county health department obtains the names of your sexual contacts and informs them that they are at risk and need testing.

Contact tracing is an uncomfortable but essential technique of infectious disease control, because it attempts to bridge a real information gap. The February 1998 *Archives of Internal Medicine* revealed that four out of every ten HIV-infected persons failed to warn partners of their status and that only 43 percent of these silent carriers use a condom. Blacks—men or women—are even less likely than whites to alert partners of their HIV-positive status. Prominent public-health officials such as Surgeon General David Satcher warned almost a decade ago that contact tracing was essential to the early testing and tracking that can reverse the pandemic. In 1996, Satcher observed, "We're getting to the point where we have to have a better form of identifying and treating AIDS, but to be successful we have to treat it like other STDs." However, he added, "We have to be able to ensure confidentiality."

Patient confidentiality is a medically sacred article of faith that physicians never abandon lightly. Why, then, have these laws abandoned the concept? "The CDC was affected by pressure from conservatives who control the budgets on Capitol Hill," explains attorney Mario Cooper, a Harvard AIDS Institute adviser and the founder of Leading for Life, an advocacy group for blacks with AIDS. "But they have made a huge mistake in aggressively pushing it without a fundamental understanding of its impact on people of color. Many in our community don't get tested for STDs and AIDS. They see such programs as monolithic institutions that grew out of Tuskegee experiments." Notification laws were also problematic because they relied upon overburdened public-health departments.

This curiously pathologizing stance toward infectious disease indicts African American behavior as criminal rather than addressing health behaviors supportively, in the more usual public-health mode, which utilizes intervention. Today epidemiological discussions focus on the high rate of AIDS in African Americans and in Africans, which is necessary and appropriate. But these discussions also pair the high rates with drug use and profligate sexual activity in the face of a resounding silence on other important issues such as lack of access to medication and medical care, an inequitable economic and human-rights climate, and even dangerous medical practices, which are discussed later in this chapter. The dearth of consistent high-quality care for HIV infection in inner-city areas is simplistically ascribed to black fear and distrust of medical treatment and research. Such problems as limited access to lifesaving antiviral drugs get short shrift. Overburdened or bankrupted AIDS Drug Assistance Programs that are charged with distributing effective AIDS medications sometimes find themselves unable to do so, even though the cost of these drugs has fallen dramatically over the past eight years. There is little discussion of how best to lower the high rate of HIV infection in children. Silence governs those risk factors that cannot be laid to a blame-the-victim paradigm that emphasizes patients' high-risk behaviors.

This blame-the-victim approach to AIDS control has backfired by instilling denial or a false sense of security in many African Americans. HIV infection has been saddled with so much cultural baggage that many people believe it strikes only the sexually promiscuous, drug-addicted, desperately poor, or "immoral" people. Many black people cannot believe diseases such as AIDS or hepatitis C can affect "someone like me." News accounts feed this misconception by focusing on black people with HIV who live in squalor, have lost custody of their children, and who turn to crimes such as prostitution to feed a drug habit. So do many narrative-driven medical journal accounts. These tragedies are real, but they are far from the whole story. Because a single act can transmit infection, sexually transmitted diseases (STDs) can affect anyone who is sexually active, not just the promiscuous. Churchgoing grandmothers can be infected as surely as club-hopping Romeos, but they may not realize this and so may not take steps to protect themselves.

AIDS IN THE LABORATORY

Poorly performed medical research has fed the high rates of infection among African Americans, and it also has fed the low rates of appropriate treatment that have plagued blacks from the first days of the epidemic. The U.S. medical establishment has failed to provide African Americans with equitable attention, testing, medications, and recruitment for medical trials, but these failures have been ascribed to African Americans themselves in the medical literature and provide another manifestation of the blame-the-victim mentality.

Misguided research has caused HIV therapy to be withheld from blacks even as it has heavily ladled guilt for the spread of AIDS upon their shoulders. For example, in the early 1990s, a Johns Hopkins study revealed that HIV-positive whites, but not blacks, were doubling their survival time by taking AZT.[13] Conventional wisdom has long laid this disparity at the feet of African Americans by insisting that blacks resisted taking AZT (later to be known as zidovudine) because of fear and distrust engendered by the U.S.PHS syphilis study at Tuskegee.[14] With a singular myopia, scientific and social science researchers have ignored the appalling wealth of other pharmaceutical and infectious-disease experimentation with blacks to seize instead upon a single PHS study with very imperfect parallels to the HIV crisis. Celebrated surveys did not ask open-ended questions to determine the roots of black aversion to AZT; instead, they asked specifically whether the Tuskegee Syphilis Study was "the" factor.[15] Popular coverage widely conveyed the assumption that the emotional overreaction of blacks to this single investigation abuse was at fault.[16]

But this monomaniac focus upon the Tuskegee Syphilis Study as the catalyst for AZT aversion ignores some pertinent research history. In February 1991, soon after azidothymidine was embraced as the first effective drug against HIV infection and AIDS, Department of Veterans' Affairs researchers informed the FDA that AZT did not work well for black patients, as it did for whites. The VA researchers also suggested that because AZT's side effects could imperil health, and even life, AZT should be withheld from blacks as an inefficacious and possibly dangerous medication.[17]

Alarmed physicians were loath to prescribe AZT to blacks in the face of such ominous findings. The prohibition against using AZT to treat blacks quickly became entrenched in the therapeutic canon. However, the VA study had utilized a relatively low number of African American patients and had not been designed to ferret out racial differences: This dramatic racial disparity generated research results that were a fluke, rather than an authentically disparate racial response. Later, rigorous research unmasked salient errors in the study and revealed that AZT was indeed efficacious for blacks. But this proved too little, too late: Physicians remained slow to prescribe AZT to their black patients, and these patients were slow to accept it. No government or medical entity undertook the large-scale public-relations effort that would have been necessary to repair the damage done to AZT's image. The reputation of AZT was permanently tarnished in the minds of African Americans and, for a while, in the opinions of the physicians who cared for them.

As a result, HIV-positive blacks quickly progressed to AIDS, promptly developing the severe opportunistic infections, cancers, neurological damage, and decimated immune system that heralded the syndrome. Medical researchers and physicians, not fearful black patients traumatized by the Tuskegee Syphilis Study, are responsible for blacks' aversion to AZT.

In 1997, the Centers for Disease Control and Prevention issued some long-overdue good news about AIDS: a heartening 13 percent decline in the death rate, the first in the fifteen-year course of the epidemic. What's more, new combination drug therapies were slowing the progression from HIV to AIDS. These included protease inhibitors such as Invirase, Crixivan, and Norvir. For most HIV-positive people, protease inhibitors promised to parallel insulin use for diabetics—not a cure, but effective management.

But once again, African Americans had not shared equitably in either the declining death rate or the distribution of the new drugs. The AIDS death rate for whites fell 21 percent, but the black death rate dropped only 2 percent, and the rate for young black women actually rose. At the Sixth Annual HIV Conference, San Francisco's mayor, Willie Brown, warned conferees, "We are now on the threshold of a new set of problems generated by success, because the drugs are terribly expensive, and a whole forgotten class of people are not getting them, including people of color." Dr. Wilbert Jordan, director of the AIDS clinic at Martin Luther King/Charles Drew Medical Center in Los Angeles, predicted, "Protease inhibitors are very expensive—about $14,000 a year—and the majority of people who won't get them are drug users, especially in the black and Latino populations."

The new drugs were too expensive for people on Medicaid, which imposed a monthly cap on drug expenses; HMOs often restricted pharmacy benefits to an average of three thousand dollars a year; and the demand for the drugs quickly overwhelmed the pharmaceutical companies' stores of free drugs for compassionate use. Despite the pharmaceutical companies' healthy profits, states were finding themselves strapped by the costs of supplying medication to the poor. The $200 million in federal and state AIDS Drug Assistance Programs (ADAP) that was set aside to provide the drugs to those not poor enough to qualify for Medicaid was half of what was needed. ADAP funds varied from state to state: New York and California residents enjoyed expansive programs, but only 10 percent of the HIV-positive in Florida qualified. Some states, such as Kansas, resorted to a waiting list.

Valerie Papaya Mann, executive director of the AIDS Project of the East Bay, validated fears of inequitable distribution: "In San Francisco, on every other corner, there's information about the latest therapies; but in the East Bay we have people of color, low wage earners and less AIDS information. Many doctors serving the indigent are not prescribing the protease inhibitors. My clients, 85 percent of whom are African-American, are still dying and will still die unless there is a loud outcry that says we all should have access to the drugs."

Nor was money the only barrier. Early protease inhibitors were taken according to complicated schedules and they fostered drug resistance when inexpertly prescribed or taken erratically. Physicians and policy makers frequently worried aloud that if the poor and homeless were given protease inhibitors and proved noncompliant, they would abet drug-resistant strains, which would prove impossible to treat. Instead of focusing on education and other routes of increasing compliance, doctors routinely withheld protease inhibitors from people in lower socioeconomic groups, such as the homeless and drug abusers, among whom African Americans were disproportionately represented. Mario Cooper complained, "Doctors are selecting people out because of racial issues. Some won't even offer drug abusers the option of taking these drugs."

One African American physician responded: "My patients with drug problems are all compliant. . . . It's ridiculous to withhold medication from drug users on the assumption that they won't adhere to the treatment schedule: Who understands the importance of taking drugs on time better than an addict?"

The prices of life-sustaining HIV medications have fallen dramatically since the fall of 2000 because of international competition between generic and proprietary drug manufacturers. Now the price of AIDS therapy costs as little as $140 annually and is within the reach of all African Americans.

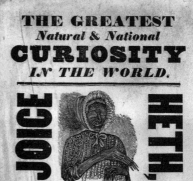

This flyer for Joice Heth, the purported 161-year-old "mammy" of President George Washington, trumpeted her December 1835 appearance at Barnum's Hotel in Bridgeport, Connecticut. Heth was regularly examined by physicians and laypersons alike, and when she died her autopsy was attended by 1,500 paying spectators. *(Reproduced with the kind permission of the Somers Historical Society and Museum.)*

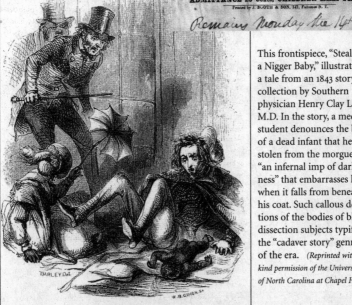

DARLEY Del.   W. B. GIHON Sc.

" My cloak flew open as I fell, and the force of the fall bursting its envelope, out,
in all its hideous realities, rolled the infernal imp of darkness."—*Page* 137.

This frontispiece, "Stealing a Nigger Baby," illustrates a tale from an 1843 story collection by Southern physician Henry Clay Lewis, M.D. In the story, a medical student denounces the body of a dead infant that he has stolen from the morgue as "an infernal imp of darkness" that embarrasses him when it falls from beneath his coat. Such callous depictions of the bodies of black dissection subjects typify the "cadaver story" genre of the era. *(Reprinted with the kind permission of the University of North Carolina at Chapel Hill.)*

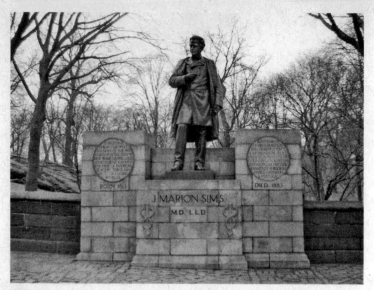

This marble colossus pays homage to James Marion Sims, M.D., "whose brilliant achievement carried the fame of American surgery throughout the entire world." It graces the eastern perimeter of New York's Central Park, just across from the New York Academy of Medicine. *(Photograph by Harriet A. Washington.)*

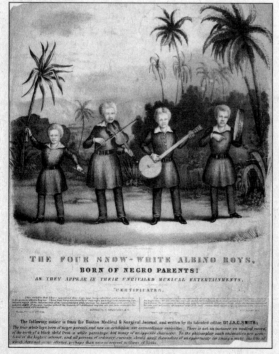

This broadside advertising 1844 Boston concerts by "The Four Snow-White Albino Boys, Born of Negro Parents!" stressed, as was usual with such "white negro" attractions, that the subjects were not of mixed race but anomalies born of black parents. The advertisement carried testimonials by several examining physicians, including the editor of the *Boston Medical and Surgical Journal*, who attested to the subjects' "pure" racial lineage. *(Lithograph by B.W. Thayer and Co., New York Public Library.)*

In 1850, Harvard biology professor Louis Agassiz, M.D., commissioned Joseph T. Zealy to produce daguerreotype images of fifteen nude or seminude African Americans in Columbia, South Carolina. The scientific rationale for these detailed images of Africans and their first-generation offspring, which emphasized physiognomic features such as head shape, profile, and stance, was to provide graphic evidence that blacks constituted a different species from whites. The frontal image is of Renty, a slave who was born in "Congo." The profile image of Delia, Renty's American-born daughter, emphasizes not only physical racial characteristics but also uses the device of partial nudity, pulling her clothes below her waist to signal her lower social status and implied sexual availability.

(© 2006 Harvard University, Peabody Museum of Archaeology and Ethnology, 35-5-10/53037 T1867.)

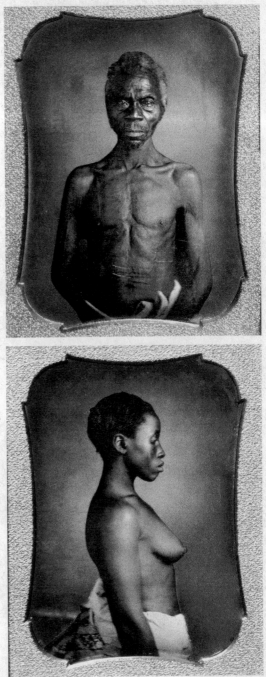

This portrait of Grandison Harris, a "resurrection man" charged with stealing black bodies for dissection, probably was drawn from life by a doctor at the Medical College of Georgia. *(Reproduced with the kind permission of the Medical College of Georgia's Greenblatt Library.)*

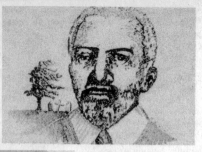

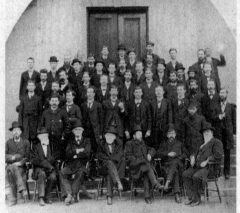

In this 1880 portrait of the Medical College of Georgia's graduating class, the dark figure at the right rear, with his arm raised, is a black porter *cum* resurrection man, possibly Grandison Harris. *(Reproduced with the kind permission of the Medical College of Georgia's Greenblatt Library.)*

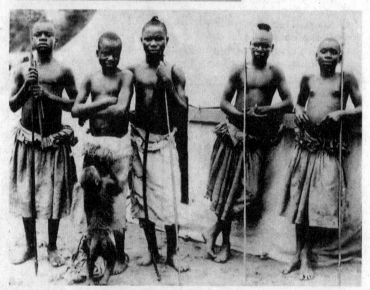

Ota Benga (second from the left, with monkey), a widower from what is now Zaire, was exhibited in New York's Bronx Zoo in 1910. Here he appears with other African men who were exhibited to the public and studied by psychologists at the 1904 St. Louis World's Fair. *(Reproduced with the permission of the South Caroliniana Library, University of South Carolina.)*

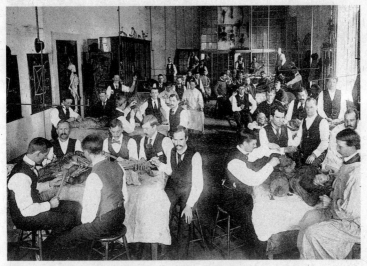

This nineteenth-century photograph shows medical students performing dissections at the Medical College of Georgia in Augusta. *(Reproduced with the kind permission of the Medical College of Georgia's Greenblatt Library.)*

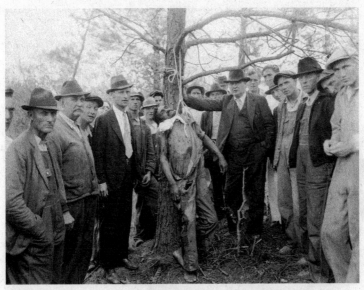

The April 28, 1936, lynching of forty-five-year-old Lint Shaw in Royston, Georgia, demonstrates parallels to anatomical portraits. The murderers and spectators are semi-formally dressed and gaze unself-consciously into the camera with their victim, who is displayed with bloody injuries visible and partially nude, his clothes having been rent into rags. *(Associated Press photograph.)*

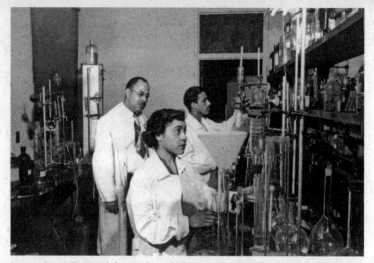

In 1956, Dr. H. D. West, left, president of Meharry Medical College, supervises two students in its biochemistry laboratory. The Nashville, Tennessee, school, founded in 1876, was one of only two black medical schools spared by Abraham Flexner's 1910 report judging medical education in the United States and Canada. *(Associated Press photograph.)*

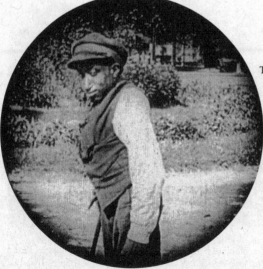

This image of a disabled black child introduced a panoply of dysgenic "undesirables" in Dr. Harry Haiselden's 1917 feature film, *The Black Stork.* *(Reproduced courtesy of Martin Pernick, Ph.D., and John E. Allen.)*

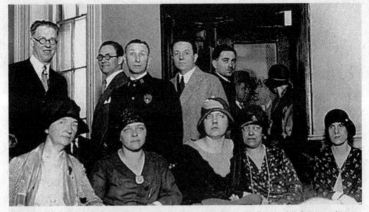

On April 24, 1929, Margaret Sanger, head of an illegal New York City birth control clinic, sits (at far left) in the Chief Magistrate's Court with her fellow defendants. They are, left to right, Dr. Hannah M. Stone, Sigrid Brestwell, Antoinette Field, and Marcelia Sideri. That same year, Sanger began researching birthrates in Harlem and planning the Negro Project, an experimental initiative to reduce births among blacks. *(Associated Press photograph.)*

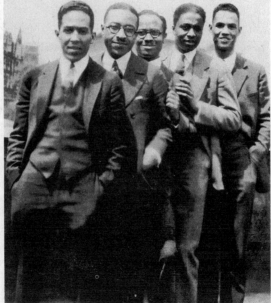

In 1924, five rising luminaries of the Harlem Renaissance posed on the rooftop of 580 St. Nicholas Avenue. From left: Langston Hughes, Charles S. Johnson, E. Franklin Frazier, Rudolph Fisher, M.D., author of the first African American mystery novel, and Hubert T. Delaney. Fisher, a Columbia-trained radiologist, died of radiation-induced illness in 1932. *(Reprinted by permission of the New York Public Library Schomburg Center for Research in Black Culture.)*

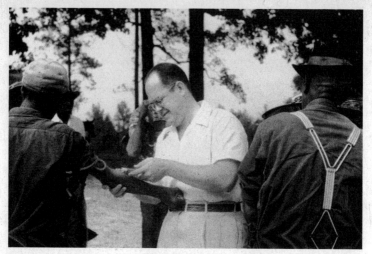

In Tuskegee, Alabama, a U.S. Public Health Service study subject receives an injection from a PHS physician. The men were not injected with syphilis, but they were administered injections and underwent other procedures that maintained the illusion that they were undergoing treatment for syphilis. *(From the National Archives and Records Administration.)*

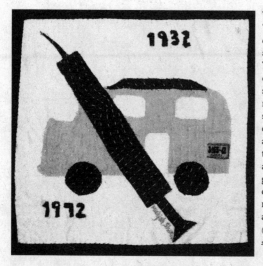

This quilt, entitled "Annual Roundup," was created by Muhjah Shakir, an assistant professor at Tuskegee University, to commemorate the PHS syphilis experiment that rounded up and tested syphilitic black subjects every year between 1932 and 1972. Shakir directs the Bioethics Quilt Project at Tuskegee, Alabama, a group of women who design quilts inspired by medical-ethics issues that affect black Americans. *(Reproduced by the kind permission of Muhjah Shakir.)*

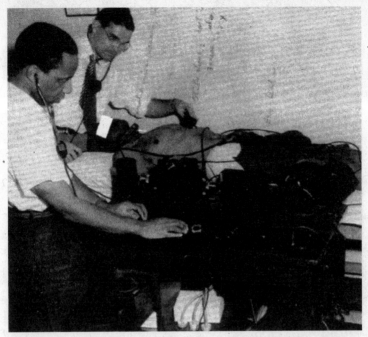

Mr. William Bouie (left) assists Dr. Stanley H. Shuman in administering a cardiographic examination to a PHS syphilis study subject in the early 1950s. *(Photograph courtesy of the Centers for Disease Control.)*

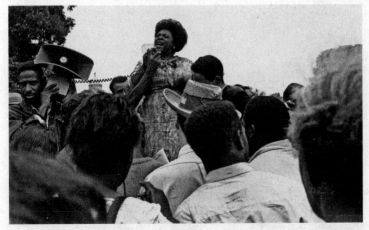

On September 17, 1965, Fannie Lou Hamer speaks to Mississippi Freedom Democratic Party sympathizers outside the Capitol in Washington, D.C., where they had gone to file a legal complaint that blacks were excluded from the election process in their home state. At nineteen, Hamer was subjected to a "Mississippi appendectomy"—a nonconsensual sterilization—to which she ascribed her political awakening. *(Associated Press photograph.)*

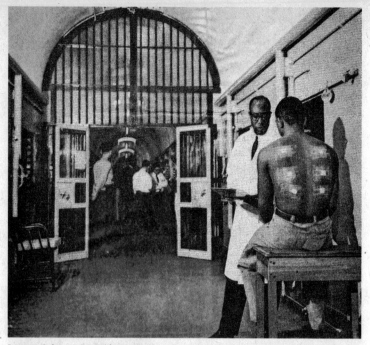

In 1966, Solomon McBride examines an incarcerated subject wearing skin patches impregnated with various experimental pharmaceuticals in H block of the Holmesburg Prison complex. *(Reprinted with the kind permission of the Temple University Urban Archives, Philadelphia.)*

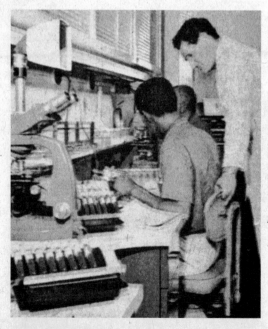

Until the early 1970s, physicians and researchers supervised experimentation with scores of inmates, most of whom were black, at sites such as the Holmesburg Prison complex in Philadelphia. Some inmates, such as those pictured seated here, worked as technicians despite their scant education and lack of training. *(Reproduced with the kind permission of the Temple University Urban Archives, Philadelphia.)*

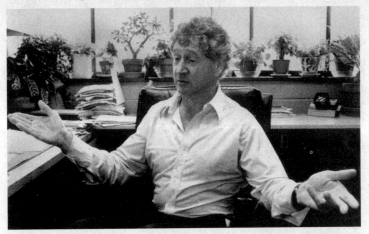

Dr. Albert Kligman earned fame and millions of dollars by conducting medical research using prisoner subjects at the Holmesburg Prison complex until the 1970s. Despite the complaints of research subjects that they were deceived and injured, he has never faced criminal charges or professional censure; instead, he has been lauded for elevating the specialty of dermatology. *(Reprinted with the kind permission of the Temple University Urban Archives, Philadelphia.)*

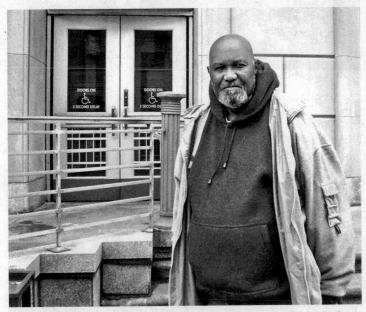

Jesse Williams is one of scores of U.S. prison-research survivors who seek legal redress for the chronic diseases, including cancers, skin conditions, and, in some cases, mental illnesses, that they ascribe to their experiences in Holmesburg Prison's research programs. *(Photograph by Harriet A. Washington.)*

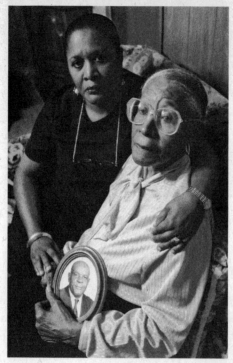

Elmerine Whitfield Bell, daughter of radiation subject Elmer Allen, comforts her mother, Mrs. Fredna Allen, at their home in Italy, Texas. Mrs. Allen holds a photograph of her deceased husband, who was one of at least eighteen Americans surreptitiously injected with plutonium by government scientists.
(Photograph by Carol Powers, reprinted with the permission of the Dallas Morning News.*)*

In June 1996, U.S. Secretary of Energy Hazel O'Leary spoke to journalists outside the Rocky Flats Environmental Technology Site near Golden, Colorado. Secretary O'Leary ushered in a new era of openness by declassifying records of radiation experimentation on unsuspecting American citizens, many of whom were black.
(Associated Press photograph by David Zalubowski.)

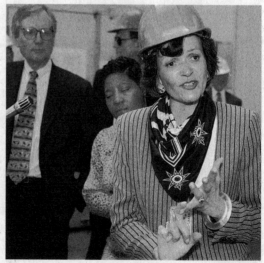

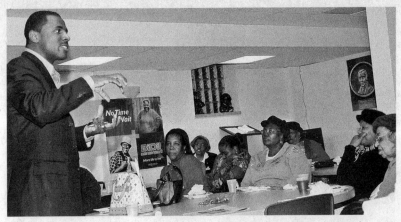

Rudell Christian, a "medical science liaison" for the pharmaceutical company NitroMed, maker of the "blacks-only" heart-failure medication BiDil, extolls the drug's virtues to members of Detroit's Trinity AME Church in March 2006. *(Associated Press photograph by Amy E. Powers.)*

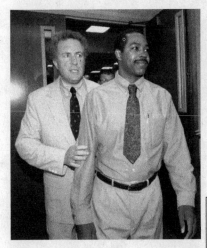

Calvin Johnson, Jr. (right), smiles as he leaves a Jonesboro, Georgia, courtroom a free man in June 1999, accompanied by his attorney, Peter Neufeld, a founder of the Innocence Project. Johnson spent sixteen years imprisoned in a work camp for a brutal rape, but he was exonerated by DNA evidence that proved another man committed the crime.

(Associated Press photograph by John Bazemore.)

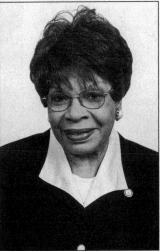

Former Savannah, Georgia, legislator Dorothy Pelote became a fierce advocate for black Florida and Georgia residents whose communities were visited by swarms of disease-carrying mosquitoes released by the CIA during the 1950s and 1960s. CIA documents suggest that scientists in its MK-ULTRA Project experimented with such biological exposures in black communities in order to determine whether such releases would be effective against foreign enemies.

(Reprinted with the permission of the Savannah Morning News.)

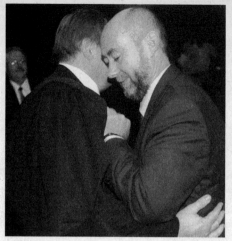

Wouter Basson, M.D. (right), is embraced by his defense counselor, Jaap Cilliers, in the Pretoria, South Africa, High Court after being acquitted of all charges against him on April 11, 2002. Basson, former head of South Africa's Chemical and Biological Weapons Program, faced hundreds of counts of murder in the deaths of poisoned black Africans, as well as numerous conspiracy, fraud, and drug possession charges, to which his former underlings confessed. Basson once said, "I must confirm that the structure of the [CBWP] project was based on the U.S. system. That's where we learnt the most." *(Associated Press photograph by Themba Hadebe.)*

On March 14, 2000, FBI agents removed a cache of illegal machine guns, thousands of rounds of ammunition, volatile explosives, and drums of poisonous chemicals from the grounds of Dr. Larry Ford's Irvine, California, home. Ford, who frequently gave racial-poisoning seminars at South Africa's Roodeplaat Research Laboratory (RRL), had killed himself on March 2 as police closed in. *(Associated Press photograph by Damian Dovarganes.)*

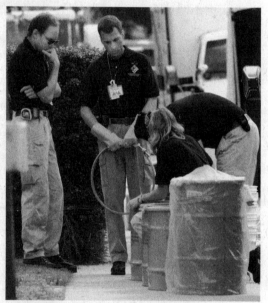

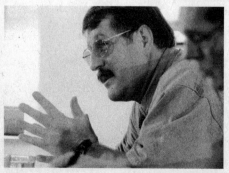

At the Cape Town offices of the Truth and Reconciliation Commission on June 11, 1998, veterinarian Daan Goosen, who headed the military-run Roodeplaat Research Laboratory, describes his scientific team's search for a bacterium that would harm only blacks. "We were in a war situation, and a weapon is a weapon." The RRL relied upon the expertise of several U.S. scientists. *(Associated Press photograph by Benny Gool.)*

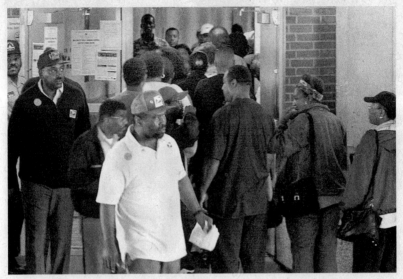

Postal employees await anthrax contamination screening in the waiting area of D.C. General Hospital. Four and a half years after the 2001 deadly anthrax attacks that left five people dead, those responsible remain at large. *(Associated Press photograph.)*

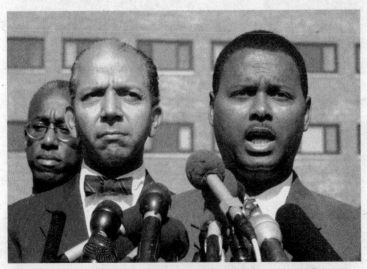

In October 2001, Washington, D.C. Department of Health director Ivan Walks, M.D. (right), is accompanied by Mayor Anthony Williams (center) as he discusses the deaths of two postal workers and the sickness of two others from anthrax inhalation. *(Associated Press photograph by Ken Cedeno.)*

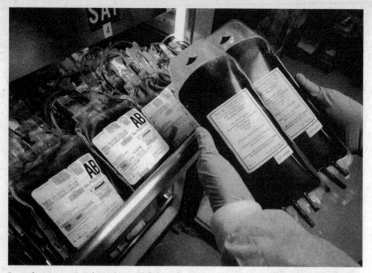

In early 2004, at Michigan's Northfield Laboratories, a technician holds two intravenous bags filled with the blood substitute PolyHeme against a rack of bags filled with expired blood. For years, at least twenty U.S. emergency rooms have tested various types of artificial blood without patient consent. Detroit hospitals have infused PolyHeme at random into severely injured, usually unconscious ER patients who cannot give or withhold consent.   *(Associated Press photograph by M. Spencer Green.)*

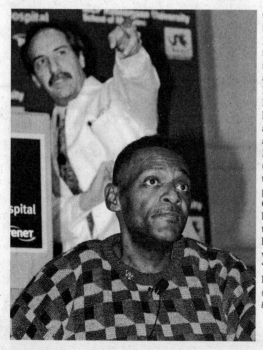

On December 6, 2001, fifty-one-year-old James Quinn (in the foreground) took part in a news conference at Philadelphia's Hahnemann University Hospital a month after he was implanted with an experimental Abiocor artificial heart. Louis Edward Samuels, M.D. (rear), directed the cardiac transplant team that performed the surgery. Quinn later insisted that he had been misled by the physicians and lamented that his life with the heart was "Nothing, nothing like I thought it would be." *(Associated Press photograph by Dan Loh.)*

THE ABANDONED VACCINE

But new barriers to effective treatment threaten to replace the old ones, and many suspect that at least one is being driven by research biases against black patients. Many African Americans and their medical advocates responded with outraged disbelief in 2003 when AIDSVAX, the first vaccine to enter Phase III trials (see chapter 10 for a description of Phase I, II, and III clinical trials), was dismissed as worthless and abandoned even though some data indicated that it actually protected blacks and Asians from HIV infection quite efficiently.[18]

The *New York Times* joined other major newspapers in lamenting the trial's "failure." Its headline read LARGE TRIAL FINDS AIDS VACCINE FAILS TO STOP INFECTION, and the trial's dramatic success in African Americans and Asians was buried within the story, surrounded by qualifications and vague expressions of skepticism.[19] No stories asked why the trials of AIDSVAX, developed by VaxGen of Brisbane, California, were being halted when its efficacy in minority groups ranged from 67 to 78 percent. Among minorities, principally blacks and Asians, only 3.7 percent of vaccinated participants became infected with HIV, in contrast to 9.9 percent of minorities who took a placebo. The vaccine cut the infection rate in blacks by 78 percent—66.8 percent after statistical refinements. Among the 314 African American volunteers, 9 of the 111 subjects who took the placebo (8.1 percent) became infected, compared to 4 of the 203 African Americans who received the vaccine. VaxGen said the vaccine protected two-thirds of African American, Asian, and mixed-race volunteers. Just 500 minority subjects participated, but the results were still statistically significant and carried, at most, a 2 percent possibility that the heartening results arose by chance.[20] "The statistics look impressive," said Dr. Anthony Fauci, director of the National Institute of Allergy and Infectious Diseases, the nation's top infectious-disease professional.[21]

But among whites, no statistically significant change emerged between vaccinated and nonvaccinated groups of subjects.[22] Researchers did not yet understand this disparity with regard to the vaccine, but such disparate effects are not unheard of: In clinical trials, a recently tested herpes (HSV-2) vaccine worked much better for women than for men, although researchers are not sure why.

But although the gender disparities in the herpes vaccine efficacy were accepted, the racial disparities emanating from the HIV vaccine trial were not. This led a team of researchers from the NIH/CDC/University of Washington to review the data. Dr. Dean Follman of the National Institutes of Health (NIH) reanalyzed the data and determined that a significant result could be obtained by chance about 22 percent of the time when the data from the fifteen subgroups, including African Americans, were evaluated. The researchers concluded that the VaxGen data indicating protection for African Americans were spurious.

This contradicted VaxGen's claims that it had tested the minority-group data and found only a 2 percent possibility that the figures showing protection against HIV could have arisen by chance. Follman explained this by alleging that VaxGen had never performed the necessary tests that would allow it to make this claim. The Follman study seems to have laid African American hopes for a benefit from the Vax-Gen vaccine to rest. Experts largely agree. For example, the International AIDS Vaccine Initiative (IAVI) Report for February–April 2004 included an article entitled "VaxGen Denouement: No Efficacy in Racial Subgroups, No Efficacy in Thai Trial."

These experts may well be right and the vaccine's hoped-for effectiveness against HIV in black and Asian segments of the population may be chimerical, a mere statistical mirage. But there is room for doubt, and it is important medically and socially to commission more exhaustive studies before deciding that the benefits are illusory. Also, compare the rapid dismissal of this purported special racial benefit with the uncritical acceptance of BiDil's supposed special racial efficacy, as detailed in chapter 13. One can then understand why some wonder if factors other than scientific rigor are driving the decisions.

Incorporating larger numbers of African American participants could help resolve any ambiguity. Despite the widespread assumptions that African Americans will not participate in clinical trials, especially HIV trials, some researchers are very successful in recruiting black subjects. Emory University professor Otis Brawley, M.D., consistently recruited a large percentage of black research subjects while he was director of the Office of Special Populations Research at the National Cancer Institute. Drs. LaSalle L'Enfant and Clarence Grim, among others, regularly meet or exceed their ambitious goals for minority recruitment in clinical trials. A *New York Times* article by Linda Villarosa has documented successes in African American recruitment by scientists such as Dr. Beryl Koblin, principal investigator of Project Achieve, and Elmerlene Robertson, an outreach worker at the University of Illinois at Chicago: They recruited hundreds of HIV trial subjects, 84 percent of whom were black women. Such programs demonstrate that even more blacks can be recruited when others invest in the trust-building that has worked for them and adopt large-scale recruitment efforts.[23]

Social justice demands continued evaluation of AIDSVAX, even if it does help "only" minorities. After all, African Americans do not represent a minority in the AIDS crisis; they constitute the majority of the people with AIDS in this country. Also, research abounds for infectious-disease therapies that work well for whites and not for blacks. For example, beta interferon research escalates steadily despite the fact that the drug is much less likely to rid infection from African Americans with hepatitis C than from their white counterparts. Funds and resources are constantly spent on refinements of the drug, as they well should be, because doing so helps protect a good proportion of the population. However, more research and resources should go into finding therapeutics that work for African Americans, who suffer disproportionately from HIV infection.

Also, should the factor that heralds AIDSVAX success in minorities prove real, not an artifact, it may not be biological or "racial" at all. It may well be a behavioral or environmental factor that can be adapted to other ethnic groups, as well. Therefore, if this vaccine is ultimately shown to work for minority-group members, a way might be found for it to protect whites. Even should the effectiveness prove to have a biological basis, it will probably, like most "racial" features, prove to be very imperfectly correlated with race: Whites will benefit from it, too.

Finally, the world is watching our decision on AIDSVAX. The World Health Organization mounted a "3 by 5" initiative to treat 3 million people with AIDS by 2005, and an effective vaccine would be an essential tool in the global struggle with AIDS. But we have an ugly history to overcome. The United States has consistently tested candidate medications tailored exclusively to the needs of the developed world by using the bodies of poor Third World denizens, who are desperate for any type of medical attention. We have a moral obligation and a redeeming moral opportunity to ensure that the vaccines we design and adopt are vaccines that work for the most endangered populations. Enabling the production of such vaccines for the medically underserved at home is a good place to start.

CHAPTER 14

THE MACHINE AGE

African American Martyrs to Surgical Technology

. . . . it was cheaper to use niggers than cats, because they
were everywhere and cheap experimental animals . . .
—HARRY BAILEY, M.D., C. 1977, ON HIS NEUROSURGICAL
RESEARCH AT TULANE UNIVERSITY

It has become appallingly obvious that our technology
has exceeded our humanity.
—ALBERT EINSTEIN

James Quinn was only fifty-two when he died in 2002, but he had suffered as no man had ever suffered before. No one had ever been implanted with the same version of an experimental artificial heart and no
one had suffered his constellation of dread sequelae.[1] He was apparently
doomed by heart failure within six months, so on November 5, his
wife, Irene, said that Quinn had agreed to be implanted with an artificial
heart that was intended to make him freely mobile and that was described to him as his last chance at a meaningful life. His surgeon, Dr.
Louis E. Samuels, spoke triumphantly of Quinn having lived with his
AbioCor artificial heart longer than anyone had expected—nine
months.

But Irene remembered James's postsurgical experience as a life extended but overrun by pain, disappointment, and despair. Quinn suffered a stroke the very next month that weakened his left side and left
him with a tentative, halting gait. He soon grew unable to walk even
short distances. A deeply religious man, he had hoped to go home to his
wife, family, and church, but instead he remained tethered by exhaustion
to a bed in a hospital suite, bound by a medical lifeline that sustained
him, after a fashion, through a series of strokes and pneumonias. Quinn
himself, when asked about his life with an artificial heart, was unambigu-

ous: "This is nothing, nothing like I thought it would be. If I had to do it over again, I wouldn't do it. No ma'am. I would take my chances on life."[2]

Finally, Quinn lay brain-dead, which, as the doctors explained to Irene Quinn, simply meant dead. Her husband's brain was already gone, dooming any attempt to resurrect his body, they said, and the AbioCor heart still beat only because it was a machine whose computerized power source fueled its futile rhythm. All that remained, the doctors told Mrs. Quinn, was to unplug the machine from the insensate body that would never again think, move, feel, see, or speak. So Mrs. Quinn gathered her minister, friends, and family to join the surgical staff in the eighth-floor cardiac ICU. After Quinn's minister gave a brief eulogy, his cousin sang the Lord's Prayer and Dr. Samuels had his nurse turn off the console that supplied power to Quinn's heart.

Suddenly, Quinn sat bolt upright and thrust his arms out as if to the heavens before crossing his hands and lying back down. "You're killing him!" screamed Irene Quinn. "He wasn't ready!"[3]

Mrs. Quinn maintains that she and her husband had been deceived by the AbioCor Corporation, by the doctors who implanted the heart, and even by the patient advocate who was charged with helping them to negotiate the experimental-treatment procedure. The advocate was supposed to explain to the Quinns what life would be like with the experimental device implanted. But Mrs. Quinn now says that the patient advocate was actually an advocate for the hospital and the company, not for her husband. She sued AbioCor, and in June 2003, she and the company reached a $125,000 settlement.[4]

Hope and Artifice

James Quinn was the second of six patients to be implanted with Abio-Cor hearts and the second to suffer strokes. Robert Tools, who was also black, received the first model in the Jewish Hospital in Louisville, Kentucky, and died in July 2001, five months after the implantation.[5] The medical coverage of Tools's implantation stressed his role as a pioneer because he was the first to receive an artificial heart that was fully self-contained and implantable. The AbioCor device, like the heart, is a softball-size pump that, like the heart, resides fully within the chest, without any protruding tubes or wires. But the AbioCor is a machine, powered by batteries, and an experimental one at that. Although the coverage of Tools's new heart was almost universally positive, many African American news media took a divergent stance, asking whether Tools had been selected for an exceedingly risky and untried surgery *because* he was black (and by implication, expendable).

However, no media outlets asked another important question: Should self-contained artificial hearts become FDA-approved and go on the market with a hefty price tag, will African Americans be able to afford them, or will they be shut out of the technology that they helped to perfect? The same question can be asked of other bionic technologies being devised to replace diseased or damaged eyes, ears, and limbs. Geography, tradition, and culture intersect to make blacks likely research subjects for new technologies, but race and economics tend to place them outside the marketplace for these same technologies when they are perfected.

This is a consistent pattern with novel surgical technologies. Marion Sims's vesicovaginal-fistula research subjects were black slaves, and today groups of poor black women are least likely to benefit from the surgery. Today's highly visible role of blacks in testing heart-transplantation technology parallels a deluge of medical-journal articles documenting how blacks are less likely than whites to receive high-tech cardiac interventions once they are perfected and become the standard of care.[6]

The media coverage has also failed to question the significance of two successive trials with black patients. When Quinn's heart was implanted, media outlets treated his story separately from the experience of Robert Tools, thus ignoring its significance as part of a pattern. At this point, African Americans, who make up 12.3 percent of the population, constituted 33 percent of the implantees—almost three times their representation in the population. It is interesting that the incipient pattern was all but ignored in the United States, because other countries plagued by black-white racial tensions, such as South Africa under apartheid, have faced the same questions. Pioneering surgeons there are well aware of the suspicions raised by such use of black subjects. For example, the first potential donor for the world's first heart transplant, chosen by South African surgical pioneer Christiaan Barnard,[7] was a black man, but Barnard's colleagues warned him that if the experiment went awry, he would go down in history as an Afrikaner Mengele, so he waited for the heart of a white subject.

AbioCor's experimental protocol permits it to recruit its subjects from patients with end-stage heart failure whose chance of dying within thirty days is a least 70 percent. The company is supposed to approach only those people who have no other treatment options. By June 2005, all fourteen patients implanted with the heart had died, two immediately following surgery. The AbioCor heart failed in two cases. Twelve patients survived for two to seventeen months, but even for those who lived past a few months, doubts reigned about the quality of their extended lives. Yet Abiomed asked the FDA's permission to sell the heart as a "humanitarian device exemption" under a program that allows the sale of devices to patients who have no other options. When the FDA advisory panel denied this request, its chief, Julie Swain, questioned whether the AbioCor was actually "prolonging life, not prolonging death." Proponents see it as the subject's chance, however slim, for a longer life, and as a necessary step toward a device that may one day save millions from heart failure, which kills African Americans at the same rate as whites. Critics point to the dismal postsurgical record of crippling strokes and pneumonia and the poor quality of life inflicted upon its subjects. Finally, there is the fact that some, like the Quinns, were obviously expecting a very different postsurgical experience.

Such expectations are an unaddressed feature of experimental remedies that, like the AbioCor artificial heart, are offered to desperate patients with only months to live: Patients may find any chance at life irresistible and may not hear caveats about the limitations of the therapies, even if they are offered.

But are such warnings offered in a fair and intelligible manner? AbioCor's consent form warned the Quinns that death and disability are possible outcomes, but so do consent forms for gallbladder removal, nose jobs, and many other procedures that are considered relatively safe and routine. Other elements of AbioCor's consent form could be read as encouraging the hopes that the Quinns entertained.

The informed-consent process consists of much more than obtaining a patient's signature on a piece of paper. Informed consent is an ongoing process of patient notification and education. The investigator must explain the process in exhaustive detail to the patient, must divulge any financial or other interests that she has in the experiment and must answer all the subject's questions. The scientist must also make sure the subject knows all the known risks and must inform the subject of new risks as such emerge or become known. The researchers must also tell the subject that he can quit the experiment at any time, but such a guarantee is meaningless in an all-or-nothing experimental venture such as the AbioCor tests: Quitting the experiment means dying.

Several studies have revealed that certain flaws tend to characterize consent forms. The forms use technical language and scientific jargon, which makes patients further dependent upon an interpretation by the investigators conducting the study. The forms tend to exaggerate benefits and to underplay risks, presenting an overly optimistic view regarding quality of life during and after the experiment. Such understatement is typical of how the medical jargon helps to distort the portrayal of the likely quality of life. For example, the use of such words as *discomfort* and *fatigue* may mask the potential for severe pain and crippling exhaustion, Such errors can mislead patients like James Quinn into unmet expectations from their experimental devices.

But most of all, when the desperately ill are confronted with extreme measures and heroic experimental ventures, they risk confusing research with therapy, and so do their doctors. Patients rarely understand that physicians conducting the research are primarily interested in the research, not an individual patient's survival and quality of life. Witness the disparity between James and Irene Quinn's despairing assessment of Quinn's tenure on the AbioCor heart ("This is nothing, nothing like I thought it would be") and his physician's buoyant claim that Quinn had survived for nine months.

AbioCor also took a step that escalates the ethical debate. It asked the FDA to approve the experimental implantation of artificial hearts *without the informed consent of the patient.* The company wished to expand its pool of subjects by widening the experimental criteria to include patients who suffer massive heart attacks, even if they are unconscious or otherwise unable to consent. The AbioCor company said it will encourage patients to select a health proxy, who is usually, but not always, a relative, to offer consent on the part of the patient.

This, however, is not consent by the patient, and moreover, it is an unprecedented and wholly inappropriate role for a health proxy, who assumes responsibilities that devolve around therapeutic-treatment decisions, not those that relate to radical experimental devices. African Americans are at least 20 percent less likely than whites to select a health proxy or to elect any type of advance directive. Therefore, even in the scenario promulgated by AbioCor, an African American is more likely than a white to be implanted with an experimental artificial heart unwittingly and without input from any trusted person who speaks for him.

Such a step would be an unconscionable erosion of informed consent and it would disproportionately affect African Americans, who are least likely to have a health proxy and are most likely to be treated in an emergency room. It would also be dangerous, because although the company had hoped to begin marketing the heart in 2005, technical problems haunt the AbioCor heart.

The hazards of the AbioCor heart were illustrated by the September 2004 death of Don Graham, the thirteenth person implanted. After only five months of implantation, Graham, a white subject, died as a result of "an unspecified malfunction of the device," according to AbioCor official Andrea tenBroek. The fourteenth patient implanted died in 2004. The implantees lived for six months, on average, and only one ever left the hospital. An FDA committee ruled against the heart's approval in 2004.[8]

Involuntary Infusion

AbioCor's request to conscript unconscious patients in extremis as experimental subjects is not unprecedented. At least twenty U.S. emergency rooms have been using another new experimental technology, artificial blood, for years without patient consent.[9] Detroit hospitals have been quietly experimenting with a commercial blood substitute called PolyHeme, which is derived from human blood. To test this substance, emergency medical technicians and participating hospitals infuse it at random into severely injured, mostly unconscious ER patients who cannot give consent. Patients who require a blood infusion alternately receive PolyHeme and blood during their first twelve hours in the ER. A similar blood substitute called Hemopure, consisting of purified hemoglobin[10] derived from cow's blood, was first tested on moribund emergency room patients, but in South Africa. Hemopure's manufacturers say it is screened for the "mad cow" prion that causes bovine spongiform encephalopathy (BSE) and Creuzfeldt-Jakob disease (CJD) in humans, but there are concerns about other emerging diseases. Nevertheless, it was approved for South African use in 2001 and is used principally in hospital emergency departments that serve black-township patients.

A safe blood substitute is devoutly to be wished because it would enable transfusions without the need to match types, and it would allow patients to avoid the risk of illnesses such as HIV, HCV, and other blood-borne pathogens. People with sickle-cell anemia who need transfusions will face no hemoglobin incompatibilities, and surgery will become safer for Jehovah's Witnesses, whose religion prohibits the ingestion or infusion of blood. A safe blood substitute will replenish the stores of blood banks, which run low with regularity in large cities, and will serve ambulances that cannot stock blood because of its forty-two-hour shelf life: Hemopure lasts for two years at room temperature.

But administering substances such as PolyHeme at random to accident victims and to emergency room patients without their permission is a troubling step. First, if PolyHeme, like the earlier substitute, proves injurious or fatal to some, this result will be unnecessary, because human blood would have treated them without experimental risk. Any injury will have been compounded by the failure to have sought the patient's permission. Also, the random administration serves the experiment's needs for randomization but does not constitute good medical care, which should be predicated upon the individual patient's needs. Such emergency room research is likely to be conducted with blacks, not whites. In the 1980s, Department of Health and Human Services data confirmed that black Americans are more likely than other Americans to use emergency departments for their medical care, and both a 2001 study in the *Yale Journal of Health Policy, Law and Ethics* and a September 2002 study in *Academic Emergency Medicine* confirm that this trend continues.

Early test results revealed that subjects who received PolyHeme instead of blood suffered more adverse effects, such as shock, respiratory failure, and pneumonia—and a 49 percent higher death rate. Despite this deeply troubling finding, in May 2007, the federal government launched much more of the same—a $50 million, five-year, eleven-site project to be managed by the Resuscitation Outcomes Consortium. It will subject approximately 21,000 patients to medical experiments without first asking their permission.

The FDA has approved at least fifteen such nonconsensual research projects since 1996, when it began to allow researchers to dispense with asking patient consent for experimental treatment in life-or-death scenarios. This disproportionate use of black bodies to perfect cutting-edge medical technology is hardly novel. Even medieval medical lore entertained the belief that black bodies were suitable for use in experimental treatments. For example, a medieval engraving by fifteenth-century artist Girolamo da Cremona entitled *Saints Cosmas and Damian Transplanting a Leg* shows the transplantation of a black leg onto a white body. The story focuses upon the miracle of a saint made whole by the amputation of an infected leg and its replacement by another, but some who view it will focus instead upon the black grafted leg, wondering about its provenance: Did it come from a truly dead body? In the background of the painting, which still hangs in the museum of the Church of San Marco in Florence, the artist is painting a black man with one leg entombed in a casket.

Five hundred years later, in 1935, University of Pennsylvania School of Medicine gastroenterologist William Osler Abbott was developing a way to rapidly intubate the human intestine by inserting a tube from mouth to rectum that would enable doctors to treat intestinal disorders more efficiently. Testing the device entailed getting men to swallow twelve feet of rubber tubing, then submit to radiation scans to track the intubation. Jobless white men turned their noses up at the disgusting work and paltry pay, but through his black janitor, "Harry," Abbott found poor black men who would submit for fifty cents an hour, possibly because he failed to explain how dangerous the repeated radiation exposures were. Abbott consistently referred to his subject pool as "my animals," as when he cackled during a postprandial speech to Philadelphia's Charaka Club (a group of physicians with an interest in literature): "I'm sure my animals had a larger intake of corn liquor, pork chops, and chewing tobacco than the white rats in the medical school, but at least they were human."[11]

Abbott went on to describe how, once, a fluoroscopy revealed a bullet lodged in a subject's muscle, leading the doctor to muse, "Such events led me to wish at times that I could keep my animals in metabolism cages. Those boys may have been short on morals but they were long on gut."[12]

At least Abbott's despised subjects were consenting, if not informed. Researchers have also tested cutting-edge technologies without the permission and sometimes without the knowledge of the subject.

For example, in his memoir *As I Remember Him: The Story of R.S.*, Harvard microbiologist Hans Zinsser recalls that when he needed specimens of live lice for his research on typhus, he approached a Boston policeman, who obligingly arrested "the old coon that sells pencils down near the South Station," forcibly taking the vendor to the station house. There, Zinsser retrieved his lice at leisure. Despite the man's protests that "I'm an American citizen and I got my rights. I dunno what youse all talkin' bout de cause of science," the police threatened him with jail if he did not permit Zinsser to harvest his lice for medical research.[13]

The use of engineered human cells for medical treatment is another example of medical technology devised through research on blacks but from which they benefit less often than whites. In 1951, the science of cell-line culture was founded with usually long-lived cervical cells from black Baltimore housewife and cancer patient Henrietta Lacks. (Her cells were conventionally nicknamed HeLa, after the two initial letters of her first and last names.) Without the knowledge or consent of Lacks or her family, George Gey, M.D., of Johns Hopkins Hospital, harvested her cells and used them to transform medicine. Vaccines could now be tested and lengthy experiments completed that would have been unthinkable a few months earlier. One advance was immediate and dramatic: The Salk polio vaccine was tested and perfected with HeLa cells produced by Tuskegee Institute Laboratories in 1952, only a year after Henrietta Lacks died. Today, the science of cell-line culture has enabled cultivation and therapy with stem cells, immature cells that can develop into many other types of needed cells, including red blood cells, white blood cells, and platelets. Today, many Americans and most scientists hail research with stem cells as the key to taming disease; the only identified group to oppose stem-cell research are African Americans, 44 percent of whom are opposed to their use. This attitude may be driven by the racial disparity in current stem-cell treatments such as bone-marrow transplants, because African American patients are less likely than whites to match with a donor.

In the 1950s and 1960s, some surgeons still were quite candid about using black bodies bought cheaply for testing for new technologies. In 1955, Dr. Harry Bailey was a promising and ambitious young Australian psychiatrist, who is remembered by friends and foes alike as possessed of a prominent arrogant streak. As a World Health Organization traveling research fellow, Bailey had worked in several countries and in Chicago before he arrived in New Orleans for a fateful collaboration with Dr. Robert Heath at Tulane University.

Dr. Heath offered Bailey a researcher's dream: bold, adventurous projects, a surfeit of docile black subjects, a cadre of researchers as ambitious, arrogant, and ruthless as himself, and a deluge of funding, courtesy of the Central Intelligence Agency, which equipped, oversaw, and bankrolled their research.

The CIA charged the researchers with conducting extensive, ambitious mind-control research because it was concerned that the Soviet Union and other U.S. enemies might have learned to control behavior via "brainwashing."

Among their many science-fiction neurosurgical exploits was the array of electrodes that Bailey and Heath devised and then implanted into the brains of black subjects for as long as three years each. The team used the electrodes to deliver charges to the limbic system of the brain. This group of related brain structures includes the amygdala, the hippocampus, and the septum, which are key to emotions and judgment. By stimulating these areas, Bailey evoked pleasure, pain, joy, anger, sexual arousal, and other powerful emotions in his black subjects at will. The electrodes were designed to facilitate stimulation of the brain's "pleasure centers" either by a remote operator or by the subject himself, using a transistorized "self-stimulator" unit worn on the patient's belt. Bailey did some of these experiments on black prisoners in New Orleans's Louisiana State Penitentiary but made no mention of how he gained access to other hospitalized patients for such experiments or whether any sort of consent had been sought. Neither he nor Heath ever mentioned what they told the patients. But Bailey reminisced about his methods at Tulane when speaking to a group of nurses in Chelmsford, back in his native Australia, twenty years later,

> Well now, this goes back to America, when I was working in America in New Orleans, there was experimental work being done there on cats, where they found that if you put electrodes down on the anterior part of the brain, in the septal region between the two hemispheres and down, right deep down, sort of here, put electrodes in here, that you struck a [inaudible] which had something to do with screwing and orgasm and pleasure and satisfaction. And if they put a wire in this and took it out and put it on to a push button, the cat would very quickly know that if it pressed the button, it got a little "chop," and this was a sort of a little orgasm. And

so the cat would go "pop" again, and get the taste of it, and the cat would go "pop, pop, pop, pop." Here was something important. What did you make of it?

So, in New Orleans, where it was cheaper to use niggers than cats, because they were everywhere and cheap experimental animals—there wasn't much working there, the people we have been picking for the operation has [*sic*] really been at the bottom of the can. Nothing is going to help them—shoot them is the only thing—so they started to use them, Negroes—patients in hospitals—and so, the same area, little box, was put on their paws with a button. They just went around, "pop, pop, pop," all the time, continuous orgasms. . . .

Bailey also tested LSD and the drug bulbocapnine, which can cause "catatonia and stupor," on African American prisoners at the Louisiana State Penitentiary. According to one CIA memo, the Agency wished to know whether bulbocapnine could produce aphasia (the loss of speech), anesthesia, memory loss, or a sabotaging of willpower "in persons with a weak type of central nervous system." Decades later, some survivors sued the federal government and the CIA, which settled out of court and agreed to pay $750,000 to seven former mind-control victims.

After his return to Australia, Bailey opened a "deep sleep therapy" clinic for depression and a wide variety of other psychiatric complaints at Chelmsford Hospital in Sydney, which he operated between 1963 and 1979. The deep sleep therapy technique is a misnomer for patient abuse that Bailey practiced by placing thousands of patients with a wide variety of psychiatric symptoms into a barbiturate-induced coma for two weeks, during which time he administered repeated electroshock therapy and implanted electrodes and even metal plates into many of their brains, without their knowledge or consent. Many patients deteriorated dramatically, but they learned only years later from news accounts what their doctor had done to them. He sexually abused some of the women patients. Scores of patients died, although Bailey concealed the true number by arranging for many worsening patients to be shipped off to other hospitals, where they died without ever regaining consciousness.

Australian courts attributed at least sixty-five of his patients' deaths to "unlawful and negligent treatment." But rather than face a criminal trial, Bailey committed suicide in 1985, with Tuinal, a barbiturate that he had used to destroy the minds of his victims.[14]

In his 1967 work *Human Guinea Pigs,* physician Maurice H. Pappworth chronicled the use of black subjects to perfect new medical technologies. For example, he described an event in the 1962 experimental perfection of the new technique of translumbar aortography:

> A thirty one year old negress had abdominal pains and urinary symptoms and because the diagnosis was in doubt, it was decided to submit her to aortography. However the needle instead of entering the abdominal aorta, was accidentally pushed into the spinal canal and the contrast medium was injected into the meninges [the protective covering of the brain and upper spinal cord]. Forty-five minutes later, severe lumbar pain was followed by convulsion and the patient died in two hours. Post-mortem showed a tuberculous left kidney which could have been successfully treated.[15]

This chapter has described how, in a sparsely examined subtext of surgical research, African American bodies have served to refine technologies from vesicovaginal fistula to artificial hearts, but unfortunately, once perfected, the distribution of that technology has not been colorblind. Blacks are likely to have less access to the technology.

Safe, nonexploitative research into surgical technology is in everyone's best interest, but for African Americans to remain open to such research, medical policies and practice will have to do a better job of shielding black Americans from abuse.

CHAPTER 15

ABERRANT WARS

American Bioterrorism Targets Blacks

*The development of molecular medicine based on our new under-
standing of genomics will allow a vast range of new weaponry to be
developed. Among that range could be biological weapons specifically
targeted at particular ethnic groups.*

—PROFESSOR MALCOLM DANDO, BRADFORD UNIVERSITY,

SCOTLAND, 1999

*I must confirm that the structure of the [Chemical and Biological
Warfare] project was based on the U.S. system. That's where we
learnt the most.*

—WOUTER BASSON, M.D., THE "MENGELE OF SOUTH AFRICA"

During segregation, the long last gasp of American apartheid, the legal
standard of "separate but equal" meant more than racial separation. It
meant inequality sanctioned by law and enforced by violence and terror.
In southern states such as Florida and Georgia, segregation meant inferior education, nearly nonexistent health care, and dilapidated housing
that was infested by vermin, glazed with lead, and for blacks only. But as
the multiracial civil rights movement gained momentum, proud symbols of the dawning new age rose. In Miami, Florida, the state built a spa-
cious modern 466-unit addition to a sprawling 1946 housing complex in
the summer of 1951. Unlike the older portions of the complex, it was
opened to blacks. This pristine symbol of hope was named Carver Village, after Dr. George Washington Carver, America's best-loved scientist.[1]
The glistening new buildings, in a fledging town of the same name, remained black-only dwellings in the summer of 1951, but Carver Village
was the largest, most impressive new minority-housing development in
the nation.

This distinction was quickly eclipsed, however, by the complex's prominence as one of the bloodiest battlegrounds of the civil rights movement. Carver Village amounted to a desegregation of the larger housing complex, and this precipitated Klan organizing drives in Miami, white motorcades accompanied by rock throwing, and the shooting of a black man. On September 22, two one-hundred-pound boxes of dynamite blasted an untenanted building at the complex. In October, three bombs tore through Jewish schools and synagogues in the city. When threats, rallies, lynching, and drive-by shootings failed to keep Carver Village residents from demanding places at the local polls and lunch counters, the Ku Klux Klan escalated its murderous assaults.

On November 30 and December 2, 1951, more dynamite blasts rocked Carver Village, leaving huge areas bombed out and uninhabitable. Another bomb was left on the steps of a Catholic church that was the spiritual home of antisegregationists, and the *Miami Herald* reported, "Floggings were reported in Orange County."

December was a particularly bloody month: Dynamite blasts blew out windows and leveled walls of the Miami Hebrew Synagogue and Tifereth Israel Synagogue to punish Jewish sympathizers, and this incendiary violence was followed by the Christmas Day bombing assassination of Harry T. Moore, head of the Florida NAACP. Open racial warfare in the streets began to punctuate the exchange of acerbic racial rhetoric. But by 1960, unnoticed amid Carver Village's raucous racial strife, the dramatic bloodletting had been married to another, silent, species of violence, this time at the hands of the U.S. government.

The U.S. Army and the CIA, like the Klan, had Carver Village in their sights.

Despite U.S. insistence that it was only developing defensive biological weapons, the Central Intelligence Agency in 1952 entered into a partnership to produce chemical and biological weapons with first-strike capability. The Army's Special Operations Division laboratories at Fort Detrick, Maryland, served as the site of the joint army-CIA program dubbed MK-NAOMI.

Fort Detrick's Army Chemical Corps laboratory bred more than four million mosquitoes *per day* and released them in hordes around Florida, including near Carver Village. This was an experiment to determine whether these droning syringes on the wing—disease vectors, in medical parlance—could be used as first-strike biological weapons to

spread yellow fever and other infectious diseases, ostensibly among foreign troops during wartime.[2] This was not the government's first local
exercise in such biological "friendly fire." A similar 1955 experiment had
also targeted a black area, but because it bordered a white development,
people of both races were sickened: Such exposures had already tripled
Florida's whooping cough cases within a year, resulting in a dozen deaths
after a whooping cough virus was released in Palmetto, on Florida's west
coast. Carver Village was more precisely targeted and was subjected to
the same strain, which drove up 1955 infection and death rates; and 8
percent of these 1,080 whooping cough cases affected children nine years
old and under.[3] By 1960, Carver Village residents had been plagued by a
rash of mysterious illnesses, including the symptoms of dengue and yellow fever, and deaths.[4]

An analysis of the records of MK-ULTRA, of which MK-NAOMI
was a part, suggests the Agency released various biological agents, from
mosquitoes to bacteria, in hundreds of such dispersals, and the large
number of exposures makes it less surprising that mosquitoes were also
unleashed upon another all-black site called Carver Village, this one in
Georgia's Chatham County (Savannah is the county seat).[5] Longtime
Carver Village, Georgia, resident Dorothy Pelote, former president of the
Carver Heights Mission Improvement Organization, recalls that in 1955,
"young white men came to our house and talked with me and my husband. They said they were doing a study on mosquitoes and wanted to
place a trap in our backyard to see how far they had spread in our area,
but they didn't go into detail. They lied. They said one thing when they
were really doing something else. I [had] figured that they were from the
Health Department.

"Later, when people started getting sick and dying, I spoke with several people who recalled those boxes being placed in their backyards. After the study, they came back and got the boxes from our backyard."

In 1979, Pelote also told the *Atlanta Journal*[6] that between April and
November 1956, the army conducted a survey of residents to determine
how many had been bitten by mosquitoes. "But nothing was revealed to
us until the '80s: I could not believe it, but those people used us as guinea
pigs."

After the story broke in the 1980s, victims came forward, but news
accounts tended not to name them. In 1956, for example, one unnamed

black woman had fainted after a swarming "dark cloud of mosquitoes" covered her thickly. She had to be taken to a hospital, where medical workers wondered at the bite marks covering her body. Twenty years later, she still could not walk unassisted.

The phrase "human guinea pigs" is frequently a prelude to hyperbole, but Dorothy Pelote sounds far too businesslike to be a conspiracy theorist. Her speech is crisp and her responses are unfailingly concise and on point, even impatient, as she recalls the events of half a century ago without hesitation or ambiguity. But then, she has relived those events often. In the 1960s, she organized the residents in an attempt to understand the mosquito experiments, twenty years before evidence of their true nature surfaced.

The spikes in local disease and deaths convinced the army-CIA consortium that the infected mosquitoes would indeed make an effective biological weapon against the Soviets, who had no medical capability for organizing massive vaccination programs.[7]

But for years, the CIA denied that it had unleashed such biological agents against its own citizens, despite the dramatic leap in illnesses and death rates and despite the testimony of Pelote and other Georgia Carver Village residents. The government agents could plead innocence because they knew that there was no evidence.

In 1973, MK-ULTRA's director, Dr. Sidney Gottlieb, decided to sweep up the program's paper trail, citing his agency's "burgeoning paper problem." One can argue that he really intended to erase all traces of MK-ULTRA's nefarious experimentation in the wake of the intense media and popular scrutiny of Cold War medical aggression by the government against its own people. During the late 1960s and the 1970s, as has been detailed in earlier chapters, the media revelations of the government's unethical prison experimentation, the Tuskegee Syphilis Study, and the XYY experiments with black boys in Baltimore outraged the nation. Such research scandals were generating headlines and restrictive new laws. Reporters were alive to the news value of just the sort of Frankensteinian research that Gottlieb's team had been promulgating with tax dollars, from the electrodes implanted in the brains of black prisoners by Harry Bailey, M.D., to the mosquitoes that invaded Carver Village. Gottlieb was not eager to join his erstwhile colleagues in the klieg lights. Also, the new legal restrictions had ended the carnival-like laissez-faire research atmosphere marked by generous funding and few questions.

These developments had driven most MK-ULTRA researchers to search for other, less controversial sources of federal money, and others, such as Bailey, were no longer active in America.

It was in this atmosphere that Gottlieb oversaw the destruction of Agency and individual case files. In 1975, CIA director William E. Colby acknowledged that the Agency discarded most MK-ULTRA documents, including those of its subset MK-NAOMI, by 1973, rendering them "very incomplete."[8] With them vanished not only the proof but the institutional memories of yesterday's research abuses; it was as if they had never existed.

But some residents of the Florida and of the Georgia exposure sites had not forgotten. They knew they had suddenly begun to sicken and some had died of mysterious ailments after 1953 and some remembered being visited by government representatives who made unusual requests around that time the sicknesses began. Something was amiss. Dorothy Pelote put the two occurrences together and became the point woman, seeking answers to what she was convinced was the poisoning of her community.

However, she had no proof. That is, she had no proof for more than a quarter of a century, when American Citizens for Honesty in Government, a subcommittee of the Church of Scientology, launched a dogged, ambitious investigative report into MK-ULTRA's activities. American Citizens for Honesty in Government collected the heavily censored documents and collated them with known biological exposures, then released a report that included copies of the damning originals. They repeatedly used Freedom of Information Act requests to obtain the detritus of Gottlieb's purge, only to discover that all that escaped destruction were some folders full of the most mundane material imaginable.[9] Train schedules, restaurant checks, and receipts from a wide variety of drugstores, laboratory and biological supply houses, hardware stores, and restaurants were all that remained of the top secret activities for researchers. But the few receipts for biological agents inspired the resourceful, detail-oriented reporters to decipher the more ordinary receipts in order to retrace the trail of domestic bioterrorism. They showed how circled train timetables and train ticket receipts corresponded to journeys made to Carver Village, Florida, the CIA headquarters, and the repositories of biological agents. Receipts for test animals, chemicals, and even the hiring of a crop duster dovetailed with the spread of biological agents. For example, signed, itemized receipts were issued for such items as cultures of *Hemophilus pertussis*—a whooping cough pathogen—in January 1955, the year that Florida whooping cough cases tripled. The documents also include physicians' bills for attention to injuries suffered by laboratory workers who handled bacteria, as well as receipts for formaldehydė and lime for burying dead lab animals, Lysol for decontaminating protective gear, nasal filters for handling microbes, and the aforementioned crop duster for field dissemination. Some receipts were stamped MK-NAOMI. Others bore the signature of scientists who were managing the project. Despite a 1969 presidential order prohibiting the production or storing of biological-warfare agents, MK-ULTRA receipts for biological and laboratory supplies revealed that the dissemination of disease-carrying mosquitoes in Florida beginning in 1955 and 1956 triggered a long history of domestic bioterrorism by the U.S. government against its own citizens through at least 1972.

Not until nearly 1980 did the Scientologists' research group finish piecing together its research and publish a report, which detailed, among other things, how in 1955–1956 the residents of Florida's Carver Village has been visited with a plague of *Aedes aegypti* mosquitoes. Swarms bred by the Army Chemical Corps at Fort Detrick, Maryland, carried, among other things, yellow fever and dengue fever. A surviving November 9, 1962, MK-ULTRA document described payments for "drugs & other materials," including the "development & testing of . . . BW [biological warfare] harassment systems" and for "large scale production of microorganisms."

Despite the checkered reputation of the Church of Scientology, regarded by many as more cult than church, the extrapolations made by subcommittee members, linking the innocuous-looking MK-ULTRA receipts to the deadly campaign against black Floridians, were so meticulously drawn that the rigor of the reporting gained the respect of the nation's premier periodicals. In 1979, the story was taken up by the *New York Times,* the *Christian Science Monitor,* and the *Washington Post,* which on March 11, 1980, described how "disease-causing agents, one that could touch off undulant fever [brucellosis] and another that could bring on tularemia, were mass produced. And there were many opportunities to utilize such germs—with unwitting American citizens serving as 'test subjects.' "

These newspapers supplied some additional evidence of how these Americans had become targets of domestic bioterrorism research. As in many other terrorist incidents, MK-NAOMI targeted an ethnically distinct group—African Americans. The *New York Times* wrote that the Army Chemical Corps also deployed contaminated homing pigeons in the area during the 1950s and had mounted biological-warfare tests on oat crops in the (predominantly black) Virgin Islands. According to the *Times*, "at least one test caused oat crops to be infected with cereal rust, a destructive grain disease."[10]

Contrast reports on the egregious assaults on the health of black Floridians, Georgians, and Virgin Islanders in the 1950s and 1960s to a 1969 report that details how the government abandoned its plans to test zinc cadmium sprays in northern Virginia to determine the extent of fallout in chemical and biological warfare—the same ostensible purpose as the Carver Village exposures. In the latter case, concern about the possible health effects upon another group of residents—bald eagles in their nesting area—stayed the hand of government scientists.[11]

Unfortunately, these southern exposures were no isolated incidents. For decades before and after, blacks have been subjected to U.S.-mediated bioterrorism perpetrated by American scientists at home and abroad.

Lately, the word *terrorism* has been bandied about widely. It has come to encompass anything from a frank physical assault to an enforced political agenda that differs from the subject's. But terrorism is best defined more narrowly—as a threat or the use of violence (including kidnapping, extortion, assault, and murder) by an individual or organization that targets innocent civilians. In contrast to mere criminality, terrorism is employed to further ideological, political, or religious goals.[12]

Living Weapons

Bioterrorism employs chemical or biological agents such as microbes and poisons in the service of terrorism. Biological weapons often consist of disease-causing organisms, usually microorganisms such as bacteria, viruses, fungi, or derivatives from humans, animals, or plants. These may exist in nature or may be produced by labs; either way, they sicken or kill via infection or poisoning. But nuclear weapons and other chemical agents are also agents of bioterrorism because they can poison biological entities—for example, via radiation poisoning—as well as kill them outright. Bioterrorism can kill people directly, or it can kill by destroying or polluting the water, animals, and plant life upon which people depend.

During World War II, the United States and Great Britain undertook the training of South African military personnel in chemical and biological weapons (CBW) development and strategy, a relationship that was to deepen and continue with ominous implications for black South Africans. Even during the Korean conflict, the United States armed forces unequivocally documented its efforts with regard to psychological and biological warfare. Maj. Gen. Robert L. Lee, director of plans, U.S. Air Force, noted on March 17, 1953, that "the psychological warfare division will direct and supervise covert operations in the scope of unconventional BW weapons (biological warfare) and CW (chemical warfare) operations and programs."[13]

The postwar American agricultural program produced a large amount of weaponized agents. The 1950s scientists favored distribution in bombs filled with a chemical and feather mix, which gave way to aerosol methods. These, however, were dwarfed by the effectiveness of the Soviets' hoof-and-mouth, rinderpest, and African swine fever mixtures, which targeted livestock.[14]

During this period, as we have seen, the Floridian communities of Palmetto and Carver Village[15] were army targets of disease-carrying mosquitoes. Research and development on the use of wheat rust, rice blast and rye blast, foot-and-mouth, and rinderpest against plants and animals was supplemented by the experimental development of porcine brucellosis, anthrax, and psittacosis to be used against humans. But by 1969, the United States would declare that it had ceased development of new biological-warfare agents.[16] The defoliant Agent Orange constituted a biological friendly-fire incident when its use backfired by triggering a variety of persistent health problems in American servicemen and servicewomen in Vietnam.[17]

The Geneva Convention banned CBW in 1963, but evidence suggests that some nations, such as South Africa, never ceased using these weapons. The refinement of weaponized biological and chemical agents by South Africa, the Soviet Union, Israel, and Iraq ushered in the current age. Throughout the 1970s, South Africa was accused of unleashing anthrax against Zimbabwe in the Rhodesian civil war and the Soviets were reported to have used glanders against Afghanistan in the 1980s.[18]

Race and Ricin

Bioterrorism is often a murderous expression of ethnic hatred. In the United States and in South Africa under apartheid, this hatred has been racial in nature, whether white Rhodesians poisoned communities of its black majority or white American "Christian" supremacists modeled on the Klan targeted African Americans. Sometimes the ethnic element lurks below the ideological surface, but U.S. groups with frankly racial political agendas[19] often mount baldly racial attacks. The chief aims of today's violent cults are not only political and social fanaticism but also genocide.[20]

Unsurprisingly, right-wing extremists devise most domestic acts of bioterror against blacks. For example, in 1987, the Arkansas white Christian supremacist group known as the Covenant, the Sword, and the Arm of the Lord amassed thirty gallons of potassium cyanide to poison urban water supplies throughout the nation. They relied upon God, they said, to ensure that only blacks, Jews, and nonbelievers would expire. Their stated aim was to topple the federal government and hasten the Second Coming of the (presumably white, Gentile) Messiah. Before the Covenant could complete this curious act of biological faith, the FBI infiltrated it and arrested its ringleaders.[21] In 1989, yet another group of violent racial extremists deployed a gas bomb that injured eight people in the Atlanta office of the NAACP. These acts of domestic bioterror continued unabated through the end of the century. FBI infiltrators foiled the April 1991 attack on the nation's water supply that the right-wing Patriot's Council of Minnesota planned to undertake with ample stores of the deadly toxin ricin it had manufactured from castor beans. In 1995, yet another American neo-Nazi group stockpiled bubonic plague, apparently purchased from a Maryland firm that provides biological agents for scientific research. But even leftist radicals have targeted blacks through CBW. In fact, the first legally proven fatality from domestic bioterrorism was the 1973 murder of West Oakland school superintendent Dr. Marcus A. Foster, an African American, who was felled by a cyanide-tipped bullet from the arsenal of the Symbionese Liberation Army.[22]

According to the *Bulletin of the Atomic Scientists,* the FBI had mounted 74 investigations involving domestic chemical and biological warfare and nuclear attacks by 1997. The next year, cases ballooned to 181 investigations. Approximately 40 of these were deemed credible threats.[23] But the press reports have tended not to characterize such coordinated domestic genocidal aggressions as bioterrorism, but merely as bizarre weapon attacks by the lunatic fringe. Small violent groups of every stripe embrace CBW as the poor man's nuclear weapon, easier, cheaper, and churning more pervasive anxiety than a gun or a bomb.[24]

Today, the most notorious pathogens that threaten humans are *Yersinia pestis,* which causes bubonic plague; *Bacillus anthracis,* which causes anthrax; and viruses such as variola, the cause of smallpox, and hemorrhagic fevers such as Lassa, Marburg, Ebola, and Hantaan. Most of these have been considered for weaponization.[25]

The Color of Counterterrorism

The terrorists' felling of the World Trade Center towers and concomitant attack upon the Pentagon were followed a month later by anthrax attacks in which five people died and thirteen were sickened.[26] When anthrax was found in mail addressed to several congresspersons and contamination was suspected, Congress was immediately shut down and lawmakers fled the buildings, which were immediately closed and sealed, then decontaminated.

But at the Brentwood Mail Processing and Distribution Center facility in Washington, D.C., where 92 percent of the 2,646 workers were black, letters contaminated with *Bacillus anthracis* spores were processed by both machines and human handlers.[27] Four U.S. Postal Service workers at Brentwood fell ill with what was tardily diagnosed as inhalational anthrax; two died.

Many African Americans perceived a clear racial disparity in how the black and white victims of the anthrax attacks were treated. Thousands of D.C.-area postal workers may have been exposed to anthrax spores from contaminated letters such as those mailed to Senators Thomas A. Daschle and Patrick Leahy. Although inhaled anthrax is 89 percent fatal, a three-day delay intervened before these workers were treated with a sixty-day course of antibiotics.[28] Afterward, postal workers were offered the same experimental anthrax vaccine that was being tested on U.S. soldiers without their consent, which is discussed in the Epilogue. But instead of a clear recommendation from government physicians, postal workers were told that making the complex decision to risk the experimental vaccine and its possible side effects was their own responsibility. Prominent epidemiologists gave conflicting advice. Some cited the dangers of side effects and other experts stressed the need for additional protection, such as adjunct vaccine to discourage the development of anthrax in the exposed, because the antibiotics offered protection only up to sixty days.

But no one had warned the workers that the sixty-day course of antibiotics they accepted would not be sufficient to protect them, and when workers were belatedly told of this and offered the experimental vaccine to supplement the antibiotics, this fed, rather than damped, their suspicions. This offer of a vaccine also seemed to contradict government assurances that the facilities were perfectly safe. When HHS Secretary Tommy Thompson finally officially recommended the vaccine, suspicion reigned among the black staffers that experimentation, not treatment, was the real goal of vaccine administration. The situation was not improved when Washington, D.C., health director Ivan C. A. Walks and Mayor Anthony Williams advised workers to shun the vaccine because of its side effects and unproven efficacy. "There was a public perception that people on Capitol Hill got treated quickly and effectively and lost no one, while the perception at Brentwood was that people were ignored and lost two co-workers," said Walks. The coverage by *Black Enterprise,* a highly respected financial magazine, was entitled "Cures for the Privileged?"[29] Nor did the *Washington Post* shrink from reporting the racial nature of the distrust:

> Using words like "guinea pigs" and references to the Tuskegee experiments, postal workers, many of whom are African American, said that two times now the Bush administration has relegated them to second-class status. "These are the same guys that told us when the Daschle letter went through that it was perfectly okay to go into Brentwood," said Azeezaly Jaffer, the Postal Service's vice president for communications.[30]

Meanwhile, four machines at New York City's Morgan Station Center tested positive for anthrax, prompting the union to demand its closure and decontamination before workers returned. They, too, cited the alacrity with which congressional representatives had been evacuated and Congress was adjourned to nullify the risk of contamination. But the USPS responded with a ten-day supply of Cipro, latex gloves, paper masks, and a refusal to test the employees or to close the facility. "It's absurd. It's criminal. There are live spores in these machines," protested one union representative who refused to return to work. By November, 30 percent of the facility's employees had joined him in boycotting the postal facilities. In the end, only the machines, not the building, were decontaminated.

The New York Area Metro Postal Union's president, Willie Smith, an astute and plainspoken everyman, laid the case of resentful postal workers, many of them black. "We're simply asking the post office to close the building and make sure it's safe," Smith told the *New York Times.* "I realize that Morgan employees are not Supreme Court justices or senators or congressmen, but they are God's children. . . . They have the same right to life as the aristocrats. No one piece of mail is worth a human life."

It remains to be seen how much of the Defense Department's Domestic Preparedness Program's forty-million-dollar allocation for 120 U.S. cities will be used to protect the largely African American postal workers who believe themselves on the front line of domestic bioterrorism threats.[31]

White Weapons

The racial nature of CBW attacks is hardly confined to U.S. borders, and neither is the key role of U.S. scientists. Iraq's chemical warfare against the Kurds is often given as the most recent use of ethnic bioterror on the global stage, but it is not. The most recent biological warfare was the South African apartheid government's decades-long CBW terror campaign waged against its black majority and against neighboring black states.[32] The physicians who headed South Africa's Chemical and Biological Warfare Programme (CBWP) were able to carry out their genocidal bioweapons campaign only with the help of American scientists.

The current media obsession with bioterrorism focuses upon violence perpetrated by the politically marginalized upon developed nations. But this focus has obscured the vigor with which powerful governments can wield biological weapons against weak, racially distinct groups. For example, by the 1980s, the South African apartheid regime felt increasingly threatened by opposition abroad. As its scientists and universities were cut off from the global community by academic boycotts and economic divestitures, the black antiapartheid movement was being joined by persons of other races and the multiethnic African National Congress (ANC) was gaining power and influence.

In response, apartheid politicians and scientists funded research and development into exotic biological and chemical weapons for use against the black majority so that the power of weaponized biologicals might help the white minority to destroy its opponents without firing a shot. Some apartheid-era scientists were skeptical at first,[33] but others were certain that biological weapons could cripple and even kill enough antiapartheid activists to allow them to control the nation's black majority. Not one of the scores of CBW-scientists was black or Colored.[34]

South Africa's systematic murders via biological agents are important to this book because so many of the scientists involved in crafting South Africa's racist bioterror were Americans. In fact, the science of apartheid could not have existed without the avid participation and guidance of a handful of American scientific renegades.

The existence of this genocidal medical program was dragged from the shadows only in 1999, when police arrested Dr. Wouter Basson, the most powerful medical man in apartheid-era South Africa, on a Johannesburg street for the illicit sale of one thousand ecstasy pills.[35] Prosecutors allege that he had financed a bizarre assortment of racist bioterror activities by the sale of illicit drugs. But Basson was not merely a crazed drug dealer; as head of South Africa's CBWP, he was a highly respected scientist, a confidant of the surgeon general, and he held administrative positions at several major hospitals, supervising staff who were shocked to read of his biologic Doomsday schemes in the pages of Pretoria newspapers.

On October 4, 1999, Basson stood trial in Pretoria. Although he was accused of murdering, by the most conservative count, 229 people, all black, with poison, he was charged with only 67 deaths. His accusers included all of his surviving former confederates. Each testified at his trial that Basson had engineered South Africa's rampant, far-ranging campaign of chemical and biological warfare against its own black citizens and against black denizens of neighboring African states. Basson also faced scores of other fraud, murder, and drug-related charges, which South African newspapers and trial transcripts recounted daily. These charges, which are far too numerous to list in their entirety, included accusations that Basson supervised cadres of government scientists who grew cholera cultures for use in black townships and against antiapartheid demonstrators; directed the production of huge quantities of narcotics, including Ecstasy, to be sprayed upon antiapartheid demonstrators to pacify them; and supervised the development and use of poisoned foods for use in assassinations.

Basson's James Bond armamentarium included umbrellas that fired poisonous darts and hypodermic needles housed within screwdrivers. However, Basson was no lone renegade: As head of South Africa's CBWP, he operated under the aegis of his personal friend, South African surgeon general Niels Knobel. The CBWP's most dramatic political function was as an assassin of antiapartheid heroes.

One former security police officer testified to the Pretoria High Court that in 1989, Basson poisoned the Rev. Frank Chikane of the South African Council of Churches, a charismatic antiapartheid activist, by picking the lock of his suitcase and powdering the reverend's underpants with toxins.[36]

No black South African leader was safe from Basson. According to testimony by former CBWP scientists at Basson's trial, Nelson Mandela was still imprisoned when Basson's cadre of scientists plotted to poison him slowly with the heavy metal thallium to render him mentally incapable of managing the nation's antiapartheid resistance. Chillingly, the well-connected Basson once cooked dinner for an unsuspecting Mandela at a mutual acquaintance's dinner party.[37]

But Basson was most adept at designing large-scale weapons of mass destruction specifically tailored for blacks. Basson concocted a plan to saturate T-shirts with chemical agents, then to distribute the shirts gratis throughout impoverished black townships. Equally reprehensible was the CBWP research on an agent that would temporarily turn a white man's skin black in order to allow agents of the South African Defense Force to infiltrate black groups.[38]

Dr. Basson's chemical grasp exceeded the borders of South Africa, targeting blacks in other African countries. In just one incident, Basson's erstwhile lieutenants described how they forced two hundred Namibian prisoners onto a plane, injected them with an experimental muscle re-laxant that collapsed their lungs, then dumped their bodies from the plane into the sea. The death of activist Steven Biko is attributed to sim-ilar poisoning, administered after he was beaten by South African secu-rity police and deprived of medical care.

The *Washington Post* even traced the 2001 U.S. anthrax attacks to the South Africa's CBWP. Evidence taken from a Frederick, Maryland, pond by the FBI suggests that perpetrators handled the deadly bacterium un-derwater without infecting themselves or releasing the anthrax spores indiscriminately. This technique was devised by the CBWP.[39]

The South African bioterrorist campaign depended upon very close relationships with U.S. scientists. Despite the supposed isolation im-posed upon South African scientists by the international embargoes of the 1980s and 1990s, Basson and his minions could not have undertaken biological warfare without the support of the U.S. government. From 1981 until 1993,[40] the United States supported Wouter Bassoon's weapon-ization programs by financing close collaborations with U.S. scientists and by sponsoring Basson's sojourns to the United States for conferences and education. For example, in 1983, Basson attended a closed Depart-ment of Defense conference on biological and chemical warfare in San Antonio.[41] During his trial, Basson recounted his participation in a 1981 federal conference in San Antonio with army officers from the United States, West Germany, Japan, Britain, and Canada. He declared, "I must confirm that the structure of the [CBWP] project was based on the U.S. system. That's where we learnt the most."[42]

Basson says he was also grateful for expert American consultants, be-cause the CBWP was dependent upon a colorful assortment of Ameri-can scientists, especially Larry Ford, M.D., of California. Ford and Basson shared strange research proclivities, acerbic racist sensibilities, and a fascination with scientific genocide. Extant medical and legal doc-uments and the testimony of Basson's former confederates under oath describe their shocking joint-research projects.[43]

According to Ford's lawyer, he was a chemical-weapons researcher for the U.S. government in the 1980s, In 1987, the United States sent him to South Africa to train microbiologists at the military-run Roode-plaat Research Laboratory (RRL), a key component of South Africa's chemical-weapons program and a front for the apartheid South African

Defense Force.[44] Ford returned often to teach RRL scientists how to produce biological agents such as anthrax and botulinum toxin for use as weapons against antiapartheid forces and against blacks in general. He also taught apartheid's defenders how to transform innocuous objects such as doilies and tea bags into biological weapons. His seminar series, a master class for poisoners. proved popular among South African scientists, who dubbed it "Project Larry." Lt. Gen. Lothar Neethling, head of the apartheid regime's police forensic laboratory, was in attendance. So was RRL microbiologist Dr. Mike Odendaal, who recalls, "Ford spent an entire day showing us how to contaminate ordinary items and turn them into biological weapons." He says Ford gave them "ideas about how to infiltrate innocuous objects such as perfume or household items" and place them in close proximity to a potential target.

Ford's expertise in the toxicology of everyday life was put to use as South African physicians busily set about eliminating the enemies of apartheid. Ford was warmly welcomed within the nation's top echelon of medical politicians: For example, the home of former surgeon general Dr. Niels Knobel is graced by a prominently placed framed photograph of him and Ford posing with a lion that Ford had shot.

Back in the United States, Ford's California friends and neighbors praised him as a "Good Samaritan" and "devout Mormon" to South African journalists who descended in the late 1990s to inquire into his prominent role in the recently revealed science of genocide.

However, his neighbors had occasion to revise those warm sentiments on March 11, 2000. That weekend, four dozen area families had to be evacuated when police searching the grounds of Ford's Irvine home discovered twenty-eight containers of firearms, deadly biological agents, and live ammunition. Ford himself was dead, having shot himself on March 2 as police closed in to question him about the attempted murder of his business partner Patrick Riley. Ford's suicide, the discovery of his biological weapons cache, and the unveiling of his ties to Basson, Knobel, and Project Coast (described below) all raised FBI suspicions that a multitude of American crimes utilizing bioweapons had been committed in South Africa by Ford and other U.S. scientists. Accordingly, the FBI has undertaken a "weapons of mass destruction" investigation.

Ford's suicide spared him from his scheduled appearance to give testimony at the U.S. leg of Wouter Basson's trial, where Basson faced sixty-one charges, which encompassed murder, drug trafficking, and fraud.[45]

The CBWP's ultimate goal was the development of a "pigmentation weapon" that would kill or harm only black people. As apartheid waned and the legal web closed upon Basson, his former associates say that he feverishly turned his attention to the production of the unthinkable—a deadly virus that would infect only blacks. The CBWP dubbed this key endeavor "Project Coast." But was this ever a real threat? How practicable were Basson's hopes to tailor biological weapons against blacks?

Very. There is strong evidence from credible sources that the unthinkable has been achieved. The active development of bioweapons against specific ethnic groups—including those specifically tailored to injure blacks—may already be an industry. As early as 1970, the respected armed forces journal *Military Review* discussed the possibility of devising bioweapons to target racial groups.[46] Dr. Carl A. Larson, head of the Department of Human Genetics at the University of Lund in Sweden, discussed the past targeting of racial minorities and the relative ease with which many of these weapons could be tailored to the genetic vulnerabilities of specific ethnic groups. In fact, a report entitled "Biological Testing Involving Human Testing" by the Department of Defense's Senate Select Committee on Health and Scientific Research indicates that the United States may have sought to develop such weapons thirty years before the *Military Review* article. The committee's report documents how a U.S. Navy contract supported the University of California's 1940s tests of airborne fungal spores to spread valley fever. The spores can cause deadly illness by seeding in the lungs and then infecting other body organs. Valley fever kills half of those it sickens and the university's research found that African Americans and Asians were more susceptible to the deadly fungal infection than whites. Dr. Gerald Horne of Brooklyn College claimed that the army and navy investigated the fungus's possible deployment as an "ethnic weapon" as early as the 1940s, and decades later, at a 1977 congressional hearing, an unnamed Pentagon official recalled how the armed forces spread fungus in the Norfolk Naval Shipyard in Virginia and on a loading dock in Mechanicsburg, Pennsylvania. In both worksites, most of the laborers were black and the official specified that the Mechanicsburg docks were particularly chosen because "Negroes are more susceptible to the fungus than whites."[47]

Throughout the Cold War, Western newspapers were peppered with sporadic accounts of ethnic and racial bioweapons being developed by

South Africa with U.S. assistance. U.S. news media broadly maligned all such reports as "misinformation" disseminated by the Soviet Union to embarrass the United States.[48] However, in 1999, a decade after the dissolution of the USSR, the British Medical Association (BMA) warned against ignoring the diverse reports that such weapons were being widely developed. The BMA insisted, "Weapons could theoretically be developed which affect particular versions of genes clustered in specific ethnic or family groups." Its January 1999 report, "Biotechnology, Weapons and Humanity," added that the pending completion of the gene-identification arm of the Human Genome Project would carry the adverse effect of facilitating the production of such weapons. This warning took on new urgency in the wake of the September 11 attacks and after the completion of the HGP project in 2002. However, interested scientists and nations had not waited for these milestones. A 1998 London *Sunday Times* story alleged that Israel already has used South Africa's research to develop a genetically specific weapon against Arabs.[49]

Such weapons development is not nearly so far-fetched nor so difficult as it sounds. Already London police have used American scientific expertise to tailor a nonlethal weapon—the mother of all stink bombs—to specific ethnic groups.

> In 1998, the Pentagon commissioned scientist Pam Dalton, from the Monell Chemical Senses Centre in Philadelphia, to test disgusting odours. One question she was trying to answer was whether there were different cultural reactions to bad smells. She tested the odours on five ethnic groups. . . . [And she] said that the malodorous weapons made volunteers scream and curse after just a few seconds of exposure. "If these were released, they would clear an area in seconds."[50]

But most ethnic weapons under discussion are less benign. Some could be effectively crafted merely by exploiting existing variations in genetics, lifestyle, habits, health profile, and even diet. Even a low-tech approach can be quite selective. For example, approximately 82 percent of African Americans live in urban areas, and predominantly black urban areas have an extremely low density of white residents, so simply striking certain areas of Harlem, East St. Louis, East Palo Alto, or Chicago's

South Side would target blacks with near-surgical precision. One could also lace particular "ethnic" foods marketed to African Americans with biologic toxins. Infusing malt liquors, fortified wines, and African American ethnic delicacies would target blacks, as well. Such scenarios may be redolent of paranoia, but the ease with which they could be realized was brought home in 1968 when the *Pittsburgh Courier,* a black newspaper, reported on incidents that were inspiring a fear of "racial genocide" among black Americans. In 1967, it reported, a white Sacramento millionaire was convicted of plotting to poison two batches of cut-rate gelatin destined for the shelves of stores in black neighborhoods. When arrested, he divulged his plans to pump cyanide through the air-conditioning systems and into the water supplies of exclusively black institutions.

But most discussions of bioweapons center on the strategy of selecting toxicants that affect only a selected group or that affect them far more adversely. Such agents do exist. Although toxicologists do not agree about the extent of difference, poison centers, when contacted about an instance of a child eating mothballs, will sometimes ask, "Is he African American?" because G6PD deficiency, an enzymatic variation that is more common among African Americans than whites, enhances the toxicity of naphthalene, the active component in mothballs. Weapons could easily exploit such vulnerabilities. Similarly, if medications marketed to African Americans, such as hydroxyurea (for sickle-cell anemia) or BiDil (for blacks in heart failure), were tainted, many blacks but almost no whites would constitute the victims. Weaponizing the 1A genotypes of the hepatitis C virus (HCV) coupled with geographic distribution could target African Americans, and other physiological differences between whites and African Americans could provide a fulcrum for targeted weapons. For example, as chapter 1 explained, more than 70 percent of African Americans (and 95 percent of sub-Saharan Africans) lack the Duffy gene,[51] which is almost universal in white Americans. Therefore, developing a poison that is harmless in the presence of this gene would also target most African Americans, while sparing their white compatriots.

Project Coast

Under apartheid, a staggering variety of ethnic biowarfare initiatives eclipsed all the tentative musings about racial targeting. South Africa's Project Coast long ago moved from theory to selective racial murder via bioweapons—with the critical assistance of American scientists. "In the early 1980s, fears of a black tidal wave drove white scientists to try to develop a variety of means that could ensure the survival of white South Africa. Plans were devised to build a large-scale anthrax production facility at RRL, "observed the *Bulletin of the Atomic Scientists.*[52]

From 1981 to 1993, Wouter Basson placed Project Coast under the direction of Daan Goosen, M.D. Goosen told the *Washington Post* that his division was under orders to perfect agents that would preferentially sabotage blacks' fertility, and to devise a "silver bullet" biological weapon, designed to kill only black Africans.

Goosen supervised a multitude of biological assaults on black townships, including the release of pathogens and their vectors, such as mosquitoes, to seed disease epidemics there, just as the army and the CIA had released them over Carver Village. Those involved in Project Coast also laced flyers, chocolates, letters, and cigarettes with anthrax and saturated T-shirts with poisons. Goosen, Basson, and their deputies investigated the use of Mandrax, an amphetamine, and Ecstasy for crowd control, infused township water supplies with treatment-resistant strains of cholera, and deployed napalm and phosphorus against blacks in Namibia and Angola during the 1980s.[53]

Basson also ordered Goosen to suppress black reproduction surreptitiously and suggested the clandestine addition of contraceptives to townships' drinking water. Basson stressed that this was a direct edict of the South African surgeon general.[54]

Project Coast also set up international shop, according to a 1989 price list that included salmonella-infused sugar cubes, pesticide-laced beer and peppermints, and a now chillingly familiar threat: envelopes sprinkled with anthrax spores.

Only the fall of apartheid cut Basson's efforts short. In its aftermath, the United States and Great Britain asked F. W. DeKlerk's apartheid government not to hand over the fruits of Dr. Basson's labor, the biological warfare technology, to the new ANC government. Instead, DeKlerk met with Nelson Mandela, who ended the program.[55]

After the U.S. anthrax attacks in October 2001,[56] Goosen tried not only to sell Project Coast's research documents but also to interest the U.S. Department of Defense in a partnership for developing South Africa's repertoire of anthrax vaccines and antisera specialized antidotes. According to the *Washington Post*, Goosen's other offerings to the FBI included modified plague, salmonella and botulism agents, and antisera intended to strengthen resistance to any future bioterrorism attacks. The DOD set up a January 2002 meeting between Goosen and Bioport Corp., a Michigan company that has the sole license to produce military anthrax vaccines, but no agreement was reached. The Americans demurred when confronted with Goosen's voluminous demands, which included a five-million-dollar cash disbursement, amnesty, and immigrant status for a wide assortment of apartheid-era researchers, family members, and hangers-on. The United States did, however, quash the sale of the biological weapons to Middle Eastern nations.[57]

Thus, Goosen and the other apartheid scientists were forced to take a less lucrative route to amnesty. They confessed their crimes to the South African Truth and Reconciliation Commission (TRC), and in this way, they escaped the sort of public high-stakes trial that threatened Basson with the loss of his medical degree, wealth, and freedom.[58]

Pretoria bioengineer Dr. Jan Lourens, who later headed the biotech firm Protechnek, was one of the scientists who confessed and applied for amnesty to the TRC after the fall of apartheid. By doing so, he and his confederates escaped the fines and imprisonment, to say nothing of the death sentences, that had befallen their Nazi counterparts a half century earlier. Faced with ruin or confession, the Project Coast and CBWP scientists admitted their years of heinous research in the service of racial genocide. Basson, their boss, was the lone holdout. He refused to confess or to apologize, evidently hoping that he could beat the charges, even with his former subordinates arrayed against him, giving reams of damning testimony.

Despite the implicating confessions by his colleagues and a slew of eyewitnesses to genocide, Judge Willie Hartzenberg dropped the murder charges against Basson in 2002 and rejected the testimony of all 153 witnesses against him. Only Basson had testified in his own defense, and Basson's was the *only* testimony that the judge accepted. Hartzenberg dismissed all the evidence against him and found Basson innocent of forty-six charges—including murder, drug trafficking, fraud, and theft involving some R37 million ($3.7 million in U.S. currency), but he did not stop there: For good measure, Hartzenberg also granted Basson amnesty.

The trial, South Africa's longest, had lasted thirty months and cost the state R20M ($2 million in U.S. currency). In 2002, the prosecutors' request for a retrial was denied.[59]

Standing between Basson's many accusers and a conviction was Hartzenberg, an apartheid-era judge who was widely viewed as a holdover, nursing, as he did, a strong nostalgia for white-minority rule. He had remained on the bench despite an attempt to recuse him before the trial started. Once the trial began, court journalists alleged, Hartzenberg "made no secret of who he most admires in his court room."[60] Hartzenberg likened Basson to "the Virgin Mary" in open court and threw out conspiracy and murder charges that legal analysts insist should have been prosecuted.[61]

However, one needs no legal expertise to wonder how Basson could be innocent when so many of his key lieutenants testified in detail and with consistency about crimes they committed together.[62] Basson's innocent verdict had been predicted by news analysts, based upon the all-white courtroom players and the pro-Basson bias of the judge. So Basson was right to gamble that he would be convicted of no crime and serve no sentence. The judge, the barristers, the journalists, and the scientists, both South African and American, as well as the trial analysts were all white, leaving one to wonder, Who speaks for the black victims of Dr. Death? ANC official Smuts Ngonyama resorted to understatement: "The justice system has let us down on this case."

A September 2005 appellate court decision raised hopes that this bleak failure of the South African legal system may yet be mitigated by some measure of justice. The appeals court found that Hartzenberg had erred in throwing out charges related to the deaths of hundreds of blacks outside of South Africa—those in Namibia, Mozambique, Swaziland, and the United Kingdom—between 1979 and 1989. Citing a "real and substantial connection," the court granted South African prosecutors permission to reopen six charges of conspiracy and murder against Basson in the deaths of ANC members, South West African People's Organization (SWAPO) members, and others marked as enemies of the apartheid state. However, in late November 2005, South Africa declined to prosecute, citing the prohibition against double jeopardy. South African prosecutors have abandoned hopes of trying Basson again, but in 2006 as this book went to press, the legal systems of neighboring nations such as Namibia were considering attempts at extradition and trial.

As for bioterrorism back in the United States, a similar campaign for the truth against government-sponsored bioterrorism was proving equally futile for its black victims. As mentioned earlier, MK-ULTRA, the CIA mind-control program that began in 1953, had been exposed by investigative reports as the culprit in the biological assaults on black Floridians, Georgians, and Virgin Islanders.

Of course, this was not news to Georgia legislator Dorothy Pelote, whose descriptions of her frustrated attempts to attract governmental recognition of the atrocities at Carver Village opened this chapter. Pelote's grateful neighbors elected her county commissioner, then state representative in 1984, and she never stopped trying to get an acknowledgment of the government's actions in Carver Village and some compensation for her neighbors. In 2004, she explained to me that the exposure by the Church of Scientology[63] and the national news media had failed to bring justice to Carver Village's victims. "We had several meetings that were very regularly attended by representatives of various organizations and the EPA [Environmental Protection Agency] and our congressman sent someone. We talked about it, but because we were lay people, we needed expert advice . . . [and] some people we needed to dialogue with did not show. . . . Later, some people from the government approached me, saying they were going to have congressional hearings, but they never did. They never called me back when I called about it."[64]

Pelote is passionate about health issues, large and small, that pollute the lives of those residing in forgotten small black communities like Carver Village. Although she may appear unprepossessing to the uninitiated, Pelote has accrued a great deal of political power because her constituents trust her, and she has not been reluctant to wield that power in what she considers their best interests. This has earned her some political enemies and she has been ridiculed for some of her legislation. For example, she introduced a bill to prevent supermarket baggers from licking their fingers to open recalcitrant plastic bags while packing customers' groceries. Much was also made of murky claims Pelote made regarding the fate of Chandra Levy, the twenty-two-year-old intern who disappeared in 2001. Reports of her affair with California representative Gary Condit were disclosed at the time. (Levy's body was found thirteen months later, in a wooded area, as Pelote had predicted.)

But the Scientologists' report and subsequent mainstream news media accounts of biological agents at Carver Village validated Pelote, and later news reports revealed some projects of which Pelote had never dreamed. For example, MK-ULTRA scientists had utilized technology in the form of a machine they devised called a Biogen. It mass-produced pathogens, including cranking out huge vats of cultures that could cause fatal illnesses. The CIA financial archives include invoices for the maintenance and repair of the machine over a period of thirteen years. During that period, the *Washington Post* speculated, MK-ULTRA scientists "may have produced hundreds of pounds of various biological agents and microorganisms."

The biological agents used as friendly fire to test the vulnerabilities of blacks in Carver Village represented just the first wave of governmental domestic bioterrorism. *The Biology of Doom,* a book by Ed Regis, described how whites as well as blacks were targeted by government-produced pathogens in other cities. In San Francisco, lightbulbs filled with purportedly benign bacteria were purposely disseminated in public areas, where they were dropped in the subway system so researchers could study how effectively the pathogens would spread. The Special Operations Division used custom-fitted suitcases in 1964 and 1965 to spray bacteria onto unwitting passengers in Washington, D.C.'s National Airport and in Greyhound bus terminals. The Special Operations Division scientists counted the tickets sold at the time of exposure and thus were able to determine that the "infected passengers" spread the bacteria to more than two hundred cities. These tests were undertaken to determine the results of using smallpox or other deadly biological agents in public places, but unlike what occurred with the Carver Village exposures, the agents substituted purportedly harmless bacteria called *Bacillus subtilis* (a bacillus ia a rod-shaped bacterium that grows in the presence of air). However, *B. subtilis* is not harmless: We now know that it triggers respiratory infections, blood poisoning, and food poisoning.

Other major cities were not spared. A 1979 report exposed Operation Big City, the CIA's 1956 secret biological warfare experiments that were conducted in the New York subway system in partnership with U.S.

Army personnel. These exposures were more democratic than those detailed here, and affected people of every race. But still other projects that targeted the Northeast demonstrated the CIA scientists' special interest in targeting African Americans.

For example, another round of tests in various East Coast cities sought to validate claims that a species of fungus caused lung disease in blacks more often than in whites. It was sprayed throughout an area where more blacks than whites worked. An army report stated that the purpose of this exposure was to test this vulnerability, because "within this [supply] system, there are employed large numbers of laborers, including many Negroes, whose incapacitation would seriously affect the operation of the supply system." Senator Paul Wellstone (D-Minn.) commented, "No one should ever have been subjected to these tests,"[65] and he helped to mount a congressional investigation into the project's health effects on the subjects. None of these large-scale biological assaults on black Americans has been formally acknowledged by the government.

Dorothy Pelote retired in 2001 after nearly three decades in public life, although she remains active in attempting to protect the health of her community. But as she leaves the government arena and as the affected residents of the nation's Carver Villages age and die, a real danger looms that the memory of government-mediated bioterrorism will die with them—unless it happens again.

EPILOGUE

Medical Research with Blacks Today

The voluntary consent of the human subject is absolutely essential.
—THE NUREMBERG CODE

In this book, I have traced the long, unhappy history of medical research with black Americans. I have detailed how blacks have been convenient, powerless, maligned, and abused subjects of profitable medical research and also how their treatment has changed over the years. Slaves were physically forced into painful medical bondage, their bodies were forced onto the stage of medical experiments to lend credence to claims of black inferiority and difference, and black bodies were even conscripted for anatomical dissection after death. Blacks were made subjects of experimentation that served to denigrate their intelligence or to provide distorted justifications for their enslavement. The reproductive rights of blacks also have been subjugated via fraudulent research up to the present day. Groups of vulnerable blacks, including children, soldiers and prisoners, have been consistently targeted. Both the federal government and private corporations have devised large-scale research abuses that range from radiation experiments to biological-weapons development. This medical ill-usage has not strictly paralleled scientific knowledge: Rather, it has mirrored the larger American cultural beliefs as well as politics and economic trends.

Once, black Americans enjoyed the sparsest of legal and social protections, nearly universal abject poverty, and few health-care options. But this social and legal landscape has changed dramatically, and so have research practices.

Where We Are Today

Today, the worst abuses are mostly memories, although some forms of abusive research persist, and a few new issues have arisen. However, today's offenses pale beside those our forebears survived. Today, much medical research is more than safe for African Americans; it is necessary. This may seem a strange message for a book that has described so many racial research abuses, but this volume's frankness is an essential prerequisite for asking African Americans to consider participating in medical research. No one can dismiss blacks' historically grounded fear of research and retain any credibility. We must acknowledge the past in order to regain trust and to seize the future.

But medical abuse is more than historical fact. Although less rife, it remains a contemporary reality, and an ever-present possibility. The challenge is to prepare the way for a new openness to medical research on the part of African Americans while maximizing their protections from abuse. I do not see how this can be accomplished without candor, because the traditional strategy of ostrichlike denial merely heightens mistrust.

To gain trust, we must first acknowledge the flagrant abuses of the past and the subtler ones of the present, yet much of the popular argument around medical experimentation and African Americans is dictated by culture and politics, not historical fact. The scientific camp includes most physicians, medical researchers, and others of all racial groups who pride themselves upon their educational sophistication. They tend to deny all present research dangers and most past ones, dismissing fears as emanating from those who are uneducated about the legal protections governing research or so credulous as to believe unsubstantiated rumors about the medical targeting of blacks. Mainstream medical scientists, journals, and even some news media fail to evaluate these fears in the light of historical and scientific fact and tend instead to dismiss all such doubts and fears as antiscience. The potentially damping effects on medical research, not the facts, become the focus of most discussions of troubled experiments. Like the medical school professor whose horror at my choice of topics I described in the introduction, many claim that any acknowledgment of abuse will drive African Americans from sorely needed medical care. However, a steady course of lies and exploitation has already done this. A 2002 *American Journal of Law and Medicine* article estimated that as many as twenty million Americans have enrolled in formal biomedical studies—but fewer than 1 percent are African American.[1] Yet the focus on African American fears is misplaced.

A January 2006 *Public Library of Science* study entitled "Are Racial and Ethnic Minorities Less Willing to Participate in Health Research?" examined the consent rates of twenty research studies that reported consent rates by race or ethnicity for more than 70,000 individuals. It found only slightly lower consent rates for blacks compared to (non-Hispanic) whites. The investigations ranged from interviews to drug treatment to surgical trials. Yet blacks are significantly less likely to be included in clinical trials, which suggests that some factor other than consent is implicated. Studies such as those mentioned in chapter 11 already show that black children are more likely to be used in nontherapeutic, harmful studies than in therapeutic investigations. Future research may document that this is true for black adults as well.

In short, many scholars such as Tuskegee Bioethics Center director Dr. Vanessa Northington Gamble aver that the true focus should not be on the aversion of black subjects but rather on the untrustworthiness of American medical research when it comes to studies involving blacks. This book certainly documents this ethical deficiency.

Although the focus of this book is clearly on experimental abuses of a vulnerable population, I do not want to leave the impression that I am advising people to avoid potentially beneficial medical experimentation. Quite the contrary. African Americans desperately need the medical advantages and revelations that only ethical, essentially therapeutic research initiatives can give them. The reticence of African Americans is the reasonable and understandable result of a horrendous history, but it lags behind progress. African American absence from research reflects the realities of yesterday, not today. More to the point, this aversion is a reaction black Americans can ill afford.

For this book to have the most value, I ask readers to hold two seemingly contradictory but actually complementary facts in mind. The first is that African Americans must welcome and embark upon medical research as a bridge to fording the gulf that yawns between the health profiles of sickly enfranchised blacks and those of healthy, long-lived whites.

The second fact is that African Americans must remain wary of research abuses. They are rarer, but the potential for exploitation and abuse still looms.

Physicians, patients, and ethicists must also understand that acknowledging abuse and encouraging African Americans to participate in medical research are compatible goals. History and today's deplorable African American health profile tell us clearly that black Americans need both more research and more vigilance.

The worst abuses no longer occur and others are becoming far rarer, in part because the media exposure of racial research scandals has led to public condemnation. This, in turn, has helped to support the enactment of stiffer laws carrying real penalties rather than yesterday's toothless codes, such as that written at Nuremberg. This matrix of legislation is not perfect, but it reduces the unabashed use of African Americans as duped or unwitting research subjects. Sociopolitical changes have also helped in this regard. There are no more "separate but equal" hospitals to provide powerless research fodder. There are no more nakedly vulnerable black people without the protection of the law; there are no more hospitals devoid of those black physicians who can protest racial dichotomies in patient treatment. Black physicians, researchers, and journalists now join the white professionals of conscience who have brought such abuses to attention and to a stop. The news media may not always discern and detail the patterns underlying problems with new therapies, but they do regularly expose research abuses.

Government has shown itself more likely to close down entire university research programs under the aegis of the FDA when embarrassed by federally sponsored abuse. Closure is a fate that has been suffered by even premier universities, from Duke to Johns Hopkins. Most universities have heeded the message.

All this amounts to a limited but real success story. African Americans are no longer the primary targets of research, exploitation, and abuse. Research ethics and policies have evolved to the point where the worst abuses of blacks are but a bad memory. That's the good news.

Africa: Continent of Subjects

The bad news is that the racial mythology, the medical exploitation of black bodies for profit, and even the instances of medical sadism that threatened African Americans in the past have been exported to Africa. The recent history of medical research in Africa parallels closely that of African Americans in the United States a century ago. Colonialism and its residual racial and class separations have isolated blacks in hospitals or hospital wards away from whites, just as segregated hospitals once provided exclusively black subjects for white doctors. Laws that offered few or no protections for abused blacks have emboldened unscrupulous physicians and researchers who put curiosity and profits above the rights and welfare of their black patients. Western physicians, scientists, and pharmaceutical companies need large pools of people for Phase I trials, and they have swarmed Africa as they once flocked to prisons.

U.S. researchers who can no longer conduct trials at home without intense scrutiny from the FDA and the news media have moved their operations to sub-Saharan Africa to exploit the public-health vacuum that once condemned black Americans.

"To get around consent forms and a skeptical public, many researchers are turning their attention to African and other developing countries," Robert F. Murray, Jr., M.D., chief of the Division of Medical Genetics at Howard University, has observed. "I would say the greatest chance for injury is in the Third World, where people don't even know research is going on and don't have a clue."

The long history of how Western investigators have taken their more questionable research initiatives to Africa is well documented in works such as Dr. Wolfgang U. Eckart's *Medizin und Kolonialimperialismus.* In it, Eckart details how, in a ghastly dress rehearsal for Dachau, nineteenth-century German scientists conducted genocidal experiments on Africans, especially the Herero of Namibia.[2] The United States, like Europe, has long used its nonwhite colonies and territories as its laboratories. For example, Richard Strong, M.D., used prisoners in the Philippines to conduct deadly malarial experiments, and chapter 8 relates how Brazilian, Mexican, and Puerto Rican women have more recently been used for birth-control trials that maimed and killed many.[3] Warwick Anderson, M.D., documents how colonizing nations, including the United States, have used often-mythical racial differences, including the purported infectious-disease immunities of Africans, to further colonial aims and to justify the use of natives as workers in dangerous environments—just as U.S. slave owners once did. In much of Africa, Asia, and South America, a wide understanding has reigned that ethical rules governing medical experimentation were not "for natives."

Henry Louis Gates, chairman of African American Studies at Harvard University, recalls encountering such persistent racial myths during his undergraduate studies. "I was premed at Yale and took a year off to work at a mission hospital in Tanzania, where the doctors were all Australians. I was only twenty-one years old and I gave anesthesia to patients. I was shocked by the fact that when patients were writhing in pain, the doctors would say, 'They don't experience pain the same way we do.' I was totally disgusted. I complained loudly and called them all racists, of course. But this illustrates how it is always easier to distance oneself from the pain of 'the other.'"

The use of poor people of color abroad by American scientists today enables researchers to escape both the strictest scrutiny of institutional review boards and the gaze of the FDA, says Murray, who issued a prescient warning in 1994: "People are going overseas trying to do research in Africa. They are saying, 'We don't have to go through all that IRB stuff to study AIDS, sickle cell and other diseases. This sort of questionable research is now going on in Africa and Third World countries because there are plentiful patients and the scientists are not subject to the same restrictions they are now subjected to here."

The Third World has become the laboratory of the West, and Africans have become the subjects of novel dangerous therapeutics. In 2002, the hormones of "Bushmen" were mined for potential weight-loss therapies;[4] human growth factor was tested on Pygmies before being used on Western children;[5] and Depo-Provera, although a carcinogen, was tested on Zimbabwean women before it was introduced into the United States as a reproductive injection. American firms tested artificial blood on unsuspecting black South African hospital patients, at the cost of at least twenty deaths. Harvard tested HIV therapies through research that would have violated ethical requirements for Americans.

Some of the research on Africans by Western scientists has been more subtle but equally troubling from an ethical perspective. For example, trypanosomiasis, or sleeping sickness, kills as many as half those it infects in the central African regions of Uganda, the Democratic Republic of Congo, Sudan, Ethiopia, Malawi, and Tanzania. Melarsoprol, the only effective treatment, is a very toxic compound of arsenic and antifreeze that kills one in five people who take it. By 1995, the pharmaceutical firm Aventis had completed research demonstrating that its drug eflornithine was effective against sleeping sickness, although not against cancer, as the firm had hoped. But the company decided to abandon its use against trypanosomiasis, due to high production costs and low profits. It began seeking other profitable uses for the drug, and U.S. researchers soon found one: Eflornithine effectively banished facial hirsutism in women. Aventis and later Bristol-Myers Squibb began marketing the drug as Vaniqa, because many American women were able to part with fifty dollars a month to keep their faces free of hair, while few Africans were able to pay fifty dollars monthly to save their lives. It is completely understandable that the firm should focus its resources upon the profitable depilatory use of their medication, but it is disappointing that it chose not to make the drug available cheaply to Africans in order to vanquish sleeping sickness. Doctors Without Borders forged a coalition, which included Bristol-Myers Squibb, Bayer, and the Bill and Melinda Gates Foundation, to provide drugs to Africans through 2006, but although sleeping sickness threatens sixty million people, only 7 percent of these have access to adequate medical treatment.[6]

Medications considered far too dangerous or too hopelessly tainted for testing in the West have been introduced into clinical trials with unsuspecting African patients. Within the past decade, even the infamously teratogenic drug thalidomide has been tried on Africans as a treatment for leprosy—forty years after it produced twelve thousand horribly deformed babies around the world. FDA researcher Frances O. Kelsey, M.D., refused to approve thalidomide as a treatment for morning sickness in the 1950s because she determined that clinical trials did not demonstrate its safety; her caution saved most American infants the fate suffered by English and Europeans whose mothers took the drug. (Only those U.S. babies whose mothers received thalidomide samples from their physicians were affected.)[7] But Third World women subjects of thalidomide trials for leprosy and AIDS were not warned of the horrible birth defects the drug can cause.

African experimental subjects, like the slaves of antebellum America, are legally vulnerable, relatively powerless, and racially distinct. Like black Americans after the Civil War, Africans' poorer health and vanished health-care infrastructure make it easier to pass off nontherapeutic research as medical therapy or to impose participation in research as a condition for therapy.

The U.S. physician-researchers who descend upon Africa in search of subjects frequently characterize their work as therapy, offering experimental solutions for medical disasters. When physicians offer Africans the same therapeutics they offer Westerners, they can lay claim to unalloyed beneficence. But the Western standard of care is not being offered; usually poor black Africans with no access to medical attention are offered treatments that are new or untried. Sometimes U.S. researchers appear in the midst of an epidemic against which the stricken Africans have no medication and offer experimental treatment.

During the height of a 1996 meningococcal meningitis epidemic, for example, scientists offered Pfizer's experimental drug Trovan (floxacin) to terrified parents in Kano, Nigeria. Nigerians desperate for medical attention grasped at Trovan's straw. By the time the experiment ended, two hundred children were left severely disabled and eleven were dead. In 2001, at least 211 Nigerian parents sued New York–based Pfizer, Inc., alleging that non-FDA-approved experiments had killed or injured their children; that Pfizer failed to obtain the requisite approval from local leaders; and that the pharmaceutical giant failed to administer standard therapies with proven efficacy, such as Pfizer's own ceftriaxone to those children who continued to deteriorate after being given Trovan. Peter Ebigbo of Childrights Africa told Inter Press Service, "Our leaders must not allow Nigerians to be used as guinea pigs by any company to make money."

Pfizer counters that it treated ninety children with Trovan and ninety-seven with ceftriaxone, and that it obtained all the necessary approvals. However, Dr. Sadiq Wali, chief medical director of the Aminu Kano Teaching Hospital, says the hospital's medical ethics committee never gave Pfizer the required approval to use the drug at the infectious-disease hospital in Kano. "Pfizer did not do that. I am not sure if they had the consent of the people used as guinea pigs, because that means informed consent in medical parlance. Such consent has to do with the patients being told the good as well as the side effects of the drugs to be administered," said Dr. Wali.

But documenting Trovan's effects on these patients for the lawsuit would prove tricky: The medical records of 350 meningitis patients treated between April and June 1996 have disappeared from the hospital.[8]

The dearth of health care in much of Africa and the Third World makes its peoples vulnerable to experimental abuse.

One cannot generalize about a continent as large and diverse as Africa. There are wealthy countries as well as poor ones, and a few health-savvy nations, such as Cameroon, could teach us a thing or two about providing health care to all our citizens. But much of sub-Saharan Africa has been devastated by colonial rape and depletion. These have left poor health, a ravaged health-care infrastructure, and few physicians in their wake. A mere 750,000 health workers care for the continent's 682 million people. The Organisation for Economic Co-operation and Development estimates that this represents a health-care force that is as much as fifteen times lower than in OECD countries.

Only 1.3 percent of the world's health workers practice in sub-Saharan Africa, but the region harbors fully 25 percent of the world's disease.[9] A bare minimum of 2.5 health workers is needed for every one thousand people, but only six African countries meet this standard. Instead, the average in sub-Saharan Africa is 0.8 health workers per one thousand people—less than one-third the minimal standard. To achieve the minimum health-care staffing level will require an infusion of one million health workers into the continent.

Safe devices are as scarce as doctors. Reused SUDs (single-use devices) and unsterilized needles help to spread AIDS and other infectious illnesses throughout Africa. The medically damaging injection practices and use of ethically suspect research has fomented a loss of trust in vaccines in Nigeria. Much of the news coverage focuses upon the contentions by suspicious Africans that the administration of Western vaccines spreads HIV and causes sterility.[10] But no matter whether these fears are correct or imaginary, the practical result is unambiguous: suspicious patients avoid care, and this iatrophobia means that "conquered" diseases such as polio are seeing a resurgence on the continent.

A burgeoning research culture is thriving in the midst of this desultory public-health activity and therapeutic vacuum. While the continent's wounds go unbound, research is big business in Africa. Seventy billion dollars is spent each year on medical research, but only 10 percent is devoted to diseases that cause 90 percent of the global health burden.[11] This dichotomy provides an incubator for research abuses. Surrounded by pain, death, and infection, desperate, medically ignored Africans are confronted with a Hobson's choice: experimental medicine or no medicine at all.

Western researchers who conduct investigations in the Third World are supposed to elicit the approval of their home medical institutions. For example, most university policies align with FDA regulations that require treatments given to the control-group members must be the standard of care for the treatment of the illness. Thus if one wanted to test Trovan in Connecticut, the protocol or research plan would stipulate that researchers must give the control group the best drugs known to treat meningitis, a drug such as ceftriaxone. Under some conditions, generally when no effective treatment for a condition exists, control-group members receive a placebo, an inert substance or a sham technique that does not offer any intrinsic therapeutic value but allows scientists to compare results between a treated and an untreated group.

But placebo studies, which are falling out of favor in the West, are completely inappropriate for serious diseases for which effective treatment exists. You cannot ethically justify withholding, for example, an efficacious drug such as AZT from HIV-positive people or people at high risk of contracting HIV just to determine whether protease inhibitors work better than nothing. You must give the tested group protease inhibitors and the control group either AZT or the best-known standard therapy. Tossing the people in the control group placebos, vitamins, or antibiotics would doom the control group and so would be an unacceptable ethical breach—at least in the West.

However, American IRBs treat Africans as second-class subjects and employ different standards for evaluating study designs in Africa than those used in the United States. Requiring evidence that the drug being administered meets or exceeds the standard of medical care is de rigueur for Western trials, but university IRBs now employ an ethical sleight of hand to stipulate that the tested drug must meet or exceed the standard of care *in the country where the study is being evaluated.* In impoverished, medically underserved sub-Saharan African countries, that standard of care has historically tended to be nothing.

Americans who conduct research in African venues are supposed to seek the consent of their subjects. But this has never been a popular move, as the exasperated 1964 complaint of Dr. Francis D. Moore, a Harvard surgeon whose photograph had graced the cover of *Time* a year earlier, illustrates.

> Several years ago an individual from this country went to Nigeria to try out a new measles vaccine on a lot of small children. Now how exactly are you going to explain to a black African jungle mother the fact that measles vaccine occasionally produces encephalitis but that more important than that it might sensitize the child for the rest of his life to some other protein in the vaccine? We now know that any sort of immune response excites cross reactions. For example, if a person develops a heightened immune reaction to some specific antigen such as typhoid he will be found to have other high titers against non specific antigens at the same time. In fact, there is a suspicions [*sic*] that some of the so-called auto-immune diseases are aroused by exposure of the reticuloendothelial system to completely different antigens.
>
> The possibility therefore arises that measles vaccines applied to thousands and thousands of children might excite in some of them such diseases as thyroiditis and ulcerative colitis.
>
> Can you imagine trying to explain that to a jungle mother?
>
> . . . One of the greatest assets of a good doctor is the ability to look a patient in the eye and have the patient go along with him on a hazardous course of treatment. . . . The same quality is exhibited by a medical experimenter when he looks at [a] patient and says that he thinks everything is all right.[12]

Moore avoided the troublesome task of individual disclosure and consent, and so do many researchers in Africa today, who do not want to take the time to translate their proposal into the local language and culture. They do not want to explain to hundreds or thousands of subjects such risks as iatrogenic encephalitis and sensitization—concepts that would have been as murky to a Connecticut homemaker in 1964 as they were to Moore's "jungle mother." These scientists do not want to risk having the subjects reject the experiment once they understand the possible health costs. Neither do they especially want to explain why they are testing a new therapeutic approach to HIV thousands of miles away from the millions of cases in their own country. Moore doesn't mention this sort of question in his tirade against informed consent, but I suspect that it is the more difficult of the questions his jungle mother might put to him today.

The Erosion of Consent

Unlike the disastrous Third World research trends, medical research with black Americans has lost so much of its historically abusive nature that black Americans should embrace new medical research—after judicious inquiries of their own into any study they are considering. But there are still issues that must be addressed, and until these problems are rectified, black Americans must embrace medical research warily.

These issues include the recent erosion of informed consent; the need for better-quality research into black health issues; the overemphasis upon genetic research in nongenetic issues; and the government's distortion of research with black Americans to further political and ideological ends.

"It is the most fundamental tenet of medical ethics and human decency that the subjects volunteer for the experiment after being informed of its nature and hazards. This is the clear dividing line between criminal and what may be noncriminal. If the experimental subjects cannot be said to have volunteered, then the inquiry need proceed no further." So testified Andrew Ivy, M.D., chief witness for the prosecution in the Nuremberg doctors' trial.

The Nuremberg Code was instituted in August 1947, by Americans judging twenty-three physicians and scientists, to ensure that the horrors of abusive medical experimentation never again be visited upon the world. Its very first line is unambiguous: "The consent of the subject is absolutely essential."

But American research culture increasingly disagrees.

In October 1996,[13] the Department of Health and Human Services passed 21CFR50.24, a regulation that robbed seriously ill emergency room patients of the right to informed consent. This allows researchers to legally enroll such patients in medical-research studies and test experimental therapies on them without their consent.[14]

The emergency room deaths began the very next year. On April 1, 1997, when the Occupational Health and Hygiene Plan (OHHP) suspended a U.S. clinical trial that had enrolled unwitting patients in a clinical trial of diaspirin cross-linked hemoglobin (DCLHb) for treating shock. So many more people who received the experimental treatment died than those receiving standard care that the trial had to be stopped early. These people had never given their consent to participate in the study that killed them. Yet today the practice of experimenting with nonconsenting emergency room patients continues. For example, when they need a blood transfusion, unconscious patients brought into some emergency rooms are as likely to be given an artificial substitute as blood—without their knowledge. Also, the AbioCor company proposes to implant their complication-ridden model of a self-contained artificial heart into a wide variety of heart-attack patients who are brought into emergency rooms if they meet certain (rather wide) research criteria—again without their permission or knowledge.

And informed consent is also being attacked more insidiously—in assaults upon existing laws.[15] Various ethicists who are experts in human medical experimentation, such as Jay Katz, M.D., and George Annas, J.D., worry that the vague language of federal regulations governing human medical experimentation is being interpreted in a manner that minimizes protections. At the same time, they point out addenda to these regulations that further curtail patient protection and patient autonomy while expanding the types and number of people who can become subjects.

The erosion of consent is often presented as a partial surrender or a compromise between the needs of researchers for subjects and a small loss to a patient autonomy. Or it is presented behind the mask of futility—in such scenarios, it is argued, the patient is unconscious and cannot agree or disagree to partaking of a possibly lifesaving experimental treatment, so his doctors should decide for him.

In such cases, "research" is conflated with "treatment" to justify removing informed consent from the equation. But these scenarios are false and misleading. It is not necessary to waive informed consent in order to provide the unconscious with treatment: Laws already exist that permit doctors to offer the best-available treatment to patients who are comatose, unconscious, underage, or in other ways unable to consent to treatment. But these laws do not extend to experimentation, and rightly so. Treatment focuses upon the patient's needs; experimentation focuses upon the researchers' needs, no matter how much those researchers may invoke possible or future benefits for patients. In fact, these studies are typically randomized, which means that the computer, not the doctor, determines what experimental therapy will be administered. This may not be the best treatment for the patient, nor the therapy the patient would choose.

Once one loses the right to be told what one is about to undergo, to agree or to refuse participation, research policy gains momentum on a very slippery slope. This book documents the depths to which researchers have stooped to bypass the consent of the subject. In fact, African Americans first became favored subjects because during the antebellum period they did not enjoy legal protections and researchers did not need their consent.

This vulnerability also persists today in other settings where blacks are overrepresented, such as military ground troops. In 1990, the Department of Defense (DOD) sought and obtained from the Food and Drug Administration a waiver of the informed-consent requirements for human medical experimentation. Under Rule 21 CFR 50.23(d), soldiers suddenly lost the protection of the informed-consent provisions that give other Americans the right to say no to experimental medications. The DOD forced them to accept experimental drugs, including pyridostigmine bromide, a putative prophylactic against nerve gas attack; and the pentavalent botulinum toxoid vaccine for botulism. In 1998, with FDA permission, the DOD Anthrax Vaccination Immunization Program (AVIP) also began immunizing 2.4 million soldiers against the potential threat of airborne anthrax: At least 900,000 troops have been immunized to date. But, citing devastating side effects and deaths that have been validated by amendments to the medication warning labels, hundreds of soldiers have refused to comply, at least one hundred of whom have been court martialed, and many have been forced to leave the military. One of these was Jemekia Barber, who while stationed in Colorado was ordered to accept an anthrax vaccination in preparation for a transfer to Korea. She disobeyed that order on the grounds that the vaccination may not be safe for females of childbearing age. Black soldiers such as Barber are twice as common in ground troops as in American society, and so are especially vulnerable to measures such as forced vaccinations.[16]

In late 2003, Judge Emmet G. Sullivan of the United States District Court in Washington, D.C., noted that the Supreme Court had ruled that U.S. combat troops could no longer be compelled to take the experimental anthrax vaccinations. The FDA responded by rapidly elevating the anthrax vaccine from a questionable investigational drug to an approved therapeutic, allowing the DOD to sidestep the intent of the law and restoring the soldiers to a state of investigative servitude—"investigative" because the data collection and evaluation of the anthrax vaccine risks, including death, will continue among soldiers. Fortunately, in 2004, Judge Sullivan ordered the DOD to stop forcing anthrax vaccines on U.S. military personnel. Barber's lawsuit against the army continues.

Today, African American are at greater risks than whites of being conscripted into such research without giving their consent, because blacks are more likely than whites to receive their health care from emergency rooms.

However, this coin of research vulnerability has an obverse: We also need more and better research into black health care. Such high-quality research has begun to emerge but, as chapter 14 points out, it has also taken some wrong turns. For example, research into black ailments and medications, such as that conducted in support of the black heart-failure drug BiDil, is sometimes sloppy and illogical, and in other cases it is based on the thinnest of premises.

The long history of flawed science in the service of preconceived notions is being supplemented by new, insufficiently questioned racial theories of disease. Adopting these unquestioningly while ignoring important environmental disease factors not only imperils black health; it also reinforces the idea of blacks as possessing dramatic physiologic differences.

The inclusion of blacks in quality American medical research is also important for everyone. Why? Many arguments cite the dollar savings or the reduction in disease exposure to the larger society that will emanate from better health among African Americans. However, I am often uncomfortable with arguments that focus solely on utility, especially when it comes to medicine and health. Such benefits can be elusive or hard to quantify. I believe that caring for people and maximizing their chances at health and happiness are goals that we should pursue for their own sake, because they are the right thing to do. They elevate us spiritually and socially, and reaffirm our cohesion and our humanity.

But that said, there's no denying that increasing the ethical, reasonably safe research available to African Americans will benefit everyone else. This book has repeatedly demonstrated how the poor health profile spawned by experimental abuse has not only harmed blacks but has spilled over to harm their white compatriots.

Pathogens, for instance, are notoriously democratic. Had African Americans not been excluded from early AZT therapy on the basis of flawed HIV-treatment clinical trials (that largely excluded them), would the number of HIV-infected African Americans be lower today? Would the number of all domestic AIDS cases be lower, considering that black Americans today constitute half of all the HIV-infected? It's too late to know now, but not too late to do better racial recruitment for the next HIV clinical trials.

The fallout extends beyond infectious disease. For example, Donna Christian-Christensen, M.D., who represents the U.S. Virgin Islands in Congress, has observed that the percentage of black Americans who are insured is lower than that of white Americans, and the cost of caring for these uninsured people raises the rates and health-care costs of all Americans. She said, "We're getting to the hospital late, using much more expensive care: We're really driving up the costs of health care."

In fact, a decade ago, research by Harvard School of Public Health professors Ichiro Kawachi, M.D., and Deborah Prothow-Stith, M.D., explained this public-health phenomenon in detail and even quantified it, emerging with what was popularly referred to as the "Robin Hood Index." The shorthand is that public health suffers more in the nations with the greatest inequities in wealth, and that the middle class suffers nearly as much as the poor from inequities. In the United States, which has, for example, one of the world's greatest disparities in income between the haves and have-nots, we have not only the greatest health disparities but the greatest health-cost burdens for the mostly white middle class. In short, whites should care about quality medical research for African Americans because its dearth has generated needless pain, suffering, anger, and costs that continue to permeate the fabric of our entire nation: It is not only a racial tragedy but also an American tragedy.

For their part, African Americans cannot afford passivity. Seneca said, "It is part of the cure to wish to be cured." When it comes to medical research, that wish must be awakened in African Americans. African Americans should not shun lifesaving research; indeed, they cannot afford to do so. Instead, they must carefully scrutinize research initiatives before becoming subjects. But we must do more: We must also address the dearth of therapeutic research in areas that affect the health of African American most dramatically.

What changes are necessary to achieve this?

REPAIR THE SYSTEM OF INSTITUTIONAL REVIEW BOARDS (IRBS)

IRBs judge the scientific and ethical acceptability of proposed studies on human subjects. However, a string of abusive experiments have revealed that the nation's five thousand IRBs have failed to perform their role of protecting the public, and African Americans in particular. In June 1998, a Department of Health and Human Services (HHS) report concluded that IRB staff are inadequately trained, subject to conflicts of interest, and overwhelmed by too many cases.[17]

The Office of Protection from Research Risks (OPRR) requires IRBs to have a minimum of five members, at least one of whom must have primarily scientific interests, another of whom must have primarily non-scientific interests, and another of whom must be otherwise unaffiliated with the IRB's institution. But most IRB members are scientists affiliated with the organization in question, and even the lay members tend to have loyalties to the home institution. I propose that each IRB be composed of equal numbers of scientists and of peers of the group who will be asked to participate as subjects.

Some may object that laypeople will be unable to understand enough about scientific experiments to judge their suitability and value, but as a medical communicator, I doubt this: I know many skilled and motivated scientists who routinely convey complex information to many people, although to do so may require some preparation and effort.

Moreover, if a project cannot be explained to laypersons in an IRB meeting, how does a researcher propose to explain it to the potential subjects, as he must do by law? I also propose that each IRB include a medical ethicist and, if possible, a medical historian.

STOP THE EROSION OF CONSENT

Ban exceptions to informed consent. Recognize the right of every patient to say yes or no as an absolute value and cease designating groups such as soldiers, unconscious emergency room patients, and Third World experimental subjects as appropriate subjects without their input. When physicians are faced with a patient who is unable to consent because of his or her medical condition, and whose condition requires treatment before a family member or other proxy can be consulted, I propose that the patient be treated as if the physician had no research protocol to worry about. Treat him or her, but don't enroll that patient in a study. Instead, use the best-known treatment for that particular individual.

INSTITUTE A COORDINATED SYSTEM OF MANDATORY SUBJECT EDUCATION

The NIH and the Office of Research Integrity require that every practicing medical researcher receive education in the ethical and practical conduct of biomedical research. I took such a course at Harvard Medical School in 2004 and found it factually invaluable and culturally revealing. I propose that prospective research subjects be given the same advantage. Every institution that receives government funds to perform research should be required to hold approximately three classes that equip subjects with information about how research is conducted, what risks and benefits are inherent in different types of research, what their legal rights and moral responsibilities are, what sort of questions they should ask, and how they can maximize their chances of getting the desired result from the clinical trial they enter.

Except for seriously ill or otherwise-incapacitated patients, only people who have completed this course should be eligible to participate in government-funded clinical trials, and only they should be permitted to serve on IRBs.

EMBRACE A SINGLE STANDARD OF RESEARCH ETHICS

We cannot retain moral credibility if we champion human rights in medical research at home and ignore them abroad. Researchers should be made to follow informed-consent strictures abroad that are as restrictive as those governing their research on American shores. Pharmaceutical companies should be forced to make lifesaving drugs available to people in poor countries, even when this means sacrificing their obese profits for the benefit of human welfare. Because the federal government sponsors much of the research that enables pharmaceutical companies to develop vital medications, the federal government should take advantage of its legal right either to force manufacturers to lower their prices or to suspend patent enforcement in poor countries.

However, more important than any of the above recommendations is the need for African Americans to set their own research agendas. Black patients must take ownership of medical-research issues, as they have done with so many other complex health issues, from AIDS to environmental racism. Already, expert medical organizations have taken leadership roles. The National Center for Bioethics in Research and Health Care at Tuskegee University provides not only a center for scholars but also a venue for much-needed lay education on medical research. The National Medical Association has also spearheaded patient education through its Project IMPACT, which has helped black Americans to navigate clinical trials safely by providing brochures, Web sites, and access to experts.

African American and other health organizations must continue and expand the work of these pivotal groups, and much of this can be done close to home, through church health fairs, social organizations, and community activism.

I challenge African Americans to bring medical-research education to the fore of the American health agenda. I challenge you, the reader, to familiarize yourself with the informational documents on this book's Web site and elsewhere, to join an IRB, to ask the hard questions of physicians who are recruiting in your community, and to join appropriate clinical trials once you have satisfied yourself that they are worthwhile and relatively safe. I challenge African Americans to effect a transformation of our attitudes toward medical research and to demand our place at the table to enjoy the rich bounty of the American medical system in the form of longer, healthier lives.

I challenge us to change, because as Charles Darwin once observed, "It is not the strongest species that will survive, nor the most intelligent, but the one most responsive to change."

APPENDIX

CHOOSING A CLINICAL TRIAL

This guide to finding and participating in a clinical trial can be found on the *Medical Apartheid* Web site: www.medicalapartheid.com

ACKNOWLEDGMENTS

I always assumed that composing the acknowledgments would be the easiest part of writing this book. I was wrong. It is not only easy but deeply pleasurable to thank the many people who have supported me, but space prevents me from thanking everyone, and I am troubled by the prospect of rewarding someone's generosity with silence. So I begin by thanking the people whose names do not appear here for various reasons, including their own modest wishes. You know who you are and you know that I am grateful.

I am also going to break with convention and begin, not end, by thanking my mother, Corene Marie Washington. This book, and any other meaningful endeavor I complete, owes her a great debt.

And speaking of great debts, how can I thank those who provided me opportunity, resources, and an academic home while I prepared to write this book? In 1992, long before I conceived of this work in its present form, the Fellowship for Advanced Studies in Public Health at the Harvard School of Public Health gave me the means to prepare for it. The courses, faculty seminars, and time away from the rigors of daily journalism enabled me to enrich my education and to formulate ideas, thanks to former Dean Harvey V. Fineberg (now president of the Institute of Medicine), Jay A. Winsten, Ph.D., director of the school's Center for Health Communication, and former Deputy Director Robert Meyers, now president of the Washington Journalism Center. They, Deputy Director Susan Moses, and Terri Mendoza have always made me feel part of the CHC family.

It isn't possible to note all the many people on the Harvard faculty who taught, supported, and encouraged me, but Lawrence O. Gostin, J.D., who now directs the Center for Law and the Public's Health at Johns Hopkins and Georgetown universities, has been an unwavering source of support, and serving as his teaching assistant taught me much. The late William J. Curran, J.D., professor of public health law, provided sage advice over afternoon tea, and the late Jonathan Mann, M.D., always inspired me. I am also deeply grateful to Robert Coles. M.D., professor of psychiatry and medical humanities at Harvard Medical School, and to *Harvard Health Letter* editor Patricia Thomas, now Knight Chair in Health and Medical Journalism at the University of Georgia.

I deeply value the early support given me by Professor George Annas, chairman of the Health Law Department at Boston University, and Jay Katz, M.D., Elizabeth Dollard Professor Emeritus of Law, Medicine, and Psychiatry at Yale University. I am deeply indebted to the largesse and the openness of Stanford University, which granted me a fellowship to its Professional Publishing Course in 1995 and a luxurious John S. Knight Fellowship for Professional Journalists in 1997 specifically to study human medical experimentation. The famously accomplished James V. Risser, J.D., professor emeritus, provided not only an impossibly high standard of journalistic excellence to yearn toward but also a wealth of support and guidance. So has Professor James R. Bettinger, the current Knight director, who generously made time to read a portion of this manuscript and to give me excellent advice. I also thank Carl Djerassi, Ph.D., professor emeritus of chemistry and Renaissance man, for dramatically enriching my Stanford experience by accepting me into his splendid writing course for scientists.

In 1999, the late Marion Gray Secundy, Ph.D., appointed me senior research scholar at Tuskegee University's National Center for Bioethics in Research and Health Care, and in 2005, its new director, Vanessa Northington Gamble, M.D., Ph.D., author of the comprehensive *Making a Place for Ourselves,* was kind enough to include me once again in its accomplished group of diverse scholars. I owe a debt of thanks to the National Medical Association on several fronts, not the least of which is "The Guide to Clinical Trials" on this book's Web site, which was informed in part by work I completed as a NMA consultant under James H. Powell, M.D., and Yolanda Fleming.

In 2002, program directors Walter Robinson, M.D., assistant professor of social medicine and of pediatrics, and Mildred Solomon, Ed.D., accepted me into Harvard Medical School's Medical Ethics Fellowship, which provided me with invaluable clinical medical ethics training and access to thinkers on today's thorniest ethical issues, many of which are discussed in this book. I could not have asked for a more brilliant and nurturing environment than that provided by the program director of the Division of Medical Ethics, Allan M. Brandt, Ph.D., Amalie Moses Kass, Professor of the History of Medicine, and by Bryon Good, director of the HMS Division of Medical Ethics, who generously extended my fellowship so that I could more easily complete this book. So many physicians and ethicists added to my understanding of research ethics that I cannot possibly list them all, but Robert Truog, M.D., HMS professor of anesthesia and medical ethics, graciously expanded on the intricacies of brain death in response to my endless flow of questions.

I am grateful to those who invited me to present my work in conferences and seminars and offered invaluable feedback, including June Jackson Christmas, M.D., medical professor emerita at CUNY Medical School; Lorraine Cole, Ph.D., president and chief executive officer of the National Black Woman's Health Imperative; Stephen B. Thomas, Ph.D., director of the Center for Minority Health at the University of Pittsburgh; Volker Roelcke, M.D., director of Institut für Geschichte der Medizin, Universität Giessen; David J. Rothman, Ph.D., and Sheila M. Rothman, Ph.D., directors of the Columbia University Center for the Study of Society and Medicine; and Cécile Caldwell Vulliéty and Florian Nica of the Foundation Brocher in Geneva, Switzerland; as well as Rodney J. Reynolds, founder and publisher of *American Legacy* magazine.

The expertise and generosity of various libraries and librarians have been central to the development of this book. I did much of the early research at the New York Academy of Medicine Library on Fifth Avenue, and its former director, Edward T. Morman, Ph.D., the former librarian of the College of Physicians of Philadelphia and director of the Francis C. Wood Institute for the History of Medicine, took me under his wing, providing encouragement, support, and incisive criticism. Wayne J. Furman, director of the New York Public Library Center for Scholars and Writers, gave me access to not one but two urban aeries—the Wertheim Study and a coveted berth in the Frederick Lewis Allen Room—until this book was completed. The librarians of Harvard's Countway Library of Medicine also provided esoteric papers, images, and memoirs, as did the staff of the National Archives, especially Michael P. Musick and Sharon Culley.

I also thank the staff of the New York Writers Room, that incomparable haven for scribblers, and the Alfred P. Sloan Foundation for the Science Desk Award, which subsidized the initial work on this book and several other projects.

I am sorry that space prevents me from acknowledging the scores of physicians who have helped me to illustrate the questions posed in this book. I would especially like to thank: James Bowman, M.D., professor emeritus in the Department of Pathology, Medicine, and Genetics at the University of Chicago; Benjamin Roy, M.D., of Atlanta, Georgia; Joye Carter, M.D., former chief medical examiner for Harris County, Texas; Professor Robert Murray, M.D., professor of genetics at Howard University; Clive O. Callendar, M.D., chairman of the Department of Surgery at Howard University Hospital; Victor McKusick, M.D., professor at the Johns Hopkins Hospital; Professor Martin S. Pernick, Ph.D., associate director for history and medicine at the University of Michigan; and an early inspiration, Ruth Lawrence, M.D., professor of pediatrics, obstetrics, and gynecology at the University of Rochester, who has been a role model to an entire generation of women healers. In the realm of inspiration, I perhaps owe the most to Benjamin S. Carson, Sr., M.D., humanitarian, bestselling author of *Gifted Hands*, and chief of pediatric neurosurgery at Johns Hopkins Medical School, for our many long discussions of a decade ago. In him I discerned how the spirit of scientific endeavor is perfectly compatible with faith in God, humility, and dramatic medical innovations that are devoid of any hint of exploitation.

My fellow writers have been generous and encouraging, particularly Eileen Welsome, Pulitzer Prize–winning author of *The Plutonium Files*, an elegantly written chronicle of the nuclear devastation unleashed upon unsuspecting Americans. Allen Hornblum, author of *Acres Of Skin*, invited me to Philadelphia and introduced me to the prisoner subjects on whose behalf he still labors. Martha Stephens, author of *The Treatment*, also shared her expertise with me.

From the inception of this work, Sheri L. Fink, M.D., Ph.D., fellow of Harvard's François-Xavier Bagnand Center for Health and Human

Rights and author of *War Hospital*, read versions of the manuscript and gave me unstinting support and sage advice, both as a physician and as a journalist. Harvard University's Khadija Robin Pierce, J.D., a visiting scholar at the University of Bergen, Norway, offered a plethora of perceptive feedback. Eva Winkler, M.D., Ph.D., fellow of the Department of Hematology and Oncology at the University Hospital, Munich, offered excellent feedback on my ethical arguments, and Dr. med. Frank Winkler, Department of Neurology, University of Munich, deployed his expertise to elucidate the tangled neurochemistry of fenfluramine challenge. These four also supplied friendship and warm hospitality whenever I needed a place to lay my head in Boston.

Other writers read portions of the manuscript and made helpful suggestions, including Dawn M. Bracely, Robyne Curry, and members of the peerless writing group of Annie Murphy Paul, author of *The Cult of Personality*. Its members became a providential source of camaraderie and advice just when I needed it most. Irene Billips and Lois Wolf Friend also offered feedback and much-appreciated support.

Many historians of medicine helped me, including Susan Lederer, Ph.D., associate professor of the history of medicine at Yale, a warm font of expertise and support; Evelyn Hammonds, Ph.D., professor of the history of science and of African and African-American studies, who allowed me to audit her fascinating class; Rebecca Herzig, associate professor of women and gender studies at Bates College; and Susan M. Reverby, professor of women's studies at Wellesley College, author of the breathtakingly comprehensive *Tuskegee's Truths*.

I also learned much from discussions with Vernellia R. Randall, R.N., J.D., M.P.H., professor of law at the University of Dayton, and Mario Cooper, J.D., director of Leading for Life, Harvard AIDS Institute.

This book could not have been written without the many people who courageously shared their stories with me, including Jesse Williams, Elmerine Whitfield Bell, Calvin Johnson, Dorothy Pelote, Rudy M. Brown, J.D., an advocate for some New York City experimental subjects, and the family of Henrietta Lacks, especially David Lacks.

I thank my wonderful lawyer, Zick Rubin, J.D., Ph.D., and my brilliant, vibrant agent, Lisa Bankoff of International Creative Management, whom I feel incredibly lucky to work with and to know: she believed in this book and has offered warmth, wisdom, and assistance far above and beyond the call of duty. Gerald Howard, executive editor-at-large for Doubleday Broadway, has been a trusted adviser, a wise confidant, and when needed, a deft literary surgeon: Thank you so much for caring about this book.

I thank my family for their support, especially Kate, Eric, Theresa, Khari, Wesley, Rashida, Carl, Tierney, Dustin, Jayme, and Demitrius. Death has stilled the voices of my brother Percy Cecil Washington, Jr., and my father, Percy Cecil Washington, Sr., but it will never mute their encouragement and pride, which still nourish me.

NOTES

CHAPTER 1. SOUTHERN DISCOMFORT

1. Frederick Gardiner, M.D., "A Mormon Rebel: The Life and Travels of Frederick Gardiner," Family History Records, Family Ancestral File No. 477D–4H, Pedigree Chart, Historical Department, Church of Jesus Christ of Latter-Day Saints, Salt Lake City.
2. Pathogens are disease-causing microorganisms.
3. Calomel (Hg_2Cl_2) is now used as an insecticide and fungicide.
4. Laudanum is a tincture of opium in alcohol.
5. Jalap is derived from the tuberous roots of the Mexican plant *Ipomoea purga*.
6. *Harrison's Principles of Internal Medicine* (New York: McGraw-Hill, 1998). pp. 2568–2569.
7. Ibid., pp. 2566–2567.
8. Todd L. Savitt, *Medicine and Slavery: The Diseases and Health Care of Blacks in Antebellum Virginia* (Urbana: University of Illinois Press, 1978; reprint 2002).
9. Steve M. Stowe, "Seeing Themselves at Work: Physicians and the Case Narrative in the Mid-Nineteenth Century American South," *American Historical Review* (February 1996), pp. 39–79.
10. In *Medicine and Slavery,* historian Todd Savitt coined the powerful description of slaves as "legally invisible" medical subjects.
11. R. H. Shryock, "Medical Sources and the Social Historian," *American Historical Review* 41 (1936): 465, cited in Walter Fisher, "Physicians and Slavery in the Antebellum Southern Medical Journal," *Journal of the History of Medicine and Allied Sciences* 23 (1968): 145–152.
12. Sharla M. Fett, *Working Cures: Healing Health and Power on Southern Slave Plantations* (Chapel Hill and London: University of North Carolina Press, 2002), p. 181.
13. Ibid.
14. Ibid.
15. Ammonium carbonate is an equivalent mixture of ammonium bicarbonate and ammonium carbamate.
16. Using original physicians' and planters' records, historian Sharla Fett has com-

piled an impressive dossier on the uses of medicine to abuse and punish slaves; see Fett, *Working Cures,* pp. 186–187.

17. Ibid., p. 150.

18. Wes Brady interview in *The American Slave: A Composite Autobiography,* ed. George P. Rawick (Westport, CT: Greenwood Press 1972), suppl. 2, pp. 401–402.

19. Martha Griffith Browne, *Autobiography of a Female Slave,* Electronic ed., (Chapel Hill: Academic Affairs Library, University of North Carolina, 1999).

20. John Duffy, ed., *The Rudolph Matas History of Medicine in Louisiana* (2 vols.) (Baton Rouge, 1958–1962).

21. Notably in Bruce Dain's *A Hideous Monster of the Mind: American Race Theory in the Early Republic* (Cambridge, MA: Harvard University Press, 2002), Robert V. Guthrie's *Even the Rat Was White: A Historical View of Psychology,* 2nd ed. (Boston: Allyn and Bacon, 1998), and Stephen Jay Gould's *The Mismeasure of Man* (New York: W. W. Norton, 1992).

22. Buffon, *Histoire naturelle générale, et particulière, avec la description du cabinet du roi* (Paris: Penaud, 1749). In his forty-volume encyclopedia, Buffon attempted a comprehensive description and classification of living things and made rudimentary attempts at theory for the mutation of plants and animals.

23. Klaus Hödl, *Gesunde Juden—Kranke Schwarze: Körperbilder im medizinischen Diskurs.* [Healthy Jews—Sick Blacks: Images of the Body in Medical Discourse] (Berlin: Studien Verlag, 2002). See also Dain, *A Hideous Monster of the Mind.*

24. See also Kwame Anthony Appiah, "Racisms," in *Anatomy of Racism,* ed. Gary David Goldberg (Minneapolis: University of Minnesota Press, 1990), pp. 4–5.

25. *Oxford English Dictionary,* s. v. "racialist," Oxford online edition, (2004); at http://dictionary.oed.com/

26. Todd Wingate, "Anthropology and Negro Slavery," *Medical Life* 102 (1929): 166.

27. Samuel A. Cartwright, "Report on the Diseases and Physical Peculiarities of the Negro Race," *De Bow's Review Southern and Western States* 7, no. 11 (1851): 692–696.

28. Samuel A. Cartwright, "Report on the Diseases and Physical Peculiarities of the Negro Race," *Southern Medical Reports* 2 (1850): 421.

29. Ibid., pp. 422–423.

30. Richard Allen Williams, *Textbook of Black-Related Diseases* (New York: McGraw-Hill, 1975).

31. Charles Darwin, *On the Origin of Species by Means of Natural Selection, or the Preservation of Favoured Races in the Struggle for Life* (London: John Murray, 1859).

32. Fett, *Working Cures,* p. 11.

33. W. T. English, "The Negro Problem from the Physician's Point of View," *Atlanta Journal-Record of Medicine* 5 (1903); 461; cited in Allan M. Brandt, "Racism and Research: The Case of the Tuskegee Syphilis Experiment," *Hastings Center Report* 8 (1978); 22.

34. Warwick Anderson, "Immunities of Empire: Race, Disease, and the New Tropical Medicine, 1900–1920," *Bulletin of the History of Medicine* 70, no. 1 (1996): 94–118. Anderson's article cites R. L. Bullard, "Some Characteristics of the Negro Volunteer," *Journal of Military Service Institutions, United States* 29 (1901): 29.

35. Todd L. Savitt and James Harvey Young, eds., *Disease and Distinctiveness in the American South* (Knoxville: University of Tennessee Press, 1988).

36. Hill Carter's Shirley Farm Journals, June 23, 1850, Library of Congress, Washington, D.C., cited in Savitt, *Medicine and Slavery,* p. 104

37. From the 1851 journal of K. Washington Skinner, overseer of the Gowrie planta-tion in Georgia, quoted in Jeffrey Young, "Ideology and Death on a Savannah River Rice Plantation, 1833–1867: Paternalism Amidst 'a Good Supply of Death and Pain,' " *The Journal of Southern History* 59, no. 4 (1993): 690.

38. John Duffy in Savitt and Young, eds., *Disease and Distinctiveness in the American South,* p. 37.

39. Less than 1 percent prevalence in the twentieth century. See Margaret Humphreys, *Malaria: Poverty, Health and Public Health in the United States* (Baltimore and London: The Johns Hopkins University Press, 2001), p. 9.

40. Ibid. See also James Bowman, M.D., and Robert F. Murray, Jr., M.D., M.S., *Genetic Variation and Disorders in People of African Origin* (Baltimore: Johns Hopkins University Press, 1990).

41. Philip Tidyman, M.D., "A Sketch of the Most Remarkable Diseases of the Negroes of the Southern States," *Philadelphia Journal of the Medical and Physical Sciences* 12 (1826): 315–316.

42. Humphreys, *Malaria,* p. 19.

43. Bowman and Murray, *Genetic Variation and Disorders in People of African Origin,* p. 233.

44. Humphreys, *Malaria,* pp. 15–18; Bowman and Murray, *Genetic Variation and Disorders in People of African Origin.*

45. Dain, *A Hideous Monster of the Mind,* p. 14.

46. Lathan A. Windley, "Runaway Slave Advertisements of George Washington and Thomas Jefferson," *Journal of Negro History* 63, no. 4 (1978): 373–374; "Eighteenth Century Slaves as Advertised by Their Masters," *Journal of Negro History* 1, no. 2 (1916): 163–216.

47. Joseph Graves, Jr., *The Emperor's New Clothes: Biological Theories of Race at the Millennium* (New Brunswick, NJ: Rutgers University Press, 2001), pp. 113–114.

48. Savitt, *Medicine and Slavery,* pp. 92–97.

49. Fisher, "Physicians and Slavery in the Antebellum Southern Medical Journal."

50. Frederick Douglass et al, *Narrative of the Life of Frederick Douglass, an American Slave* (New Haven: Yale University Press, 2001).

51. Eric L. McKitrick, *Slavery Defended: The Views of the Old South* (Englewood Cliffs, NJ: Prentice-Hall, 1963).

52. Bethany Veney, *The Narrative of Bethany Veney a Slave Woman, with Introduction by Rev. Bishop Mallalieu and Commendatory Notices from Rev. V. A. Cooper, Superintendent of Home for Little Wanderers, Boston, Mass., and Rev. Erastus Spaulding, Millbury, Mass.* (Worcester, MA: George H. Ellis, 1889), p. 32.

53. Thomas Jefferson to John W. Eppes, June 30, 1820, in *Jefferson's Farm Book: With Commentary and Relevant Extracts from Other Writings* (Princeton, NJ: Princeton University Press, 1953), p. 46.

54. Alexander Falconbridge, *Black Voyage—Eyewitness Accounts of the Atlantic Slave Trade* (Boston: Little, Brown, 1788).

55. Louis Agassiz, April 9, 1863, from unexpurgated correspondence found in Harvard's Houghton Library and cited in Gould, *The Mismeasure of Man,* p. 49.

56. Harriet A. Jacobs, *Incidents in the Life of a Slave Girl Written by Herself,* enlarged ed., (Cambridge, MA, and London: President and Fellows of Harvard College,

1987); Mary Reynolds's statement appears in *The American Slave: A Composite Autobiography,* ed. George P. Rawick (Westport, CT: Greenwood Press, 1972–1979), p. 242.

57. Fett, *Working Cures,* pp. 28–29; See also Savitt and Young, eds., *Disease and Distinctiveness in the American South.*

58. Browne, *Autobiography of a Female Slave.*

59. This dependence led to bitter struggles over the manner of doctors' remuneration. Medical journals condemned the slave owners' desire to save money by paying doctors a flat annual fee rather than for each case as an assault on a physician's dignity in which he, like the slave, became the landowner's hired worker. One physician responded, "When an individual asks me to do his practice by the year, I am often inclined to answer as a young friend of mine did on such an occasion—he indignantly replied: 'Whenever I am become black and am to be hired, I will let you know.' " Fisher, "Physicians and Slavery in the Antebellum Southern Medical Journal."

60. Kenneth F. Kiple and Virginia H. King, *Another Dimension to the Black Diaspora: Diet, Disease, and Racism* (Cambridge, England; Cambridge University Press, 1981), p. 163.

61. *New Orleans Medical and Surgical Journal* 4 (1848), p. 678.

62. But only 3 percent of slaves were insured. See Todd Savitt, "Slave Life Insurance in Virginia and North Carolina," *The Journal of Southern History* 43 (1977): 585.

63. See ibid., p. 593: "The North Carolina Mutual Life Insurance Company of Raleigh was probably the major insurer of slaves in the Carolinas. . . . The company approved its first policy on April 1, 1849. In early July it had issued 83 white and 45 slave policies. A year later 610 policies were in force, the majority of which were probably for slaves. By June 1857 (and probably earlier) three times as many slaves as whites were being insured annually." In 1858, 75 percent of the company's policies were written on slaves. See also Stowe, "Seeing Themselves at Work."

64. Savitt, "Slave Life Insurance in Virginia and North Carolina," p. 587

65. Work Projects Administration, "Joe Hawkins Interview," 8.3, supplement 1, p. 958.

66. Richard Toler's comments are recorded in Rawick, *The American Slave,* vol. 16, p. 99.

67. *New Orleans Medical and Surgical Journal* 12 (1855): 196–99, cited in Fisher, "Physicians and Slavery in the Antebellum Southern Medical Journal."

68. Herbert M. Morais, *The History of the Afro-American in Medicine* (Cornwell Heights, PA: The Publishers Agency, Inc., 1979), p. 12.

69. "Cesar's Cure for Poison," *Massachusetts Magazine* (1792), reproduced in ibid., p. 211; see also Louis W. Sullivan, "The Education of Black Health Professionals," *Phylon* 38, no. 2 (1977): 181–193.

70. J. E. Brown, *Blacks in Connecticut, a Historic Profile* (New Haven: Connecticut Afro-American Historical Society, 1979).

71. E. D. Fenner, "Dirt-Eating Among Negroes," *Southern Medical Reports* 1, no. 194 (1849): 436.

CHAPTER 2. PROFITABLE WONDERS

1. John Brown, c. 1854, in Louis Alexis Chamerovzow, ed., *Slave Life in Georgia: A Narrative of the Life, Sufferings, and Escape of John Brown, a Fugitive Slave, Now in England* (London: W. M. Watts, 1855).

2. Dr. Hamilton lived and practiced in Clinton, seat of Jones County, Georgia. See F. N. Boney, "Doctor Thomas Hamilton: Two Views of a Gentleman of the Old South," *Phylon* 28, no. 3 (1967): 288–292.

3. Historians tell us that Hamilton's life paralleled that of the federal Union, for he was born firmly rooted in the southern aristocracy a few years before the South joined and he died just before the secession from the Union triggered the Civil War. See Boney, ibid.

4. Brown, *Slave Life in Georgia*, p. 36

5. Boney, "Doctor Thomas Hamilton."

6. The freedom of freedmen was restrained by a number of byzantine laws that subjugated them to the will of whites and provided for their incarceration or enslavement for a variety of minor infractions and even for some medical conditions. See Todd L. Savitt, *Medicine and Slavery: The Diseases and Health Care of Blacks in Antebellum Virginia* (Urbana: University of Illinois Press, 1978; reprint 2002).

7. Claude Bernard, *An Introduction to the Study of Experimental Medicine* (New York: Dover, 1957), p. 20.

8. Todd L. Savitt, "The Use of Blacks for Medical Experimentation and Demonstration in the Old South," *The Journal of Southern History* 48, no. 3 (1982): 343.

9. Sharla M. Fett, *Working Cures: Healing Health and Power on Southern Slave Plantations* (Chapel Hill and London: University of North Carolina Press, 2002); Thomas Jefferson, cited in Savitt, *Medicine and Slavery*.

10. Although scientists often suggest that blacks shared an inherent, illogical, and atavistic repugnance for Western medicine and for medical experimentation, the facts do not bear this out: Africans often embraced new and experimental approaches to disease management. See Megan Vaughn, *Curing Their Ills* (Stanford, CA: Stanford University Press, 1991); see also David Wendler et al., "Are Racial and Ethnic Minorities Less Willing to Participate in Health Research?" *PLoS Medicine* 3, no. 2, p. 19.

11. Walter Fisher, "Physicians and Slavery in the Antebellum Southern Medical Journal," *Journal of the History of Medicine and Allied Sciences* 23 (1968): 145–152. See also Savitt, "The Use of Blacks for Medical Experimentation and Demonstration in the Old South," p. 343; Brown, *Slave Life in Georgia*; M. B. B. Gordon, *Aesculapius Comes to the Colonies* (Ventnor, NJ: Ventnor, 1949); Savitt, *Medicine and Slavery*; Robert L. Blakeley and Judith M. Harrington, *Bones in the Basement: Postmortem Racism in Nineteenth-Century Medical Training* (Washington, D.C., and London: Smithsonian Institution Press, 1997); James O. Breeden, "States-Rights Medicine in the Old South," *Bulletin of the New York Academy of Medicine* 52 (1976): 348–372.

12. Lawrence K. Altman, *Who Goes First? The Story of Self-Experimentation in Medicine* (New York: Random House, 1987), p. 333; see also Fett, *Working Cures*.

13. Cited in Savitt, *Medicine and Slavery*, pp. 301–303.

14. Within smaller regions served by hospitals, clinics, and medical schools, African Americans could constitute a much higher proportion of the population; for ex-

ample, 66 percent of those in some Virginia counties were African American. In Alabama's Montgomery County, where Dr. Sims practiced, slaves constituted 51 percent of the population in the 1830s; by 1840, they accounted for fully 63 percent. See Savitt, *Medicine and Slavery,* p. 289; see also *Southern Medical and Surgical Journal* 2 (1838): 345.

15. This chapter is indebted to Todd L. Savitt's seminal volume *Medicine and Slavery* and to his 1982 article, "The Use of Blacks for Medical Experimentation and Demonstration in the Old South." The passage quoted appears on pages 342–343 of the latter.

16. William Beaumont, *Experiments and Observations on the Gastric Juice and the Physiology of Digestion* (New York: Dover, 1833).

17. The records and Gage's skull are stored in Harvard University's Warren Museum exhibit, fifth floor, Countway Library of Medicine.

18. Bruce Dain, *A Hideous Monster of the Mind: American Race Theory in the Early Republic* (Cambridge, MA: Harvard University Press, 2002), pp. 19–25.

19. W. Montague Cobb, M.D., "Surgery and the Negro Physician: Some Parallels in Background," *Journal of the National Medical Association* 43, no. 3 (1951): 145–152.

20. Theodore Wright Weld, "American Slavery as It Is" (1839), cited in Savitt, "The Use of Blacks for Medical Experimentation and Demonstration in the Old South," p. 344.

21. The vaccine was procured through Dr. Edward Gantt of Georgetown in the spring of 1801.

22. Thomas Jefferson to Mr. John Vaughn, November 5, 1801, and to Martha Jefferson Randolph, January 17, 1802; reprinted in Robert L. Halsey, *How the President Thomas Jefferson and Dr. Benjamin Waterhouse Established Vaccination as a Public Health Procedure* (New York, 1936), p. 52; cited in Savitt, *Medicine and Slavery,* p. 296.

23. Savitt, *Medicine and Slavery.*

24. Walter F. Jones, "On the Utility of the Applications of Hot Water to the Spine in the Treatment of Typhoid Pneumonia," *Virginia Medical and Surgical Journal* 3 (1854): 108–110; cited in Savitt, *Medicine and Slavery,* p. 299.

25. John M. B. Harden, M.D., "Some Experiments to Determine the Relative Areas of the Trunks and Branches of Arteries," *Southern Medical and Surgical Journal, n.s.,* 2, June (1846): 330–333; Savitt, "The Use of Blacks for Medical Experimentation and Demonstration in the Old South," p. 347

26. This was actually a biography written by Sims's son but was based upon Sims's recollections and upon verbatim autobiographical accounts such as the one excerpted here.

27. J. Marion Sims, *The Story of My Life;* cited in Deborah Kuhn McGregor, *From Midwives to Medicine: The Birth of American Gynecology* (New Brunswick, NJ: Rutgers University Press, 1998), pp. 28–29.

28. Ibid.

29. Ronald L. Numbers and Todd L. Savitt, *Science and Medicine in the Old South* (Baton Rouge and London: Louisiana State University Press, 1989), p. 337.

30. Calcium is important for proper muscle contraction and magnesium is essential for muscle relaxation, while the body needs adequate vitamin D in order to utilize these two minerals. See R. M. Jenss and A. F. Christie, "Consideration of

Race and Sex in Relation to Growth and Development of Infants," *Journal of Pediatrics* 14 (1939): 136, and Theodore M. Bayless et al., *The New England Journal of Medicine* 292 (1975): 1157.

31. Sims, *The Story of My Life;* cited in McGregor, *From Midwives to Medicine,* p. 31.

32. J. Marion Sims, "Removal of the Superior Maxilla for Amputation of the Antrum: Apparent Cure. Return of the Disease. Second Operation. Sequel," *Journal of the American Medical Sciences* (1847): 310–314; "Osteosarcoma of the Lower Jaw," *Journal of the American Medical Sciences* 11 (1846): 128–132.

33. Sims, *The Story of My Life;* cited in McGregor, *From Midwives to Medicine,* p. 49.

34. *New Orleans Medical News* (1860), quoted in Felice Swados, "Negro Health on the Antebellum Plantations," *Bulletin of the History of Medicine* 10 (1941): 470; cited in McGregor, *From Midwives to Medicine,* p. 41.

35. "Growth in height or stature stops before full growth of the pelvic bones has been completed, so women who marry young and become pregnant early are at greatly increased risk of obstetric complications": L. Lewis Wall, "Fitsari 'Dan Duniya: An African (Hausa) Praise Song About Vesicovaginal Fistulas," *Obstetrics and Gynecology* 100, no. 6 (2002): 1328–1332.

36. The contracted pelvis was rachitic—flat and shallow. This structural insufficiency greatly impeded the passage of the child through the birth canal during labor. Additionally, Anarcha was no anomaly as a seventeen-year-old mother. Masters eager to add to their population of slaves encouraged very early childbearing. Today, rickets is still prevalent in areas where malnutrition and starvation are prevalent and so is vesicovaginal fistula. Specialized fistula hospitals are extant in areas of Nigeria and Ethiopia, and in Khartoum, the Sudanese capital; see Wall, "Fitsari 'Dan Duniya," pp. 1328–1330; see also McGregor, *From Midwives to Medicine.*

37. There was no cure for vesicovaginal fistula, but various surgical approaches to repair the injury had been attempted in America and France. "Sims' approaches were similar to some of these, but Sims did not know this because he was largely ignorant of the field of women's disorders." C. G. Haygood, "Cases of Vesicovaginal Fistula Treated by Operations," *Boston Medical and Surgical Journal* 44 (April 16, 1851): 220. Also see McGregor, *From Midwives to Medicine,* pp. 48–49.

38. Fisher, "Physicians and Slavery in the Antebellum Southern Medical Journal," pp. 146–147.

39. Despite the widespread mythology about the natural licentiousness of slaves, enslaved women lived in the sexually repressive Victorian era, just as whites did. Some medical scientists even described enslaved black women as unduly "prudish." No one asked or recorded their reactions, but the experience of these young girls must have been emotionally as well as physically painful.

40. In fact the speculum, used to view the vagina, was new and suspect. The speculum (actually its forerunner the metroscope) had been devised only a quarter-century earlier by French surgeon Joseph-Claude-Anselme Récamier, and public outrage at the implied sexual violation was suppressing its use.

41. McGregor, *From Midwives to Medicine,* pp. 49–50.

42. Seale Harris, M.D., *Women's Surgeon: The Life Story of J. Marion Sims* (New York: Macmillian, 1950), p. 109.

43. Martin S. Pernick, *The Black Stork: Eugenics and the Death of "Defective" Babies*

in American Medicine and Motion Pictures Since 1915 (New York: Oxford University Press, 1996). One biographer notes: "A number of white women were brought to him as soon as his success in curing the slaves became generally known, but they seemed unable to bear the operation's pain and discomfort with the stoicism shown by the Negroes." Harris, *Women's Surgeon*, p. 109.

44. J. Marion Sims, "On the Treatment of Vesico-Vaginal Fistula," *American Journal of the Medical Sciences* 45 (1852): 226–246.

45. J. Marion Sims, *Clinical Notes on Uterine Surgery, with Reference to the Management of the Sterile Condition* (London: R. Hardwicke, 1866), pp. 331–336. Sims also performed experimental surgeries on women afflicted with vaginismus. He surgically removed tissue from the hymen or laterally sliced the muscle tissue that caused the contraction. But he refused to perform such drastic experimental surgeries on women "of the highest social stratum."

46. Sims, "Stenosis of the Cervix Uteri," p. 66; cited in McGregor, *From Midwives to Medicine,* p. 201.

47. Such as his contemporary Dr. Thomas Addis Emmet; see Emmet, *Reminiscences,* p. 97.

48. McGregor, *From Midwives to Medicine,* pp. 50–51.

49. Fisher, "Physicians and Slavery in the Antebellum Southern Medical Journal," p. 48.

50. Ephraim McDowell, another gynecologic surgeon who used slave women as experimental subjects, was Sims's contemporary.

51. Harris, *Women's Surgeon*, p. 349; see also Weld, "American Slavery as It Is," cited in Savitt, "The Use of Blacks for Medical Experimentation and Demonstration in the Old South, p. 343.

52. Harris, *Women's Surgeon*, p. 251.

53. Sims, *The Story of My Life,* p. 236. The entire passage reads: "To the indomitable courage of these long-suffering women, more than to any one other single circumstance is the world indebted for the results of these persevering efforts. Had they faltered, then would woman have continued to suffer from the dreadful injuries produced by protracted parturition, and then should the broad domain of surgery not have known one of the most useful improvements that shall forever hereafter grace its annals." See also J. Marion Sims, M.D., *Silver Sutures in Surgery* (New York: S. S. & S. W. Wood, 1858).

54. McGregor, *From Midwives to Medicine,* pp. 64–65.

55. *Louisville Register,* vol. 1, pp. 83–89; cited in Fisher, "Physicians and Slavery in the Antebellum Southern Medical Journal." Bozeman describes using Sims's technique except that he substituted a "button" suture for a "clamp" suture.

56. McGregor, *From Midwives to Medicine,* p. 64; see also Savitt, *Medicine and Slavery,* p. 297.

57. John Peter Mettauer, "On Vesico-Vaginal Fistula," *American Journal of the Medical Sciences* (1847): 117–121; p. 121 also cited in Savitt, *Medicine and Slavery,* pp. 297–298.

58. "Scholars Argue over Legacy of Surgeon Who Was Lionized, Then Vilified," *New York Times,* October 28, 2003, pp. F7–F9.

59. Helen Buckler, *Dr. Dan* (Boston: Little, Brown, 1954), pp. 183, 191; cited in Eugene P. Link, "The Civil Rights Activities of Three Great Negro Physicians," *The Journal of Negro History* 52, no. 3 (1967): 169–84.

60. Cobb, "Surgery and the Negro Physician."

61. Even the instruments devised to perform the experimental surgeries are still in use helping women. From the Web site for Worldwide Fund for Mothers Injured in Childbirth: "Amazingly enough, Dr. J. Marion Sims' retractor is still as useful today as it was in the mid 1800's! The Sims retractor can be used for VVF and RVF repair, as well as for examination of fistula patients in an outpatient department!"

62. *New Orleans Medical and Surgical Journal* (October 1879–April 1880); *American Journal of the Medical Sciences* (August 1835), cited in Fisher, "Physicians and Slavery in the Antebellum Southern Medical Journal."

63. John L. Richwoods, *The Western Journal of Medical and Physicians Sciences* (1830); cited in Fisher, "Physicians and Slavery in the Antebellum Southern Medical Journal."

64. Harris, *Women's Surgeon.*

65. Savitt, "The Use of Blacks for Medical Experimentation and Demonstration in the Old South," p. 346.

66. H. M. Lyman, *Artificial Anesthesia and Anesthetics* (New York: Wood, 1891), p. 5. See also Altman, *Who Goes First?,* which adds: "Three years later, one of the actors in this affair told Long about the episode; the tale reportedly 'added courage to' Long's meditations."

67. Medical Association of the State of Georgia, *Transactions* 5 (April 1853); cited in Savitt, "The Use of Blacks for Medical Experimentation and Demonstration in the Old South," p. 347.

68. Crawford Long first successfully used ether in experiments with slaves, but this highly fictionalized painting depicts the first successful public *demonstration* of anesthesia on October 16, 1846, by William Thomas Green Morton at the Massachusetts General Hospital during an operation by Harvard Medical School professor John Collins Warren, M.D. For example, famous surgeons who were not actually in attendance are represented in the painting. The fact that Long published his discovery only after Morton's demonstration is usually given as the reason for crediting Morton with the discovery, not the fear that Long's experimentation with slaves would promulgate a less noble medical image. However, this rationale is unconvincing, because assigning credit was not that straightforward: There was actually a protracted battle for credit among Long, Morton, and Horace Wells.

69. Mather's avocation fit the medical culture of the day. Before 1700, twenty-six Harvard graduates were practicing medicine in New England, but only two held an M.D. degree; Henry R. Viet, "Some Features of the History of Medicine in Massachusetts During the Colonial Period," *Isis* 23, no. 2 (1935): 395.

70. Eugenia W. Herbert, "Smallpox Inoculation in Africa," *The Journal of African History* 16, no. 4 (1975): 539–559.

71. Ibid. Onesimus may or may not have been from the ethnic group of the "Guaramantese." Such specific ethnic designations were often randomly assigned to Africans by whites.

72. In some parts of Africa, it was common practice to "buy the disease": Children were sent to villages where smallpox was rife to buy scabs or crusts from patients to use for inoculation.

73. In a tract that is reproduced in G. L. Kittredge's *The Angel of Bethesda*, Mather

describes the instructions and training he was given by Onesimus. Curiously, he retains Onesimus's pidgin English: "People take the juice of the Small-Pox; and Cutty-skin, an Put in a Drop; then by'nd by a little Sicky sicky; then very few little things like *Small*-pox; and nobody dy of it; and no body have Small-Pox any more. . . ."

74. Cotton Mather wrote, "I have instructed our Physicians in the new Method used by the Africans and Asiaticks, to prevent and abate the Dangers of the Small-Pox, and infallibly to save the Lives of those that have it wisely managed upon them. The Destroyer, being enraged at the Proposal of any Thing, that may rescue the Lives of our poor People from him, has taken a strange Possession of the People on this Occasion. They rave, rail, they blaspheme; they talk not only like Ideots but also like Franticks, And not only the Physician who began the Experiment, but I also am an Object of their Fury; their furious Obloquies and Invectives." See *Diary of Cotton Mather, 1681–1724* (Boston: The Society, 1721), pp. 631–632, entry for "Sunday, 16 July."

75. Boylston, like many of his fellow physicians, held no degree, having been apprenticed to his father.

76. Viet, "Some Features of the History of Medicine in Massachusetts During the Colonial Period," p. 400.

77. Because the grenade failed to detonate, the note could be read and reproduced in newspaper accounts in all three Boston newspapers on November 20 and 21, 1721. Recent accounts include William M. Fowler, "Boston's Bouts with Smallpox," *The Boston Globe,* December 2, 2001, p. 7.

78. Ibid.

79. Ibid.

80. Richard T. Vetter, M.D., "Vaccines and the Power of Immunity," *Post Graduate Medicine* 101, no. 6 (1997): 154. See also *Philosophical Transactions of the Royal Society* 374 (1722): 215; cited in Herbert, "Smallpox Inoculation in Africa," and in *The Evolution of Preventive Medicine in the United States Army 1607–1939: The Colonial Period (1607–1775),* ed. Robert S. Anderson (Washington, D.C.: Office of the Surgeon General, Department of the Army). See also Viet, "Some Features of the History of Medicine in Massachusetts During the Colonial Period," p. 400.

81. England also happened to be in the throes of a smallpox epidemic, and Caroline, Princess of Wales and the wife of the future George IV, allowed her physicians to use six condemned men in Newgate for inoculation trials. When they survived, smallpox inoculation swept through the Continent. See Sir Hans Sloane (Royal Physicians) in *Philosophical Transactions of Britain* 49 (1753): 516; see also M. H. Pappworth, *Human Guinea Pigs: Experimentation on Man* (Boston: Beacon Press, 1967), p. 60.

82. *The Evolution of Preventive Medicine in the United States Army,* p. 5.

CHAPTER 3. CIRCUS AFRICANUS

1. Philips Verner Bradford and Harry Blume, *Ota Benga: The Pygmy in the Zoo* (New York: St. Martin's Press, 1992). See also Jerry Bergman, Ph.D., "Ota Benga: The Man Who Was Put on Display in the Zoo!" (2001), sponsored by Answers in Genesis, Gospel Communications Network, Master Books and MorningStar; at http://www.onehumanrace.com/docs/ota_benga.asp.

2. "Man and Monkey Show Disapproved by Clergy: The Rev. Dr. McArthur Thinks the Exhibition Degrading, Colored Ministers to Act. The Pygmy Has an Orang-Outang as a Companion Now and Their Antics Delight the Bronx Crowds," *New York Times,* September 10, 1906, pp. 1–2.

3. "The Pygmies of the Congo," *Scientific American,* August 5, 1905, p. 107.

4. "Man and Monkey Show," p. 1.

5. "Negro Ministers Act," p. 2.

6. "Man and Monkey Show," pp. 1–2; see also "Negro Clergy Protest; Displeased at Exhibition of Bushman in Monkey House," *New York Times,* [day and month not known], 1906.

7. "Mayor Won't Help to Free Caged Pygmy: He Refers Negro Ministers to the Zo-ological Society," *New York Times,* September 12, 1906, p. 9.

8. M. S. Gabriel, M.D., "Ota Benga Having a Fine Time: A Visitor at the Zoo Finds No Reason for Protests About the Pygmy," *New York Times,* September 13, 1906.

9. Ibid.

10. "A perversion from which most races are exempt prompts the negro's inclina-tion towards white women, whereas other races incline toward females of their own," remarked W. T. English in "The Negro Problem from the Physician's Point of View," *Atlanta Journal-Record of Medicine* 5 (1903): 463; see also Thomas Jefferson, *Notes on the State of Virginia* (Paris: privately published, 1783); Stephen Jay Gould, *The Flamingo's Smile: Reflections in Natural History* (New York: W. W. Norton, 1985), p. 286; Bruce Dain, *A Hideous Monster of the Mind: American Race Theory in the Early Republic* (Cambridge, MA: Harvard University Press, 2002), p. 13; and "Racial Anatomical Peculiarities," *New York Medical Journal* 63 (April 1896): 300–501. A representative opinion reads: "The facts known about the orang-outang indicate, says [Edward] Long, (author of *The History of Jamaica),* that the creature may be a savage man. An animal which walks erect, lives in society, builds huts, learns easily to perform menial services, and shows a passion for Negro women cannot be summarily excluded from the human family. Indeed, there is not much to choose as between Hot-tentot and an orang-outang, nor would an orang-outang husband dishonor a Hottentot female"; cited in John C. Greene, "The American Debate on the Ne-gro's Place in Nature, 1780–1815," *Journal of the History of Ideas* 15, no. 3 (1954): 387.

11. "Pigmy Chased by Crowd," *New York Times,* September 9, 1906.

12. "Ota Benga Now a Real Colored Gentleman; Little African Pygmy Being Taught Ways of Civilization at Howard Colored Orphan Asylum," *New York Daily Globe,* October 16, 1906.

13. Bergman, "Ota Benga."

14. The term *freak* is a disrespectful and insensitive way of labeling a person with a medical difference or anomaly. It is used advisedly in this chapter to convey the mores of the speakers and authors who embraced the term.

15. Charles D. Martin, *The White African American Body: A Cultural and Literary Exploration* (New Brunswick, NJ: Rutgers University Press, 2002), pp. 34–41.

16. I am indebted to Charles D. Martin for some of these particulars of Moss's self-exhibition, as well as for his evocative description of Moss's performance as a "striptease of science." See ibid.

17. Ibid., pp. 41, 44.

18. Rush's belief that blacks would prefer to possess white skin makes him ethno-centric, but no more a racist than those who interpret whites' fondness for tanning salons as a desire for black skin.

19. Martin, *The White African American Body,* p. 43.

20. Ibid., p. 149.

21. Ibid.

22. As a result of accidental shotgun fire at close range, the twentyish St. Martin received a large abdominal wound that left a sizable hole when it healed. Beaumont alternately induced and compelled St. Martin to reside with him for long periods, during which he took advantage of St. Martin's unique wound as an unprecedented window into the digestive process. The actions of stomach digestion were rendered clearly visible, and for eleven years Beaumont conducted various observations and invasive experiments that allowed him to map the process of digestion and thus attain medical fame. See William Beaumont, *Experiments and Observations on the Gastric Juice and the Physiology of Digestion* (New York: Dover, 1833).

23. Beaumont's version of the relationship is detailed in his lengthy 1833 account, *Experiments and Observations on the Gastric Juice and the Physiology of Digestion.* St. Martin's side of the affair is limited to a handful of letters protesting that, for various reasons at various times, he does not want to undergo the experiments.

24. Charles Caldwell, *Autobiography* (Philadelphia: Lippincott, Grambo, 1855), p. 269; cited in Martin, *The White African American Body.* Caldwell, *Autobiography,* p. 53.

25. Dr. Alexander D. Galt to Alexander Galt (1821), Galt Family Papers, Medical; cited in Todd L. Savitt, *Medicine and Slavery: The Diseases and Health Care of Blacks in Antebellum Virginia* (Urbana: University of Illinois Press, 1978, reprint 2002), p. 307.

26. Baartman's people are now known as the Griqua.

27. Robert Gordon, "The Venal Hottentot Venus and the Great Chain of Being," *African Studies* 51, no. 2 (1992): 191.

28. Stephen Jay Gould, "The Hottentot Venus," in *The Flamingo's Smile,* pp. 291–305.

29. Linnaeus classified them thusly in *Systemae Naturae* (1735). See also Carmel Chrire, "Native Views of Western Eyes," in Pippa Skotnes, ed., *Miscast: Negotiating the Presence of the Bushmen* (Cape Town: University of Cape Town Press, 1996), p. 35.

30. Gould, *The Flamingo's Smile,* p. 294.

31. Ibid., pp. 9, 300–301.

32. European women would soon validate Galton's observation by resorting to bustles, bustiers, and corsets to achieve the hourglass shape with which the Hottentot Venuses were endowed. See ibid.

33. Sander L. Gilman, *Difference and Pathology: Stereotypes of Sexuality, Race and Madness* (Ithaca, NY: Cornell University Press, 1985), pp. 77–108.

34. Dain, *A Hideous Monster of the Mind,* p. 177.

35. "Race: There was a tendency to call both Bushmen and Hottentots by the latter name," observes John R. Baker in his *Foundation for Human Understanding* (New York: Oxford University Press, 1974), pp. 313–319.

36. After this, slaves still entered the country illegally. The last illegal slaver, the *Clotilde,* brought a cargo of enslaved Africans to the United States in 1842.

37. Gould, *The Flamingo's Smile,* pp. 293–294.

38. "Senate Ordinary Session Number 177 of 2001–2002 (on the private bill authorizing France's restitution to South Africa of the mortal remains of Saartjie Baartman, known as the 'Hottentot Venus')," by Senator M. Philippe Richert (2001).

39. Marang, Setshwaelo, "The Return of the 'Hottentot Venus,'" at http://www .racesci.org/in_media/baartman/baartman_africana.htm; Justin Pearce, "Hope of Saartjie's Return Won't Die," at http://www.racesci.org/in_media/baartman/ baartman_m&g_ movement.htm.

40. Her death on December 29, 1815, is widely ascribed to syphilis, but without proof. Übernaturalist Stephen Jay Gould ascribed her death to "an inflammatory ailment"; see Gould, *The Flamingo's Smile,* p. 81.

41. Cuvier, quoted by Léon Poliakov, *The Arian Myth: A History of Racist and Nationalist Ideas in Europe* (London: Sussex University Press/Heinemann Educational Books, 1971), p. 220.

42. Until 1976, anyone could view the plaster cast and preserved skeleton, vulva, anus, and brain as a set of publicly exhibited medical trophies in Paris's Musée de l'Homme. But when Baartman's homeland, now the Republic of South Africa, rescinded apartheid and white-minority rule, it began vigorously requesting the return of her remains. The French responded by relegating the remains to more private rooms, where scientists were able to view them undisturbed until 2001. When I visited the museum in 2004, I was initially denied permission to view the room where the remains had been held, but officials relented a few days later.

43. Cuvier, quoted in Gould, *The Flamingo's Smile,* p. 296.

44. P. T. Barnum, *The Life of P. T. Barnum, Written by Himself* (New York: Redfield, 1855).

45. "Longevity in America Among the Negroes: Its Causes," *New York Evening Star,* reproduced in the *Boston Transcript,* September 22, 1835; cited in Benjamin Reiss, "PT Barnum, Joice Heth and the Antebellum Spectacles of Race," *American Quarterly* 51, no. 1 (1999): 78–107.

46. Ibid.

47. P. T. Barnum, "Adventures of an Adventurer, Being Some Passages in the Life of Barnaby Diddleum" (1841); cited in Reiss, "PT Barnum, Joice Heth and the Antebellum Spectacles of Race," pp. 69–70.

48. Ibid., p. 98.

49. Martin, *The White African American Body;* Constance García-Barrio, "African-Americans Under the Big Top," *American Legacy Magazine* (Fall 1999); "Circus and Museum Freaks—Curiosities of Pathology," *Scientific American,* March 28, 1908; Joel Benton, "The P. T. Barnum of the Barnum and Bailey Circus," at http://www.electricscotland.com/history/barnum/chap5.htm.

50. Barnum's "ownership" predated the Fugitive Slave Act and the Dred Scott decisions that verified slave owners' legal claim on their human property in the free states.

51. "Born into slavery in North Carolina on July 11, 1851, the Siamese twins, reported to weigh seventeen pounds at birth, were joined at the base of the spine, and

had a common nervous system below that point." García-Barrio, "African-Americans Under the Big Top"; see also Savitt, *Medicine and Slavery,* pp. 305–306, wherein Savitt notes that Millie-Christine were first exhibited nationally at the instigation of a physician, not a circus owner.

52. García-Barrio, "African-Americans Under the Big Top"; see also Allan Gurganus, "P. T. Barnum and My Great-Great-Granddad's Slaves," *Harper's Magazine* (June 2002), p. 2.

53. García-Barrio, "African-Americans Under the Big Top."

54. Johnson could speak, however, and although he was said to possess only "dull normal" intelligence, was able to care for himself. See "Zip Grins in Death, Mask Off at Last," *New York World,* April 29, 1926.

55. "The blonde loveliness of the Circassian Beauty, who delighted our unsophisticated younger days, was, of course, a case of albinoism, and the 'wild men of Borneo' and Barnum's 'what is it' we now recognize, in the maturer years of professional experience, as cases of microcephalous idiocy, gathered for the most part from the negro population of our southern plantations": "Circus and Museum Freaks—Curiosities of Pathology," *Scientific American,* March 28, 1908.

56. García-Barrio, "African-Americans Under the Big Top," pp. 38–48.

57. Brian Wallis, "Black Bodies, White Science: The Slave Daguerreotypes of Louis Agassiz," *Journal of Blacks in Higher Education* 12 (1996): 4.

58. Ibid., pp. 102–106.

59. *New York Medical Journal;* cited in "Circus and Museum Freaks—Curiosities of Pathology."

60. Robert Bogdan, *Freak Show: Presenting Human Oddities for Amusement and Profit* (Chicago and London: University of Chicago Press, 1988), p. 187.

61. Such popular displays of aboriginal peoples were not unusual. Charles D. Martin relates how in 1550 Henry II of France had entire Brazilian villages imported to the suburbs of Rouen; years later, Martin Frobisher lured the people he called "Eskimo" from Nova Scotia onto boats heading for Europe, where they were widely exhibited; see Martin, *The White African American Body,* p. 6.

62. Bradford and Blume, *Ota Benga,* pp. 94–95.

63. "African Pygmies," *St. Louis Post-Dispatch,* June 26, 1904.

64. Robert V. Guthrie, *Even the Rat Was White: A Historical View of Psychology,* 2nd ed. (Boston: Allyn and Bacon, 1998), p. 47.

65. In 1699, English physician Edward Tyson determined that a skeleton of a "pygmy" that he had studied belonged to the ape family. The skeleton he pored over was actually one of a chimpanzee, but the characterization of "pygmies" as apes proved tenacious. Gould, *The Flamingo's Smile,* p. 107. See also Bergman, "Ota Benga."

66. Dain, *A Hideous Monster of the Mind,* pp. 249–262.

67. Wallis, "Black Bodies, White Science: The Slave Daguerreotypes of Louis Agassiz," p. 4.

68. In Dain, *A Hideous Monster of the Mind,* p. 238.

69. Gurganus, "P. T. Barnum and My Great-Great-Granddad's Slaves," p. 3.

70. Charles D. Martin describes many. In 1697, an eleven-year-old former slave with prominent patches of white skin was displayed widely in England. William Byrd II published a description in "An Account of a Negro Boy That Is Dappel'd in

Several Places of His Body with White Spots," published in *Transactions of the Royal Philosophical Society*. In 1759, Colon Barns described a "negro woman four-fifths as fair as any European woman."

71. Caffre, similar to the Afrikaans term *kaffir*, is a derogatory word for a native black African.

72. William M. Ramsey, "Melville's and Barnum's Man with a Weed," *American Literature* 51, no. 1 (1979): 101–104. In the seventeenth century, Balthazar Tellez first used the term *albino* to describe white-skinned peoples along the West African coast.

73. Ibid.

74. John Allan Wyeth, "With Sabre and Scalpel: The Autobiography of a Soldier and Surgeon," electronic ed. (Chapel Hill: Academic Affairs Library, University of North Carolina, 1998); Robert L. Blakeley and Judith M. Harrington, *Bones in the Basement: Postmortem Racism in Nineteenth-Century Medical Training* (Washington, D.C., and London: Smithsonian Institution Press, 1997).

75. Gurganus, "P. T. Barnum and My Great-Great-Granddad's Slaves"; "Black Man Who Died 66 Years Ago Is Finally Buried," *Jet* (1994), p. 56; Martin, *The White African American Body*, p. 198.

76. Dain, *A Hideous Monster of the Mind*, p. 47.

77. Ramsey, "Melville's and Barnum's Man with a Weed."

78. Martin, *The White African American Body*, p. 135.

79. "Miscegenation: The Theory of the Blending of the Races, Applied to the American White Man and Negro"; cited in Sidney Kaplan, "The Miscegenation Issue in the Election of 1864," *Journal of Negro History* 34, no. 3 (1949): 274–343.

80. However, in some cases, the father was undeniably white, and these births were ascribed to the sexual licentiousness and carelessness of black women who enticed white men. See Martin, *The White African American Body*, p. 25.

81. Among Smith's especially progressive proposals for resolving racial intolerance was a proposal for a vigorous program of black-white intermarriage in western states specifically set aside for that purpose. This, he suggested, would eliminate extremes of skin color and with them, excuses for race prejudice.

82. Duc de La Rochefoucauld-Liancourt, quoted in Merrill D. Peterson, ed., *Visitors to Monticello* (Charlottesville: University Press of Virginia, 1989), p. 30.

83. Martin, *The White African American Body*, pp. 19, 21.

84. *Frederick Douglass' Paper* (Rochester, New York), August 25, 1854.

85. By calling mulattoes "infertile," Nott meant that mulattoes who married each other had few offspring and that their sickly offspring tended to die before they could mate, effectively cutting off this potential source of "white negroes." However, the inherent fertility of mulattoes did not differ from that of blacks or whites. See Josiah Nott, "The Mulatto a Hybrid—Probable Extermination of the Two Races if the Whites and Blacks Are Allowed to Intermarry," *American Journal of the Medical Sciences* 6 (1843).

86. Martin, *The White African American Body*, p. 20.

87. Jefferson, *Notes on the State of Virginia*, pp. 50, 138.

88. Charles S. Johnson and Horace Mead, "The Investigation of Racial Differences Prior to 1910," *Journal of Negro Education* 3, no. 3 (1934): 333; Jefferson cited in Martin, *The White African American Body*, p. 143.

CHAPTER 4: THE SURGICAL THEATER

1. Walter Fisher, "Physicians and Slavery in the Antebellum Southern Medical Journal," *Journal of the History of Medicine and Allied Sciences* 23 (1968): pp. 46–47, 145–152.
2. At least, it was not used by Sims for his slave patients; see chapter 2, which discusses Sims's refusal to give anesthesia to the enslaved women he was using to perfect his surgical technique for vesicovaginal fistula repair.
3. *New Orleans Medical and Surgical Journal* 3 (1846): pp. 126–129.
4. *Charleston Mercury,* October 12, 1838, reprinted in Theodore D. Weld, *American Slavery as It Is* (New York: Arno Press, 1839), p. 171.
5. Todd L. Savitt, *Medicine and Slavery: The Diseases and Health Care of Blacks in Antebellum Virginia* (Urbana: University of Illinois Press, 1978, reprint 2002); Gladys-Marie Fry, "The System of Psychological Control," *Negro American Literature Forum* 3, no. 3 (1969), pp. 72–82.
6. Savitt, "The Use of Blacks for Medical Experimentation and Demonstration in the Old South," *The Journal of Southern History* 48, no. 3 (1982): 331–348; Savitt, *Medicine and Slavery,* pp. 332–333.
7. Savitt, *Medicine and Slavery,* pp. 139–46.
8. Ibid. See also Emily Bazelon, "Grave Offense," *Legal Affairs* (July–August 2002), at http:www.legalaffairs.org/issues/July-August-2002/story_bazelon_julaug2002.msp. Robert L. Blakeley and Judith M. Harrington, *Bones in the Basement: Postmortem Racism in Nineteenth-Century Medical Training* (Washington, D.C., and London: Smithsonian Institution Press, 1997); W. Montague Cobb, "Municipal History from Anatomical Records," *Scientific Monthly* 40, no. 2 (1935): 157–162.
9. "Thomas Jefferson to James C. Cabell, May 16, 1824," in *Early History of the University of Virginia as Contained in the Letters of Thomas Jefferson and Joseph C. Cabell* (Richmond: 1856), p. 310; cited in Savitt, *Medicine and Slavery,* p. 283.
10. For a discussion of physicans' acquiescence to planters, see Savitt, *Medicine and Slavery,* pp. 283–284.
11. Savitt, *Medicine and Slavery,* pp. 281–287. Whites, unlike blacks, were protected by laws and social custom as well, but itinerant poor whites were also at risk for involuntary hospitalization because reprisals were unlikely from those who had no nearby family and friends.
12. Ibid., p. 285.
13. N. I. Bowditch, *A History of Massachusetts General Hospital* (Boston: J. Wilson and Son, 1851), pp. 91, 127.
14. Savitt, *Medicine and Slavery*; Savitt, "The Use of Blacks for Medical Experimentation and Demonstration in the Old South," pp. 331–348.
15. Savitt, *Medicine and Slavery,* p. 303. See also Linda Robinson Walker, "George Pray and the 'Wild, Rude Set of Med Students,'" *Michigan Today* (Fall 1999), at http://www.umich.edu/~newsinfo/MT/99/Fal99/mt1f99d.html. Pray wrote, "The external organs of generation formed the subject for this evening's lecture." He continued, "And the dissection showed that although as much as 16 years old or more, her hymen was nearly perfect—showing that she had never been entered—which although not an anomaly is somewhat singular. . . ."

16. Theodore P. Mayo, "Care of Nephritic Colic, with Remarks," *Virginia Medical and Surgical Journal* 5 (1855): 111.

17. At this time, *idiot* was a medical term referring to any person who suffered profound cognitive defects, but especially to those suffering from congenital problems.

18. *Savannah Journal of Medicine* 2 (1880): 354; cited in Fisher, "Physicians and Slavery in the Antebellum Southern Medical Journal," pp. 145–152. Todd L. Savitt notes: "Institutional reputations were made and broken on the basis of the availability of teaching specimens. The Transylvania University Medical Department in Lexington, Kentucky, serves as a case in point. One of the causes for its decline from eminence during the 1830s was its purported difficulty in procuring bodies for clinical teaching. . . . On the other hand, a medical school was established in nearby Louisville (Louisville Medical Institute) in 1837 owing in part to the presence of a large black (as well as a transient white) population, well suited to the needs of teaching institutions." Savitt, "The Use of Blacks for Medical Experimentation and Demonstration in the Old South," p. 38.

19. The Medical College of Virginia was called the Hampden-Sydney College Medical Department until 1854.

20. "A Plan of Organization for the Roper Hospital. Adopted by the Medical Society Jan. 3 1846," cited in Savitt, "The Use of Blacks for Medical Experimentation and Demonstration in the Old South," pp. 38, 39; "An Address to the Public in Regard to the Affairs of the Medical Department of Hampden-Sydney College, by Several Physicians of the City of Richmond, 1853," quoted in Wyndham B. Blanton, *Medicine in Virginia in the Nineteenth Century* (Richmond, 1933). Savitt indicates that "of 109 patients mentioned in the Richmond medical journals between 1851 and 1860, 63.3 percent (69) were black."

21. Savitt, *Medicine and Slavery,* pp. 335–339; Savitt, "The Use of Blacks for Medical Experimentation and Demonstration in the Old South," p. 307.

22. Sharla M. Fett, *Working Cures: Healing Health and Power on Southern Slave Plantations* (Chapel Hill and London: University of North Carolina Press, 2002), p. 153.

23. Savitt, *Medicine and Slavery,* p. 335.

24. Ibid., pp. 334–335.

25. Newspaper advertisement from the *Atlanta Weekly Intelligencer* (October 12, 1855).

26. Fisher, "Physicians and Slavery in the Antebellum Southern Medical Journal," p. 46.

27. Savitt, "The Use of Blacks for Medical Experimentation and Demonstration in the Old South," pp. 331–348.

28. Sheri L. Fink, M.D., Ph.D., to the author.

29. Charles S. Johnson and Horace Mead, "The Investigation of Racial Differences Prior to 1910," *Journal of Negro Education* 3, no. 3 (1934): 328–339. See also John Harley Warner, "The Idea of Southern Medical Distinctiveness: Medical Knowledge and Practice in the Old South," in *Sickness and Health in America: Readings in the History of Medicine and Public Health,* edited by Judith Walzer Leavitt and Ronald L. Numbers (Madison: University of Wisconsin Press, 1985), pp. 53–70. These historical beliefs about black racial distinctiveness have inspired many present-day theories of black physiological distinctiveness.

30. Rudolph Matas, "The Surgical Peculiarity of the Negro: A Statistical Inquiry Based Upon the Records of the Charity Hospital of New Orleans (Decennium 1884–1894)," *Transactions of the American Surgical Association* 14 (1894): 485–609.

31. Ibid.

32. *Richmond Daily Dispatch,* July 21, 1854, p. 2; cited in Savitt, *Medicine and Slavery,* p. 283.

33. Either James B. McCaw, M.D., or George A. Otis, M.D.; the editor declined to sign his report.

34. Savitt, *Medicine and Slavery,* p. 288.

35. Fett, *Working Cures,* p. 29.

36. Dr. William Welford, for example, performed a trephination, in which a hole is bored into a living person's skull, on an eleven-year-old slave boy to display the procedure to the other surgeons, the boy's owner, several curious doctors, three of his own students, and a crowd of curious townspeople.

37. Savitt, "The Use of Blacks for Medical Experimentation and Demonstration in the Old South."

38. Fett, *Working Cures,* pp. 146–147; 239.

39. Cobb, "Municipal History from Anatomical Records"; see also "Papers Relating to Dr. Robert Knox (1791–1862 [authors unknown])," pp. 157–162, and Blakeley and Harrington, *Bones in the Basement.*

40. Fisher, "Physicians and Slavery in the Antebellum Southern Medical Journal," pp. 45–46; Savitt, *Medicine and Slavery,* pp. 301–305.

41. Ibid.

42. Savitt, *Medicine and Slavery,* p. 304.

43. R. Carter, "Case of a Negro Woman, Who Gave Birth to Twins of Different Color," *Medical Examiner and Record of Medical Science* (1849), pp. 523–524.

44. Savitt, *Medicine and Slavery,* p. 304.

45. Evelleen Richards, "A Political Anatomy of Monsters, Hopeful and Otherwise: Teratogeny, Transcendentalism, and Evolutionary Theorizing," *Isis* 85, no. 3 (1994): 377–411.

46. Fisher, "Physicians and Slavery in the Antebellum Southern Medical Journal," pp. 43–46; Savitt, *Medicine and Slavery,* pp. 301–305.

47. Ernst Haeckel, *The History of Creation* (London: Trübner, 1906).

48. Walker, "George Pray and the 'Wild, Rude Set of Med Students.'"

49. Savitt, *Medicine and Slavery,* chapter 20; see also Fisher, "Physicians and Slavery in the Antebellum Southern Medical Journal," pp. 46–48.

50. Savitt, "The Use of Blacks for Medical Experimentation and Demonstration in the Old South"; Fisher, "Physicians and Slavery in the Antebellum Southern Medical Journal."

CHAPTER 5: THE RESTLESS DEAD

1. James Lardner, "After 4 Months, Body Found at Lab," *Washington Post,* January 5, 1978, p. 1B; see also Joseph D. Whitaker, "City Told to Pay $53,000 in Case of Unidentified Body," *Washington Post,* November 22, 1979, p. B7.

2. Lardner, "After 4 Months, Body Found at Lab."

3. Medical experts prefer the term *necropsy,* and literally speaking, they are correct. *Autopsy* derives from Greek words meaning "to see for oneself," and is less spe-

cific than necropsy, which means "to see from a corpse." However, autopsy has been a more familiar lay term for more than a century; therefore, it is used here. An *autopsy* is an exhaustive examination of a corpse to glean specific information about the deceased, often to determine his or her cause of death. A dissection is instructive in a more impersonal, pedagogical manner: It is an investigation of a corpse for the purpose of furthering the dissector's medical education.

4. Todd L. Savitt, "The Use of Blacks for Medical Experimentation and Demonstration in the Old South," *The Journal of Southern History* 48, no. 3 (1982): 337.

5. L. Ebony Boulware et al., "Whole-Body Donation for Medical Science: A Population-Based Study," *Clinical Anatomy* 17, no. 7 (September 16, 2004): 570–577.

6. Duncan Campbell, "Former Klansman Convicted of Deadly Alabama Church Bombing 40 Years On," *The Guardian* (Birmingham, AL), May 28, 2005; Chandra Temple, "1963 Bombing Victim's Family Eager to Locate Site of Grave," *The Guardian,* January 1988.

7. "White Students, Black Cadavers" (review of *Bones in the Basement*), *Journal of Blacks in Higher Education* (Spring 1988), pp. 141–142; Temple, "1963 Bombing Victim's Family Eager to Locate Site of Grave."

8. Robert L. Blakeley and Judith M. Harrington, *Bones in the Basement: Postmortem Racism in Nineteenth-Century Medical Training* (Washington, D.C., and London: Smithsonian Institution Press, 1997); "White Students, Black Cadavers," pp. 141–142.

9. Blakeley and Harrington, *Bones in the Basement,* p. 9.

10. Ibid., pp. 6–7, 13. The authors observe that ". . . the medical college obtained disproportionately high numbers of African American males and adults as cadavers for dissection. This selectivity—particularly the overwhelming numbers of African Americans—comes as no surprise: those treated unequally in life were treated unequally in death." See also "White Students, Black Cadavers."

11. Blakeley and Harrington, *Bones in the Basement.*

12. Ibid., p. 15.

13. Ibid., p. 19.

14. Ibid., p. 5, figure 1, "Drie's Birds-Eye View of Augusta."

15. Lane Allen, "Grandison Harris, Sr.: Slave, Resurrectionist and Judge," *Bulletin of the Georgia Academy of Science* 34 (1976): 198; see also "Race and the Politics of Medicine" in Blakeley and Harrington, *Bones in the Basement,* and Cates, "Medical Schools in Ante-Bellum Georgia," p. 32. On the use of blacks for dissection in an Alabama medical school, see Howard L. Holley, "Dr. Phillip Madison Shepard and His Medical School," *De Historia Medicinae* 2 (1958): 1–5; cited in Todd L. Savitt, *Medicine and Slavery: The Diseases and Health Care of Blacks in Antebellum Virginia* (Urbana: University of Illinois Press, 1978, reprint 2002).

16. Excerpts of Dr. Murphy's exploits are described in Pfinizy Spalding, *The History of the Medical College of Georgia* (Athens: University of Georgia Press, 1987).

17. Tanya Telfair Sharpe, "Grandison Harris: The Medical College of Georgia's Resurrection Man," cited in Blakeley and Harrison *Bones in the Basement*; see also Allen, "Grandison Harris, Sr.: Slave, Resurrectionist and Judge," pp. 192–199.

18. Linda Robinson Walker, "Grave Subjects," *Michigan Today* 31, no. 3 (Fall 1999); William Sumner Jenkins, *Pro-Slavery Thought in the Old South* (Chapel Hill: University of North Carolina Press, 1935); Blakeley and Harrington, *Bones in the Basement*; Emily Bazelon, "Grave Offense," *Legal Affairs* (July–August 2002), at http://www.legalaffairs.org/issues/July-August-2002/story_bazelon_julaug 2002.msp.

19. "Do the Dead Tell Tales After All? Colonial-Era Burial Project Provides Clues to Africans' Struggle for Human Rights," *NLM Newsline* 56 (2001).

20. Blakeley and Harrison, *Bones in the Basement*, pp. 12–13.

21. Erwin H. Ackerknecht, *Medicine at the Paris Hospital* (Baltimore: Johns Hopkins University Press, 1967); Michel Foucault, *The Birth of the Clinic: An Archaeology of Medical Perception* (New York: Vintage, 1973).

22. Richard H. Shryock, *The Development of Modern Medicine: An Interpretation of the Social and Scientific Factors Involved* (New York: Alfred A. Knopf, 1947), pp. 170–191.

23. Bazelon, "Grave Offense."

24. Such U.S. statutes were modeled on British law. See ibid.

25. M. B. (Bear) Gordon, *Aesculapius Comes to the Colonies* (Ventnor, NJ: Ventnor, 1949), p. 132.

26. Gladys-Marie Fry, "The System of Psychological Control," *Negro American Literature Forum* 3, no. 3 (1969): pp. 72–82: Gladys-Marie Fry, *Night Riders in Black Folk History* (Chapel Hill and London: The University of North Carolina Press, 2001).

27. Blakeley and Harrington, *Bones in the Basement*, p. 73.

28. Savitt, "The Use of Blacks for Medical Experimentation and Demonstration in the Old South," p. 337.

29. Michael Sappol, *A Traffic of Dead Bodies: Anatomy and Embodied Social Identity in Nineteenth-Century America* (Princeton, NJ: Princeton University Press, 2001), p. 347.

30. Ibid., pp. 347–348; J. C. Landenheim, "The Doctor's Mob of 1877," *Journal of the History of Medicine* 5 (1950): 23–36; see also "Do the Dead Tell Tales After All?"

31. David C. Humphrey, "Dissection and Discrimination: The Social Origin of Cadavers in America, 1760–1915," *Bulletin of the New York Academy of Medicine* 49, no. 9 (1973): 819–827.

32. Bazelon, "Grave Offense."

33. U.S. Census data, cited in Humphrey, "Dissection and Discrimination," p. 822.

34. Blakeley and Harrington, *Bones in the Basement*.

35. Savitt, *Medicine and Slavery*; Savitt, "The Use of Blacks for Medical Experimentation and Demonstration in the Old South."

36. Savitt, *Medicine and Slavery*; Humphrey, "Dissection and Discrimination"; Walter Fisher, "Physicians and Slavery in the Antebellum Southern Medical Journal," *Journal of the History of Medicine and Allied Sciences* 23 (1968): 145–152.

37. Sharla M. Fett, *Working Cures: Healing Health and Power on Southern Slave Plantations* (Chapel Hill and London: University of North Carolina Press, 2002), pp. 156–157.

38. David R. Roedinger, "And Die in Dixie; Funerals, Death and Heaven in Slave Community, 1700–1865," *Massachusetts Review* 22 (1981): 163–183.

39. E. D. Fenner, "Dirt-Eating Among Negroes," *Southern Medical Reports* 1, no. 194 (1849).

40. "How the Business Is Managed at Indianapolis: Twelve 'Resurrectionists' Engaged in It," *Indianapolis Herald* (January 1875); at http://www.hcgs.net.

41. Editorial, *Freedom's Journal* (Richmond), March 30, 1827.

42. Harriet Martineau, *Retrospect of Western Travel* (Armonk, NY: M.E. Sharpe, 2000), p. 43; Savitt, *Medicine and Slavery.*

43. *Statesman and Patriot* (Milledgeville, GA), August 16, 1828.

44. Trudier Harris, "Report on the Treatment of Some Cases of Cholera" (1839): pp. 581–585; cited in Fett, *Working Cures,* p. 154.

45. Paul F. Eve, "An Essay Read Before the Medical Society of Augusta, January 10, 1839," *Southern Medical and Surgical Journal* 3 (1839): 329.

46. L. H. Anderson, "Report on the Diseases of Sumpterville and Vicinity," *Medical Association of the State of Alabama, Transactions* 7 (January 1854): 61–66.

47. However, Bentham did not practice exactly what he preached: In accordance with his wishes, his body was reconstructed from its skeleton and preserved as a dignified "Auto-icon," ensconced in an armchair at University College, London.

48. The "Ghastly Act" referred to the Armstrong Act.

49. "How the Business Is Managed at Indianapolis."

50. Fry, *Night Riders in Black Folk History.*

51. "Burking in Baltimore," *Baltimore Sun,* December 13, 1886; Brennen Jensen, "Blood Money," *Baltimore City Paper* (1998); J. K. Gillon, "The Story of Burke and Hare," at http://members.fortunecity.com/gillonj/burkeandhare.

52. Humphrey, "Dissection and Discrimination."

53. Frederick C. Waite, "Grave Robbing in New England," *Medical Library Association Bulletin* 33 (1945): 272–294.

54. James Silk Buckingham, *America: Historical and Descriptive* 5, vol. 1 (London: 1841), p. 159.

55. Ibid.; see also Fisher, "Physicians and Slavery in the Antebellum Southern Medical Journal," p. 45; W. Montague Cobb, M.D., "Surgery and the Negro Physician: Some Parallels in Background," *Journal of the National Medical Association* 43, no. 3 (1951): 148; Waite, "Grave Robbing in New England," pp. 283–284. At least one enterprising slave, Henry "Box" Brown, transported himself to freedom by hiding in a box that he arranged to have carried by railway freight from a slave state to a free one. Perhaps railway officials' knowledge that black cadavers were often transported illicitly by train helped allay suspicions about the box's contents; see Henry Box Brown, *Narrative of the Life of Henry Box Brown, Written by Himself* (New York: Oxford University Press, 2002).

56. Robert Wilson, "Their Shadowy Influence Still Hovers About Medical College," *Sunday News Courier* (Charleston, WV), April 13, 1913; quoted in Savitt, *Medicine and Slavery.*

57. "The Executions at Charleston, Virginia," *The National Era* (Charleston, VA), December 22, 1859.

58. Humphrey, "Dissection and Discrimination," p. 824.

59. "How the Business Is Managed at Indianapolis."

60. W. Montague Cobb, "Human Material in American Institutions Available for Anthropological Study," *American Journal of Physical Anthropologists* 17 (1933).

61. W. Montague Cobb, M.D., "Municipal History from Anatomical Records," *Scientific Monthly* 40, no. 2 (1935): 157, 160.

62. John Warren and Aaron Dexter, "Memorial & Petition for the Removal of Med. Lect. to Boston," in the John Warren Papers, Massachusetts Historical Society, Boston.

63. Lyle Larsen, "Odd Volumes," at http://homepage.smc.edu/larsen_lyle/odd_volumes.htm; see also Larry Buster, personal communication to the author, including an image titled "Book Bound in the Skin of an African American" (September 8, 2001).

64. Jeffry Scott, "Woman Sues over Display of Mom's Skeleton," *Atlanta Journal-Constitution,* at http://www.accessatlanta.com/ajc/metro/0303/16skeleton.html.

65. Peter B. Wright, "An Unusual Case of Paget's Disease; Presenting an Extraordinary Degree of Osteoblastic Activity," *American Journal of Bone and Joint Surgery* 33, no. A:1 (1951): 239–244.

66. Scott, "Woman Sues over Display of Mom's Skeleton."

67. Jeffry Scott, "Daughter Loses Round in Suit over Mom's Body," *Atlanta Journal-Constitution,* December 2, 2003.

68. In July 2004, I telephoned the MCG for permission to view Wilborn's skeleton but I was told that only medical staff and students may view it; when I explained that I was a fellow at another medical school, I was told that only MCG personnel could view it.

69. The execution took place in Lewisburg on March 13, 1824. Lori Samples (transcriber), "Greenbrier County, West Virginia—160th Anniversary Booklet, Part 13" (1938), p. 3.

70. Henry Lewis Clay, *Odd Leaves from the Life of a Louisiana Swamp Doctor* (Baton Rouge: Louisiana State University Press, 1997), p. 137.

71. Henry Clay Lewis, with Felix Octavius Carr Darley, illustrator, "The Swamp Doctor's Adventures in the South-West. Containing the Whole of the Louisiana Swamp Doctor; Streaks of Squatter Life; and Far-Western Scenes; in a Series of Forty-Two Humorous Southern and Western Sketches, Descriptive of Incidents and Character. By 'Madison Tensas,' M.D., and 'Solitaire' (John S. Robb of St. Louis, Mo.), Author of 'Swallowing Oysters Alive,' Etc." (Chapel Hill: Academic Affairs Library, University of North Carolina, 1998, 2004), pp. 76–77.

72. Mark Twain, *Adventures of Huckleberry Finn* (New York: Random House, 1996), pp. 62–65; facsimile, p. 405.

73. Sappol, *A Traffic of Dead Bodies*, pp. 85, 87.

74. P. Preston Reynolds, "Dr. Louis T. Wright and the NAACP: Pioneers in Hospital Racial Integration," *American Journal of Public Health* 90, no. 6 (2000): pp. 883–892.

75. F. P. Mall, "Anatomical Material—Its Collection and Preservation at the Johns Hopkins Anatomical Laboratory," *Bulletin of the Johns Hopkins Hospital* 16 (1905): 38–39; p. 39 also cited in Humphrey, "Dissection and Discrimination," p. 824.

76. Handlin, *Boston's Immigrants: A Study in Acculturation* (Cambridge, MA: Harvard University Press, 1959), pp. 115–118; cited in Humphrey, "Dissection and Discrimination," p. 824.

77. Bazelon, "Grave Offense."

78. A. M. Sadler, Jr., and E. B. Stason, "The Uniform Anatomical Gift Act: A Model for Reform," *Journal of the American Medical Association* 206, no. 11 (1968): 2505–2506.
79. Michele Goodwin, *Black Markets: The Supply and Demand of Body Parts* (Cambridge: Cambridge University Press, 2006), pp. 126–129.
80. Bazelon, "Grave Offense."

CHAPTER 6: DIAGNOSIS: FREEDOM

1. I am indebted to historian John S. Hughes, who tells John Patterson's story in his article "Labeling and Treating Black Mental Illness in Alabama, 1861–1910," *The Journal of Southern History* 58, no. 3 (1992): 435–460.
2. Trent Alexander, "A Public Use Microdata Sample of the 1860 Census of Slave Inhabitants."
3. *Microsoft Encarta 98 Encyclopedia,* s. v. "Virginia," Microsoft Corporation.
4. J. C. Nott, "The Mulatto a Hybrid—Probable Extermination of the Two Races if the Whites and Blacks Are Allowed to Intermarry," *American Journal of the Medical Sciences* 6 (July 1843): 252–256; reprinted in *Boston Medical and Surgical Journal* 29 (August 16, 1843): 29–32.
5. By "infertile," scientists meant that mulattoes tended to have difficulty conceiving, to have far fewer children, and that these children tended to die young before they themselves could mate.
6. Samuel Adolphus Cartwright, "Report on the Diseases and Physical Peculiarities of the Negro Race," *New Orleans Medical and Surgical Journal* 7 (1851): 691–715.
7. The South did not need or want black votes, but it desperately needed its blacks for the population count. The "three-fifths compromise" (third clause of art. 1, sec. 2 of the U.S. Constitution) counted each slave as three-fifths of a man. In every election between 1790 and the Civil War, the ability to count slaves as well as freemen gave the South from a quarter to a third more representatives in Congress than that to which her free population entitled her. See Nathaniel Weyl and William Marina, *American Statesmen on Slavery and the Negro* (New York: Arlington House, 1971), pp. 50–51.
8. In 1857, statisticians Henry Chase and C. H. Sanborn observed, "It will be seen that in the late several contests in the House of Representatives, had freemen only been represented, the question would invariably have been decided in favor of the North." See Chase and Sanborn, in D. B. DeBow, *Statistical View of the United States* (Washington, D.C.: B. Tucker, Senate printer, 1854), p. 153.
9. *Idiot* is now used popularly as an insult, and in archaic medical jargon it denoted the lowest stratum of measured human intelligence. However, in the nineteenth century, *idiot* was a generic medical term denoting any person of low intelligence.
10. U.S. State Department, "Compilation of the Enumeration of the Inhabitants and Statistics of the United States, as Obtained at the Department of State, from the Returns of the Sixth Census" (1841).
11. Thomas Mays, "Human Slavery as a Prevention of Pulmonary Consumption," *Transactions of the American Climatological Association* 20 (1904): 192–197; Clovis Semmes, "Reconstruction and Freedom's Ironies," in *Racism, Health, and Post-*

Industrialism: A Theory of African-American Health (Westport, CT: Praeger, 1996), pp. 49–88.

12. Albert Deutsch, "The First U.S. Census of the Insane (1840) and Its Use as Pro-Slavery Propaganda," *Bulletin of the History of Medicine* 15 (1944): 469–482; Louis Dublin, "The Problem of Negro Health as Revealed by Vital Statistics," *Journal of Negro Education* 6 (1937): 268–275; Clayton E. Cramer, "Black Demographic Data, 1790–1860: A Sourcebook" (2003); at http://www.claytoncramer.com/black.htm (accessed January 15, 2006).

13. Seale Harris, M.D., *Women's Surgeon: The Life Story of J. Marion Sims* (New York: Macmillan, 1950), p. 29.

14. Allan M. Brandt, "Racism and Research: The Case of the Tuskegee Syphilis Experiment," *Hastings Center Report* 8 (1978): 23.

15. In the North, one of every 995 whites was mentally defective; in the South, one of every 945 whites exhibited mental illness or "idiocy."

16. Of the 2,788,573 blacks in the slave states, 1,734 were insane; of the 171,894 blacks in the free North, 1,191 were insane or idiots. See U.S. State Department, "Compilation of the Enumeration of the Inhabitants and Statistics of the United States."

17. Hughes, "Labeling and Treating Black Mental Illness in Alabama, 1861–1910," p. 439.

18. Albert Deutsch, "The First U.S. Census of the Insane (1840) and Its Use as Pro-Slavery Propaganda." Read before the New-York Historical Society, February 2, 1944. Pp. 3–5.

19. Ibid., pp. 7–9.

20. Deutsch, "The First U. S. Census of the Insane (1840) and Its Use as Pro-Slavery Propaganda," p. 472.

21. Edward Jarvis, M.D., "Insanity Among the Coloured Population of the Free States," *American Journal of the Medical Sciences* 1844, no. 7 (1843): 74–75. See also Edward Jarvis, M.D., "Preliminary Report," *Boston Medical and Surgical Journal* 27 (1843): 126–132, 281–282.

22. Jarvis, "Insanity Among the Coloured Population of the Free States," p. 83.

23. James McCune Smith, "Facts Concerning Free Negroes," in *A Documentary History of the Negro People in the United States*, edited by Herbert Aptheker (New York: Citadel, 1844); W. Montague Cobb, "The Negro as a Biological Element in the American Population," *Journal of Negro Educatiion* 8, no. 3 (1939): 336–348.

24. Smith, "Facts Concerning Free Negroes."

25. Todd L. Savitt, *Medicine and Slavery: The Diseases and Health Care of Blacks in Antebellum Virginia* (Urbana: University of Illinois Press, 1978; reprint 2002).

26. Ibid.

27. The term *colored* lumped together blacks and mulattos. *Free Colored* was the term used by the United States census from 1820 through 1860 to denote the population of free blacks and free mulattoes, who were enumerated together.

28. Cramer, "Black Demographic Data, 1790–1860."

29. Hughes, "Labeling and Treating Black Mental Illness in Alabama, 1861–1910."

30. Savitt, *Medicine and Slavery*.

31. James McCune Smith, M.D., "The Memorial of 1844 to the U.S. Senate" (1844), pp. 212–213.

32. Nosology is that facet of medicine that consists of the description and classification of diseases.

33. Jarvis, "Insanity Among the Coloured Population of the Free States," p. 83.

34. *Journal of the House of Representatives,* 28th Cong., 1st sess. (Washington, D.C., 1844), p. 471.

35. "Startling Facts from the Census," *American Journal of Insanity* 8 (1851–1852): 153–155.

36. *The Medical and Surgical History of the War of the Rebellion* (Washington: United States War Department, 1870–1888), vol. 1, part 1, chap. 10, pp. xxix–xli.

37. Specifically, between November 1, 1865, and September 1, 1866.

38. Gaines Foster, "The Limitations of Federal Health Care for Freedmen, 1860–1868," *The Journal of Southern History* 48 (1982): 365.

39. Semmes, "Reconstruction and Freedom's Ironies (230)," pp. 49–88; M. S. Legan, "Disease and the Freedmen in Mississippi During Reconstruction," *Journal of the History of Medicine and Allied Sciences* 28 (1973): 257–267.

40. When Elizabeth Hyde Boturne, a white Relief Society worker in the Port Royal area of South Carolina, begged a recalcitrant doctor to visit a dying contraband, she "resorted to an appeal to his sense of compassion for 'fellow human beings.' 'Human beings!' he retorted. 'They are only animals, and not half as valuable as cattle.' " See Elizabeth Hyde Boturne, *First Days Amongst the Contrabands* (1893); cited in Foster, "The Limitations of Federal Health Care for Freedmen, 1860–1868." Foster adds: "With physicians displaying such contempt for their patients, neither adequate supplies nor professional competence offered a reprieve from the high mortality of the camps."

41. James Hunt, "On Ethno-Climatology; Or the Acclimatization of Man," *Transactions of the Ethnological Society of London* 2 (1863): 74–75.

42. W. E. Burghardt Du Bois, "The American Negro at Paris," *American Monthly Review of Reviews* 22, no. 5 (November 1900): 576.

43. Frederick L. Hoffman, "Race Traits and Tendencies of the American Negro," *Publications of the American Economic Association* 11 (1896): 1–139; Marvin L. Graves, "The Negro a Menace to the Health of the White Race," *Southern Medical Journal* 9 (1916): 407–413; C. Jeff Miller, "Special Medical Problems of the Colored Woman," *Southern Medical Journal* 25 (1932): 733–739; L. C. Allen, "The Negro Health Problem," *American Journal of Public Health* 5 (1915): 194–203.

44. In 1937, Conrad Elvehjem and his colleagues first tied nicotinic acid deficiency to "black tongue," pellagra's equivalent disease in dogs.

45. J. B. Herrick, "Peculiar Elongated and Sickle-Shaped Red Blood Corpuscles in a Case of Severe Anemia," *Archives of Internal Medicine* 6 (1910): 517–521. See also T. L. Savitt and M. F. Goldberg, "Herrick's 1910 Case Report of Sickle Cell Anemia: The Rest of the Story," *Journal of the American Medical Association* 261 (1989): 266–71.

CHAPTER 7: "A NOTORIOUSLY SYPHILIS-SOAKED RACE"

1. After 1985, the school became known as Tuskegee University.

2. James H. Jones and Tuskegee Institute, *Bad Blood: The Tuskegee Syphilis Experiment* (New York and London: Free Press, 1981), p. 64.

3. Ibid., pp. 27, 74.

4. *Harrison's Principles of Internal Medicine* (New York: McGraw-Hill, 1998), pp. 801–803; 1023–1029.

5. He made these statements while he was still a lecturer on syphilis at the University College of Medicine at Richmond, Virginia. See Jones and Tuskegee Institute, *Bad Blood*, p. 24.

6. Ibid., p. 25.

7. Ibid., p. 26.

8. Ibid., p. 25.

9. Susan M. Reverby, *Tuskegee's Truths: Rethinking the Tuskegee Syphilis Study* (Chapel Hill: University of North Carolina Press, 2000), p. 78; see also Jones and Tuskegee Institute, *Bad Blood*, p. 27.

10. Allan M. Brandt, "Racism and Research: The Case of the Tuskegee Syphilis Experiment," *Hastings Center Report* 8 (1978): 22–23. This chapter owes a great deal to Dr. Brandt's painstakingly accurate reconstruction and insightful analyses of the Tuskegee Syphilis Study. See also Jones and Tuskegee Institute, *Bad Blood*, p. 114.

11. Brandt, "Racism and Research," p. 81

12. Reverby, *Tuskegee's Truths*, p. 78.

13. Eunice Rivers, the nurse assigned to the study, told interviewers that many of the men suffered side effects such as lost teeth from the poisonous mercury compounds. See ibid. pp. 47, 321.

14. Arsphenamine ($C_{12}Cl_2H_{14}As_2N_1O_2 \cdot 2H_2O$) is a light-yellow powder.

15. Macon County Health Department, "Letters to Subjects," NA-WNRC; cited in Brandt, "Racism and Research," pp. 22–23.

16. Ibid., p. 23.

17. Ibid.

18. Helen Dibble and Daniel Williams, "An Interview with Nurse Rivers," in Reverby, *Tuskegee's Truths*, p. 323.

19. Later, the government covered the costs of the burials.

20. Letter from Raymond Vonderlehr to Stanley H. Schuman (February 5, 1952), Tuskegee Syphilis Study—NLM, box 2; cited in Brandt, "Racism and Research," p. 26.

21. Brandt, "Racism and Research," p. 26.

22. Some local AMA chapters continued to restrict or bar blacks from membership until well into the 1960s.

23. See Thomas Parran, *Shadow on the Land: Syphilis* (New York, Reynal & Hitchcock, 1937).

24. Jones and Tuskegee Institute, *Bad Blood*, p. 179.

25. Half the remaining men were older than seventy-four and half were younger.

26. Unpublished typescript, Minutes (April 5, 1965), Tuskegee Syphilis Study—NLM, box 1; cited in Brandt, "Racism and Research," p. 26.

27. "Irwin J. Schatz, M.D., Henry Ford Hospital, Detroit, Michigan, to Donald H.

Rockwell, Venereal Disease Research Laboratory Public Health Service, Atlanta, Georgia (June 11, 1965)"; reprinted in Reverby, *Tuskegee's Truths,* p. 104.

28. Jones and Tuskegee Institute, *Bad Blood,* pp. 190–193; 203–205.

29. Ibid., p. 2.

30. Some accounts give August 28 as the date the panel was convened.

31. The other panel members were: Barney H. Weeks, president, Alabama Labor Council, AFL-CIO; Fred Speaker, J. D., attorney-at-law, Harrisburg, Pennsylvania; Jeanne Sinkford, D.D.S., associate dean, Graduate and Postgraduate Affairs, College of Dentistry, Howard University; Jean L. Harris, M.D., executive director, National Medical Association Foundation, Inc.; and Seward Hiltner, Ph.D., professor of theology, Princeton Theological Seminary. Department of Health, Education, and Welfare, *Final Report of the Tuskegee Syphilis Study Ad Hoc Advisory Panel* (1974), p. 46.

32. Author's telephone interview with Fred Speaker, July 5, 1995.

33. The initial period of the charter ended in December 1972, four months after it began, but it was renewed in January 1973 and continued until March 31, 1973. The panel and its subcommittees met twelve times between September 1972 and March 28, 1973.

34. In *Bad Blood,* Jones characterizes this delay in terminating the study differently. He accepts the government's explanation that it could not give the men medical treatment unless the Tuskegee Syphilis Study remained open.

35. Author's telephone interview with Jean L. Harris, M.D., March 6, 2000; author's telephone interview with Vernal Cave, M.D., June 22, 1995.

36. I had made several requests to speak with Secretary Brown, but had not been granted an interview before he died in a 1996 plane crash in Croatia.

37. Several minority reports were filed. Those written by Dr. Katz and Dr. Cave survive as addenda to the official *Final Report.* But Dr. Butler's dissenting report was not included in, or distributed with, the report, and has not circulated widely.

38. Author's interview with Jay Katz, M.D. See also interviews with the other surviving panel members, each of whom confirmed Butler's actions.

39. Dr. Butler died on January 9, 1996. See Wolfgang Saxon, "Broadus Butler, 75, Ex-Tuskegee Airman and College Leader," obituary, *New York Times,* January 13, 1996.

40. Author's interview with Jay Katz, M.D.

41. Jones and Tuskegee Institute, *Bad Blood,* pp. 216–217.

42. Eunice Rivers et al., "Twenty Years of Follow Up Experience in a Long Range Medical Study," *Public Health Reports* 68 (1953): 381–395.

43. Reverby, *Tuskegee's Truths.*

44. Benjamin Roy, M.D., "The Tuskegee Syphilis Experiment: Medical Ethics, Constitutionalism, and Property in the Body," *Harvard Journal of Minority Public Health* 1, no. 1 (1995): 11–15; Jones and Tuskegee Institute, *Bad Blood,* p. 124.

45. "James Lucas, M.D., Assistant Chief, Venereal Disease Branch, Public Health Service, to William J. Brown, M.D., Chief, Venereal Disease Branch, September 10, 1970."

46. Author's interviews with Benjamin S. Roy, M.D., May 2, June 22, and June 25, 1995.

47. Author's interviews with Jay Katz, M.D., March 23, 1994, and July 8, 1995.

48. Susan E. Lederer, *Subjected to Science: Human Experimentation in America Before the Second World War* (Baltimore: The Johns Hopkins University Press, 1995), pp. 3–4.

49. Ibid.; see also Margaret Humphreys, M.D., Ph.D., "Whose Body? Which Disease? Studying Malaria While Treating Neurosyphilis," a speech delivered to the New York Academy of Medicine in 2001.

50. J. A. Macintosh, "The Etiology of Granuloma Inguinale," *Journal of the American Medical Association* 87 (1926): 996–1002.

51. *Journal of Blacks in Higher Education,* September 30, 1997.

52. Humphreys, "Whose Body?"

53. Mark F. Boyd and S. F. Kitchen, "Observations on Induced Falciparum," *American Journal of Tropical Medicine* 17 (1937): 213–235.

54. Jones and Tuskegee Institute, *Bad Blood,* p. 202.

55. Susan M. Lederer, "The Tuskegee Syphilis Study in the Context of American Medical Research"; reprinted in Reverby, *Tuskegee's Truths,* p. 268.

CHAPTER 8: THE BLACK STORK

1. Jerry DeMuth, "Sick and Tired of Being Sick and Tired," *The Nation,* June 1, 1964, pp. 538, 549; see also Perry Deane Young, "A Surfeit of Surgery," *Washington Post,* May 30, 1976, p. B1.

2. Kay Mills, *This Little Light of Mine: A Biography of Fannie Lou Hamer* (New York: Dutton, 1993; reprint Plume, 1994).

3. E. A. Carlson, *The Gene: A Critical History* (Philadelphia: Saunders, 1966).

4. Paul A. Lombardo, "Medicine, Eugenics, and the Supreme Court: From Coercive Sterilization to Reproductive Freedom," *Journal of Contemporary Health Law and Policy* 13 (1996): 1.

5. Paul Johnson, *A History of the American People* (New York: Harper Perennial, 1998), pp. 660–665; 703–707.

6. Martin S. Pernick, *The Black Stork: Eugenics and the Death of "Defective" Babies in American Medicine and Motion Pictures Since 1915* (New York: Oxford University Press, 1996), pp. 6–7.

7. Lombardo, "Medicine, Eugenics, and the Supreme Court," pp. 5–7.

8. Pernick, *The Black Stork,* pp. 5–6; see also Haiselden's film *The Black Stork.* In the 1927 version of the film, the black servant is replaced by a European immigrant who would not offend the sensibilities of southerners; Pernick, *The Black Stork,* p. 144.

9. Ibid., p. 64; and Figure 14, Crippled Black Child.

10. Ibid., pp. 64, 66.

11. Garland E. Allen, "The Eugenics Record Office at Cold Spring Harbor, 1910–1940: An Essay in Institutional History," *Osiris* 2, second in a series (1986): 225–64.

12. C. B. Davenport, "Heredity of Skin Pigmentation in Man," *American Naturalist* (1910), pp. 44642–44672.

13. The Kaiser-Wilhelm Institute for Anthropology, Human Hereditary Teaching, and Eugenics.

14. Reiner Pommerin, *Sterilisierung der Rheinlandbastarde: Das Schicksal einer farbigen deutschen Minderheit, 1918–1937* [Sterilization of the Rhineland Bastards: The Fate of a German Minority of Color, 1918–1937] (Düsseldorf: Droste, 1979).

15. Hans J. Massaquois, *Destined to Witness* (New York: Harper Perennial, 1999), pp. 112–113.

16. "Reichsministerium des Innern," a document from the U.S. Holocaust Memorial Museum (June 19, 1937); cited in Clarence Lusane, *Hitler's Black Victims* (New York: Routledge, 2000), pp. 139–140.

17. Robert W. Kesting, "Blacks Under the Swastika: A Research Note," *Journal of Negro History* 83, no. 1 (1998): 84–99.

18. Most of the thirty state laws barring marriage between blacks and whites remained in effect until after World War II.

19. Richmond, Virginia, *Times-Dispatch*, February 27, 1980, and March 2, 1980; cited in Daniel Kevles, *In the Name of Eugenics* (Cambridge, MA: Harvard University Press, 1995), p. 116.

20. Pernick, *The Black Stork*, p. 47.

21. Margaret Sanger, *The Pivot of Civilization* (1999), chap. 4, p. 3; chap. 8, p. 10; at http://digital.library.upenn.edu/webbin/gutbook/lookup?num=1689.

22. Margaret Sanger, ed., *Birth Control Review* (October 1920).

23. From 1930 U.S. Census data.

24. W. E. B. Du Bois, *Birth Control Review* (June 1932), p. 166.

25. William A. Darrity and Castellano B. Turner, "Family Planning, Race Consciousness and the Fear of Race Genocide," *American Journal of Public Health* 62 (1972): 1454; Darrity and Turner, "Fears of Genocide Among Black Americans as Related to Age, Sex, and Region," *American Journal of Public Health* 63 (1973): 1029.

26. Simone M. Caron, "Birth Control and the Black Community in the 1960s: Genocide or Power Politics?" *Journal of Social History* 31, no. 3 (Spring 1998): 550.

27. "Birth Control: Losing Clinics Intended to Eliminate the Black Population, or Did They See the Threat of Negroes?" *U.S. News and World Report* 63 (August 7, 1967): 11, 24–25.

28. Pernick, *The Black Stork*, p. 55; Charles S. Bacon, "The Race Problem," *Medicine* 9 (1903): 103.

29. This resolution was renewed by a U.N. treaty in the late 1960s.

30. 1970 Chicago survey by Donald Bogue is cited in Caron, "Birth Control and the Black Community in the 1960s," p. 550.

31. The Centers for Disease Control's December 2000 *Weekly Morbidity and Mortality Report* shows that while the number of abortions dropped by more than 30,000 from 1996 to 1997, a record 36 percent of all abortions were performed on African American women, who constituted just 12.3 percent of the female population in the United States.

32. Darrity and Turner, "Family Planning, Race Consciousness and the Fear of Race Genocide," pp. 1029, 1454.

33. Harriet A. Washington, "Tracking the Risks of Birth Control," *Heart and Soul* (February 1996), pp. 54–61.

34. *Buck v. Bell*, 274 U.S. 200 (1927).

35. Terence Kealey, "Don't Blame Eugenics, Blame Politics," *The Spectator* (London): March 17, 2001, pp. 10–12.

36. Philip Reilly, *The Surgical Solution: A History of Involuntary Sterilization in the United States* (Baltimore: Johns Hopkins University Press, 1991).

37. Germaine Greer, *Sex and Destiny: The Politics of Human Fertility* (New York: Harper & Row, 1984).

38. Dorothy Roberts, *Killing the Black Body: Race Reproduction and the Meaning of Liberty* (New York: Vintage Books, 1997), p. 94.

39. Ibid., p. 93.

40. Betsy Hartmann, *Reproductive Rights and Wrongs: The Global Politics of Population Control* (Boston: South End Press, 1995), pp. 254–255.

41. Carl L. Cobb, "Students Charge BCH's Obstetrics Unit with Excessive Surgery," *Boston Globe* (1972), p. 1A.

42. Author's interview with Neil Calman, M.D., March 24–25, 2000.

43. Cobb, "Students Charge BCH's Obstetrics Unit with Excessive Surgery."

44. Linda Gordon, *Woman's Body, Woman's Right: A Societal History of Birth Control in America* (New York: Penguin, 1990), pp. 432–433; Alan Guttmacher Institute, "Facts in Brief: Contraceptive Use, 1998" (1998), pp. 17–21.

45. Malaika Brown, "Black Females Die More Often from Hysterectomy Complications," *The Sentinel* (Los Angeles), November 25, 1993: "A University of Maryland School of Medicine study found that African-American women having hysterectomies are more likely than whites to develop complications . . . and to die. . . ."

46. "Contraceptive Use in the United States, 1982–90: National Center for Health Statistics Advance Data No. 260" (1995), p. 8; National Center for Health Statistics, "National Survey of Family Growth and the 1990 Telephone Reinterview" (1988).

47. Roberts, *Killing the Black Body,* pp. 22–55.

48. Washington, "Tracking the Risks of Birth Control."

49. Roberts, *Killing the Black Body,* pp. 93–94.

50. "Hormone-Based Contraceptives Play a Possible Role in the Development of Breast Cancer," *American Medical Association Drug Evaluations* (1990); Jael Silliman and Anannya Bhattacharjee, eds., *Policing the National Body: Race, Gender and Criminalization* (Cambridge, MA: South End Press, 2002); Betsy Hartmann, *Reproductive Rights and Wrongs: The Global Politics of Population Control* (Boston: South End Press, 1995), p. 204; Monica Kuumba, "Perpetuating Neo-Colonialism Through Population Control in South Africa and the United States," *Africa Today* 40 (1993): 79.

51. Roberts, *Killing the Black Body,* p. 93.

52. The birth rate among American girls aged fifteen to nineteen declined during the 1990s, according to a report from the Centers for Disease Control's National Center for Health Statistics. The most dramatic drop was among black teens, whose rate dropped 30 percent between 1991 to 1999.

53. The Robert Wood Johnson Foundation, "Making the Grade: State and Local Partnerships to Establish School-Based Health Centers."

54. Most of the trials were conducted with poor women of color in developing nations, including Egypt, Indonesia, and Brazil. Brazil rescinded its permission for the trials in 1986.

55. Edwin G. Belzer, Jr., et al., "A Method to Increase Informed Consent in School Health Research," *Journal of School Health* 63, no. 7 (1993): 316(2).

56. Esther Oxford, "What They Learn at the Paquin School," *The Independent,* October 28, 1993, p. A28. During the author's tenure on the Rochester, New York, School-Based Clinic Advisory Board, the School-Based Clinic Support Group in Houston advised it that clinics typically waive parental consent because it interferes with the adolescents' privacy and autonomy.

57. Author's interview with an anonymous parent in Rochester, New York, in 1986.

58. Most teenaged mothers are impregnated by men who are at least five years older. As early as June 1994, the Alan Guttmacher Institute publication *Sex and America's Teenagers* cited a study showing that 60 percent of girls who had intercourse before age fifteen report being forced, as do 74 percent of girls who had sex before age fourteen.

59. Frank Dikotter, "Race Culture: Recent Perspectives on the History of Eugenics," *The American Historical Review* 103, no. 2 (April 1998): 467–478.

60. K. M. Sullivan, "Unconstitutional Conditions," *Harvard Law Review* 102 (1989): 1413–1506.

61. Albert G. Thomas, Jr., "The Norplant System: Where Are We in 1995?" *Journal of Family Practice* 40, no. 2 (February 1995): pp. 125–128.

62. "Hormone-Based Contraceptives Play a Possible Role in the Development of Breast Cancer," *American Medical Association Drug Evaluations*.

63. "Norplant: Side Effects Are More Extensive Than Originally Thought," *Iris—A Journal About Women* 32, pp. 69–67.

64. Harriet A. Washington, "For Some, Norplant Is a Mandatory Miracle," *Emerge,* June 1994.

65. Leslie Berger, "After Long Hiatus, New Contraceptives Emerge," *New York Times,* December 10, 2002.

66. Untitled article, *New York Times,* January 10, 1991, p. A20.

67. *Skinner v. Oklahoma*, 36 U.S. 527 (1942); *Whalen v. Roe,* 429 U.S. 589, 599–600 (1977); *Griswold v. Connecticut,* 381 U.S. 479 (1965).

68. "South Carolina Hospital Cited for Illegal Drug Tests," Facts On File News Services, February 24, 1994.

69. I. J. Chasnoff, H. J. Landress, and M. E. Barrett, "The Prevalence of Illicit-Drug or Alcohol Use During Pregnancy and Discrepancies on Mandatory Reporting in Pinellas County, Florida," *The New England Journal of Medicine* 322 (1990): 1202–1206.

70. Charles Krauthammer, *Washington Post,* July 30, 1989.

71. *USA Today,* June 8, 1989; *New York Times,* September 17, 1989.

72. *Washington Post,* September 17, 1989; *St. Louis Post-Dispatch,* September 15, 1990; *San Diego Union-Tribune,* February 2, 1992.

73. *Teratology* 44 (1991): 405–414.

74. Ernest Drucker, "Children of War: The Criminalization of Motherhood," *The International Journal on Drug Policy* 1, no. 4 (1990): 11.

75. Roberts, *Killing the Black Body,* p. 20; Linda C. T. Mayes, "The Problem of Prenatal Cocaine Exposure: A Rush to Judgment," *Journal of the American Medical Association* 267, no. 267 (1992): 406; Barry Zuckerman and Frank Deborah, " 'Crack Kids': Not Broken," *Pediatrics 1992* 89 (1992): 337; Robert Mathias, "Developmental Effects of Prenatal Drug Exposure May Be Overcome by Postnatal Environment," *NIDA Notes* (1992), p. 14.

76. *Washington Post,* December 15, 1989; Mathias, "Developmental Effects"; *Los Angeles Times,* September 21, 1989; M. S. Scher, G. A. Richardson, and N. L. Day, "Effects of Prenatal Cocaine/Crack and Other Drug Exposure on Electroencephalographic Sleep Studies at Birth and One Year," *Pediatrics* 105 (January 2000): 39–48; *New York Times,* May 7, 1989.

77. Roberts, *Killing the Black Body,* pp. 172, 175–178. Also see Washington, "For Some, Norplant Is a Mandatory Miracle," p. 18.

CHAPTER 9: NUCLEAR WINTER

1. United States Department of Energy, Office of Human Radiation, "Human Radiation Studies: Remembering the Early Years: Oral History of Health Physicist Karl Z. Morgan, Ph.D." (1995), p. 15.

2. Howland, an army doctor stationed at Oak Ridge, told AEC investigators in 1974 that he had administered the injection without Cade's consent.

3. The "fiendishly toxic" manmade element plutonium is medically devastating because it causes cancerous changes in bodily tissues by ejecting high-energy alpha particles from its nuclei. These alpha particles damage cells, leading to cancerous changes.

4. Eileen Welsome, *The Plutonium Files* (New York: Dial Press, 1999), p. 8; see also Robert Stone, M.D., a study architect who insisted that there were twenty.

5. United States Department of Energy, Office of Human Radiation, "Human Radiation Studies" (1995).

6. Larry Tye, author of *Rising from the Rails: Pullman Porters and the Making of the Black Middle Class,* has remarked upon the frequency of this injury among Pullman porters.

7. Howard Kurtz, "Big Scoop for a Little Paper: How the *Albuquerque Tribune* Broke the Radiation Story," *Washington Post,* January 8, 1994, p. G1.

8. "Supplementary Report of the Judicial Council," *Journal of the American Medical Association* 132 (December 28, 1946): 1090.

9. Memo from Robert Wilson, AEC General Manager, to Chairman, AEC Interim Medical Advisory Committee of Clinical Testing (April 1947), cited in Advisory Committee on Human Radiation Experiments (ACHRE), "DOE Openness: Human Radiation Experiments" (1995); roadmap to the project in "Information Report Summary Sheet on Disclosure to Patients Injected with Plutonium," p. 5. (*Openness* is an umbrella term relating to the declassification of radiation documents.)

10. The February 1995 UCSF report stated that there was never any expectation on the part of the experimenters that the injection would be of therapeutic benefit to Elmer Allen.

11. ACHRE, "DOE Openness: Human Radiation Experiments."

12. Per the UCSF's 1995 review of patient-subjects' medical charts.

13. R. S. Stone, "Summary Factsheet Human Experimentation Sfs1.001, Plutonium Excretion Studies (Plutonium Injection Experiment) Field Details" (July, 1947). One of these may have been patient CH1-3 of Chicago, who has never been identified.

14. Welsome, *The Plutonium Files,* p. 161.

15. Ibid., p. 390.

16. ACHRE, Jonathan D. Moreno, "The Only Feasible Means," *Hastings Center Report* 26, no. 5 (1996), which states: "1947 Colonel E.E. Kirkpatrick of the U.S. Atomic Energy Commission issues a secret document (Document 07075001, January 8, 1947) stating that the agency will begin administering intravenous doses of radioactive substances to human subjects."

17. *The New York American,* January 10, 1904. All the headlines in this paragraph are culled from articles in the William J. Hammer Collection, 1874–1935, Archives Center, National Museum of American History (NMAH), Washington, D.C.,

box 59, folders 2 and 3, and box 60, folder 2. They are cited in Rebecca Herzig's fascinating account of radiation epilation clinics titled "Removing Roots: North America Hiroshima Maidens and the X-Ray," *Technology and Culture* 40, no. 4 (1999): 723–745.

18. Hammer Collection, NMAH: "All Coons to Look White: College Professors Have Scheme to Solve Race Problem," *New York City Morning Telegraph,* January 22, 1904, clipping in box 59, folder 2; "Radium and X-Ray Used to Beautify," *Boston Herald,* May 8, 1904, clipping in box 59, folder 3; " 'Can the Ethiopian Change His Skin or the Leopard His Spots': Radium Light Turns Negro's Skin White," *Boston Globe,* January 25, 1904, box 60, folder 2; "Burning Out Birthmarks, Blemishes of the Skin and Even Turning a Negro White with the Magic Rays of Radium, the New Mystery of Science!" *New York American,* January 10, 1904, box 60, folder 2; "Allied Forces of Science's Latest Wonder and Mystery, Radium and the X-ray, with Their Penetrating Light Disprove the Biblical Impossibility by Turning Negro's Skin White and Bleaching Leopard's Spots. Rays to Be Used to Banish Birthmarks and Discolorations of the Skin," box 61, folder 1.

19. Undated, unidentified newspaper clipping without byline, from collection 69, Hammer Collection, NMAH, box 61, folder 1.

20. Herzig, "Removing Roots," pp. 723–745.

21. Rebecca Herzig, "In the Name of Science: Suffering, Sacrifice, and the Formation of American Roentgenology," *American Quarterly* 53, no. 4 (2001): 563–589.

22. Wolfgang Weyers, *The Abuse of Man: An Illustrated History of Dubious Medical Experimentation* (New York: Ardor Scribendi, 2003), p. 516.

23. Dr. Joseph Hamilton, cited in Welsome, *The Plutonium Files,* p. 151.

24. President Harry S. Truman prohibited the entrance of pro-Nazi scientists into the United States; as a result, references to Paperclip scientists' Nazi activities were edited from their personnel files.

25. Atomic Energy Commission, "Atomic Energy Commission Document 07075001" (1947).

26. Lawrence K. Altman, *Who Goes First? The Story of Self-Experimentation in Medicine* (New York: Random House, 1987), pp. 144–146.

27. Welsome, *The Plutonium Files,* p. 126.

28. Jonathan D. Moreno, *Undue Risk* (New York: Freeman, 2000).

29. At the hands of Nazi scientists, inmates were burned, immersed in frigid water, and subjected to a number of other hellish experiments that were meant to duplicate wartime medical hazards. See George Annas and Michael Grodin, *The Nazi Doctors and the Nuremberg Code: Human Rights in Human Experimentation* (New York: Oxford University Press, 1992).

30. Moreno, *Undue Risk,* p. 148.

31. See J. Katz, M.D., *Experimentation with Human Beings: The Authority of the Investigator, Subject Professions, and State in the Human Experimentation Process* (New York: Russell Sage Foundation, 1972); see also "In the Name of Consent . . . ," *New Scientist,* February 19, 1994, p. 33.

32. Welsome, *The Plutonium Files;* Kurtz, "Big Scoop for a Little Paper."

33. Martha Stephens, *The Treatment: The Story of Those Who Died in the Cincinnati Radiation Tests* (Durham: Duke University Press, 2002), pp. 84–86; 75 percent of the 200 were black, according to ACHRE documents. See also E. Saenger et al.,

"Whole Body and Partial Body Radiotherapy of Advanced Cancer," *American Journal of Roentgenology* 117, no. 3 (March 1973): 677.

34. Saenger et al., "Whole Body and Partial Body Radiotherapy of Advanced Cancer." See also Stephens, *The Treatment*, p. 119.
35. ACHRE, "DOE Openness: Human Radiation Experiments," chapter 9.
36. Stephens, *The Treatment*, appendix 1, pp. 293–295.
37. "Oral Histories: Health Physicist Karl Z. Morgan, Ph.D.," in ACHRE, "DOE Openness: Human Radiation Experiments."
38. Stephens, *The Treatment*, p. 109.
39. Keith Schneider, "Memo Compared U.S. Research to Nazi Experiments; Radiation Scientist Warned in '50 That Human Tests Would Be Criticized," *New York Times*, December 28, 1993.
40. Rebecca Trounson and Charles Ornstein, "Researcher Violated Rules, UCLA Says," *Los Angeles Times*, April 16, 2003; at http://www.latimes.com/la-memalaria16apr16,0,650344.story.
41. Scott Allen, "Kennedy Dropped Testing Probe: Taft's Anger Led to 1971 Decision," *Boston Globe*, February 12, 1994, p. 5.
42. Stephens, *The Treatment*, p. xxi.
43. Everett Idris Evans, M.D., "The Problem of Atomic Burns," submitted to the Surgeon General of the Army (1951).
44. W. T. Harris, Jr., "Flash Burn Studies in Volunteers" (undated memo).
45. Sander L. Gilman, *Difference and Pathology: Stereotypes of Sexuality, Race and Madness* (Ithaca, NY: Cornell University Press, 1985); see also Department of Energy Atomic Energy Commission Report, 1954.
46. Charles A. Jacobi and Don Q. Paris, *X-Ray Technology* (St. Louis: CV Mosby, 1963).
47. L. Van Middlesworth, "Radioactive Iodide Uptake of Normal Newborn Infants," *American Journal of Diseases of Children* 88 (1954): 439, B442.
48. "In the Name of Consent . . . ," *New Scientist*, February 19, 1994, p. 33.
49. *American Journal of Public Health* (June 1978).
50. Andrew Buncombe, "Nuclear Site Where Deep South's Old Attitudes Live On," *The Independent* (London), August 13, 2002, p. 2
51. Author's interviews with Elmerine Whitfield Bell, 1994, 2002, 2005.

CHAPTER 10: CAGED SUBJECTS

1. Author's interview with Jesse Williams, April 16, 2004.
2. Editorial, *Journal of the National Medical Association* 2, no. 2 (1910).
3. Jessica Mitford, *Kind and Usual Punishment: The Prison Business* (New York: Knopf, 1973), p. 140.
4. "Histoire des progrès de l'anthropologie et de la sociologie criminelles pendant les années 1895–1896," 4th Congrès Internationale d'Anthropologie Criminelle, Geneva, pp. 187–199. Lombroso went on to quote his friend Hippolyte Taine: "You have shown us fierce and lubricious orang-utans with human faces. It is evident that as such they cannot act otherwise. If they ravish, steal and kill, it is by virtue of their own nature and their past, but there is all the more reason for destroying them when it has been proved that they will always remain orang-utans." Cesare Lombroso and Henry Pomeroy Horton, *Crime, Its Causes and Remedies* (Boston, Little, Brown, 1911), pp. 428, 447–448.
5. "Resolutions Adopted by the Annual Conference of the American Prison Associ-

ation, October 20–24, 1919, Including the Declaration of Principles of the 1870 Congress," printed by the New York Local Committee and the American Prison Association (1919), p. 5.

6. Advisory Committee on Human Radiation Experiments (ACHRE), "DOE Openness: Human Radiation Experiments" (1995), chapter 9, History of Prison Research Regulation.

7. Allen M. Hornblum, "They Were Cheap and Available: Prisoners as Research Subjects in Twentieth Century America," *British Medical Journal* 315 (1997): 1435–1441; Allen M. Hornblum, *Acres of Skin: Human Experiments at Holmesburg Prison* (New York: Routledge, 1998), p. 58.

8. The federal project was established to explore the possibilities of mind control and was headed by Dr. Sidney Gottlieb. Its experiments were often conducted with unwitting subjects. The project was renamed MKSEARCH in 1964.

9. Beerman and Lazarus, *A Tradition of Excellence*, p. 132; cited in Hornblum, "They Were Cheap and Available," p. 37.

10. Rick Sarlat, "Dollars Lured Former Prisoners into Labs: Stories Detail Abuses by Researchers," *Philadelphia Tribune*, October 23, 1998, p. 1A.

11. Adolph Katz, "Prisoners Volunteer to Save Lives," *Philadelphia Bulletin*, February 27, 1996, p. 1.

12. Jonathan D. Moreno, "Lessons Learned: A Half-Century of Experimenting on Humans (U.S. Army Experiments)," *Humanist* (January–February 1974); Jonathan D. Moreno, *Undue Risk* (New York: Freeman, 2000).

13. Moreno, *Undue Risk*, p. 230.

14. ACHRE, "DOE Openness: Human Radiation Experiments."

15. Author's interview with Allen Hornblum, April 12, 2004; see also Hornblum, *Acres of Skin*, pp. 11–12.

16. Hornblum, "They Were Cheap and Available," p. 17.

17. Ibid.

18. Harriet A. Washington, "Born for Evil? Stereotyping the Karyotype: A Case History in the Genetics of Aggression," in *Twentieth Century Ethics of Human Subjects Research: Historical Perspectives on Values, Practices and Regulations*, edited by Volker Roelcke and Giovanni Maio (Stuttgart: Franz Steiner Verlag, 2004), pp. 319–334. Jay Katz, M.D., *Experimentation with Human Beings: The Authority of the Investigator, Subject Professions, and State in the Human Experimentation Process* (New York: Russell Sage Foundation, 1972). See also chapter 11 *infra* for more details about this XYY experiment.

19. "Blood Exchanger Named," *New York Times*, June 23, 1949, p. 29; "Blood-Donor Hero Rests as Girl Dies," December 26, 1949, p. 31; Howard A. Rusk, "Prisoners Play Vital Role in Scientific Experiments" (1952), p. 73; "Prisoners Help Test Drug for Malaria," *New York Times*, March 16, 1966.

20. Nathan Freudenthal Leopold, *Life Plus 99 Years* (Garden City, NY: Doubleday, 1958); Richard J. H. Johnston, "Leopold Receives Parole in 1924 'Thrill' Slaying," *New York Times*, February 21, 1958, p. 1.

21. ACHRE, "DOE Openness: Human Radiation Experiments."

22. "Digest of Official Actions, Chicago American Medical Association" (1959), pp. 617–618.

23. Benjamin Mason Meier, "International Protection of Persons Undergoing Medical Experimentation: Protecting the Right of Informed Consent," *Berkeley Journal of International Law* 20, p. 513.

24. George J. Annas and Michael A. Grodin, *The Nazi Doctors and the Nuremberg Code: Human Rights in Human Experimentation* (New York: Oxford University Press, 1992), pp. 20, 23, 174–182.

25. Nuremberg Military Tribunals, *Trials of War Criminals, Under Council Control Law No. 10, Nuremberg, October 1946–April 1949*, vol. 2 (Washington, D.C.: Government Printing Office, 1949).

26. Annas and Grodin, *The Nazi Doctors and the Nuremberg Code*.

27. "World Medical Association Code of Ethics," *British Medical Journal* 1119 (1962).

28. Hornblum, "They Were Cheap and Available," p. 19.

29. Sarlat, "Dollars Lured Former Prisoners into Labs."

30. Hornblum, *Acres of Skin*, p. 5.

31. Ibid., p. 18.

32. Hornblum, "They Were Cheap and Available," p. 6.

33. Katz, "Prisoners Volunteer to Save Lives."

34. Hornblum, *Acres of Skin*, p. 65.

35. Fewer U.S. women took the medication, because the FDA was dissatisfied with thalidomide's clinical testing and refused to approve it. Therefore, it was available in the United States only on a limited experimental basis.

36. Henry K. Beecher, "Ethics and Clinical Research," *The New England Journal of Medicine* 74 (1966): 1354.

37. Washington, "Born for Evil?"

38. Walter Rugaber, "Prison Drug and Plasma Projects Leave Fatal Trail," *New York Times*, July 29, 1969, p. 1; see also "Prisoners Help Test Drug for Malaria" and "Alabama Prisons to End Drug Tests: 'Substantial Defects' Found in Private Research," *New York Times*, May 31, 1969.

39. Hornblum, *Acres of Skin*, p. 45.

40. Solomon Jones, "Under Their Skin: Experiments Performed on Philadelphia Inmates Decades Ago Still Pack Horrific Power," *Philadelphia Weekly*, May 15, 2002, p. 1.

41. Ibid.

42. Allen Hornblum, "Subjected to Medical Experimentation: Pennsylvania's Contribution to 'Science' in Prisons," *Pennsylvania History*, G7 (Summer 2000), pp. 415–426.

43. The relevant regulations are contained in Department of Health, Education, and Welfare, 45 CFR 46, subpart C.

44. Brenda V. Smith and Cynthia Dailard, "Black Women's Health in Custody," in National Black Women's Health Project and the Congressional Black Caucus Health Brain Trust, *National Colloquium on Black Women's Health* (Washington, D.C.: April 11, 2003), pp. 97–108; Angela Davis, "Masked Racism: Reflections on the Prison Industrial Complex," *Color Lines Magazine* 1, no. 2 (1998): 11.

45. Bureau of Justice Statistics, "Characteristics of Prisoners in State and Federal Correctional Institutions, 1991 and 1997" [by Sex, Race, Age, Marital Status, Educational Attainment, and Citizenship] from *Sourcebook of Criminal Justice Statistics, 1999* (2000), p. 513.

46. Carl. P. Schmertmann, Adansia Amankwaa, and Robert Long, "Three Strikes and You're Out: Demographic Analysis of Mandatory Sentencing, *Demography* 35, no. 4 (1998): pp. 445–463.

47. Julie Bykowicz, "Study Details High Rates of Infection in Prisons: Hepatitis C Said to Hit Over a Third of Inmates," *Baltimore Sun*, March 8, 2003, p. 33.

48. Jeffrey P. Kahn, "Prison Research: Does Locked Up Mean Locked Out?" (September 6, 1999); at http://www.cnn.com/HEALTH/bioethics/9909/prison. research (accessed January 10, 2006).

49. Howard A. Rusk, M.D., "Drugs and Prisoners: Tests Among Volunteers Demonstrate Need for Penology Research, Too," *New York Times,* November 11, 1962, p. 74.

50. Paul Farmer, *Infections and Inequalities: The Modern Plagues* (Berkeley: University of California Press, 1999), pp. 32, 33, 43.

51. Ronald L. Braithwaite and Kimberly R. J. Arriola, "Male Prisoners and HIV Prevention: A Call for Action Ignored," *American Journal of Public Health* 93, no. 5, pp. 759–763.

52. "New Guidelines for Inmate Medical Studies," *New York Times,* October 16, 1999, p. 9.

CHAPTER 11: THE CHILDREN'S CRUSADE

1. Rick Weiss, "Volunteers at Risk in Medical Studies; Complex Research Projects Strain System of Safeguards," *Washington Post* (series: Science on the Ethical Frontier), August 1, 1998, p. A1.

2. Gail A. Wasserman, Ph.D., "Medical and Neurological Assessment in a Population at Risk for Antisocial Behavior," New York State Psychiatric Institute and Columbia University Department of Psychiatry Institutional Review Board Protocol, summary no. 2282 (revised, February 18, 1994), p. 3.

3. "Re: research subjects," a Department of Probation intradepartmental memorandum from Robert Stone, Branch Chief to Manhattan Family Intake and Investigation Probation Officers (August 30, 1991).

4. State Division of Human Rights, "On the Complaint of Renee L. Jackson Against the City of New York," Department of Probation Title VII federal charge no. 16G930370; Annette Fuentes, "Quick Fix: Pushing a Medical Cure for Youth Violence," *Institute for Public Affairs* 22, no. 15 (1998): 14; D. R. Cherek and S. D. Lane, "Effects of D,L-Fenfluramine on Aggressive and Impulsive Responding in Adult Males with a History of Conduct Disorder," *Psychopharmacology* 146 (1999): 473–481.

5. Information about the study has been almost solely derived from the investigators' own protocols, reports, memos, and published articles. Only one researcher, Timothy Walsh, spoke with me briefly in 1998, and when I called him back, he informed me, "I've been told not to talk to you." Phone calls and e-mails requesting interviews of several principals, including Gail Wasserman, have gone unacknowledged over a period of three years.

6. Author's interview with Charisse Johnson, December 2, 2005.

7. Heidi M. Connolly et al., "Valvular Heart Disease Associated with Fenfluramine-Phentermine," *The New England Journal of Medicine* 337, no. 9 (1997): 581–588.

8. Ibid.; Food and Drug Administration, "FDA Warns Public About Chinese Diet Pills Containing Fenfluramine" (2002).

9. "Letter from Clifford Zucker to Clifford C. Scharke" (February 12 1998), p. 2.

10. Leonard H. Glantz, "Research with Children," *American Journal of Law and Medicine* 24, no. 213 (1998): 238.

11. Gina Kolata, "Two Popular Diet Pills Are Withdrawn from the Market," *New York Times,* September 16, 1997. See also Food and Drug Administration, "FDA

Warns Public About Chinese Diet Pills Containing Fenfluramine"; Connolly, "Valvular Heart Disease Associated with Fenfluramine-Phentermine."

12. E. Balaban, J. S. Alper, and Y. L. Kasamon, "Mean Genes and the Biology of Aggression: A Critical Review of Recent Animal and Human Research," *Journal of Neurogenetics* 11, nos. 1, 2 (1996): 1–43.

13. The results of the study were widely published in such reports as "Neuro-endocrine Response to Fenfluramine Challenge in Boys," *Archives of General Psychiatry* (September 1997), (54) 9: 785–789.

14. Weiss, "Volunteers at Risk in Medical Studies."

15. Ibid.

16. Catherine Walsh, B.S., and Lainie F. Ross, M.D., Ph.D., "Are Minority Children Under- or Overrepresented in Pediatric Research?" *Pediatrics* 112 (2003): 890–895; Lainie F. Ross, M.D., and Catherine Walsh, "Minority Children in Pediatric Research," *American Journal of Law and Medicine* 29, nos. 2/3 (2003): 319.

17. 45 CFR (Code of Federal Regulations) 46, title 45.

18. Glantz, "Research with Children."

19. Haider Rizvi, "An Unscientific Method," *Village Voice*, April 11, 2000.

20. Cherek and Lane, "Effects of D,L-Fenfluramine on Aggressive and Impulsive Responding in Adult Males with a History of Conduct Disorder."

21. Despite the assertions of then HEW Assistant Secretary Robert Egeberg that the project had passed review by Johns Hopkins University, Dr. Gordon Walker, the director of Johns Hopkins Hospital's committee on clinical investigations, denied that his committee had ever given approval. See Diane Bauer "Maryland Tests for Criminal Potential," *Washington Daily News*, January 22, 1970, p. 7; see also Diane Bauer, "Criminal-Prone Tests Resumed," May 4, 1970, p. 5; cited in Jay Katz, M.D., *Experimentation with Human Beings: The Authority of the Investigator, Subject Professions, and State in the Human Experimentation Process* (New York: Russell Sage Foundation, 1972).

22. Digamber S. Borgaonkar, "Cytogenic Screening of Community-Dwelling Males," in *Genetic Issues in Public Health and Medicine* (Springfield, Ill.: Thomas, 1978); Digamber S. Borgaonkar and Saleem A. Shah, "The XYY Chromosome Male—or Syndrome?" in *Progress in Medical Genetics*, edited by A. G. Steinberg and A. G. Bearn (New York: Grune, 1974), vol. 10, pp. 135–222.

23. This can be due to nondisjunction during the meiotic phase and metaphase I. See A. A. Sandberg et al., "An XYY Human Male?" *The Lancet* 2 (1961): 488–489.

24. L. F. Jarvik et al., "Human Aggression and the Extra Y Chromosome: Fact or Fantasy?" *American Psychologist* 28 (1973): 674–682.

25. J. Rovet et al., "Intelligence and Achievement in Children with Extra X Aneuploidy: A Longitudinal Perspective," *American Journal of Medical Genetics* 60 (1995): 356–363.

26. Borgaonkar, "Cytogenic Screening of Community-Dwelling Males." Borgaonkar selectively reported on a segment of his study that included the atypical 80-percent white Edgemeade component. This conveyed the erroneous impression that whites were heavily represented in the study.

27. Ibid.

28. Katz, *Experimentation with Human Beings*. See also Rick Szykowny, "No Justice, No Peace: An Interview with Jerome Miller," *The Humanist* 54, pp. 9–20: "If you

look at the juvenile system, which is worse, and where in many states now you'll find almost exclusively black kids—at least in the state institutions."

29. Harriet A. Washington, "Born for Evil? Stereotyping the Karyotype: A Case History in the Genetics of Aggression," in *Twentieth Century Ethics of Human Subjects Research: Historical Perspectives on Values, Practices, and Regulations,* edited by Volker Roelcke and Giovanni Maio (Stuttgart: Franz Steiner Verlag, 2004), pp. 320–333.

30. Stephen Jay Gould, *The Mismeasure of Man* (New York: W. W. Norton, 1981), p. 144.

31. Jane E. Brody, "Scientists' Group Terms Boston Study of Children with Extra Sex Chromosome Unethical and Harmful," *New York Times,* November 15, 1974, p. 16; Brody, "Babies' Screening Is Ended in Boston," *New York Times,* June 20, 1975, p. 6.

32. Harriet A. Washington, "Mortal Lessons: HSPH Faculty Confront a Uniquely American Scourge," *Harvard Public Health Review* (1998).

33. James Bowman, M.D., and Robert F. Murray, Jr., M.D., M.S., *Genetic Variation and Disorders in People of African Origin* (Baltimore: Johns Hopkins University Press, 1990).

34. Gould, *The Mismeasure of Man,* pp. 144–145.

35. Ibid., pp. 146–233 passim.

36. Harriet Washington, "Of Mice and Men," *Emerge* (1995); Washington, "Born for Evil?" pp. 319–334.

37. Peter R. Breggin, M.D., "The 'Violence Initiative'—A Racist Biomedical Program for Social Control," *Rights Tenet* (Summer 1992).

38. Andy and his colleagues also performed hemispherectomies, in which they literally cut the brain in half by severing the connecting structure, the corpus callusum, not as therapy, but for behavior control. It should be noted that their surgeries differed acutely from such contemporary therapeutic surgeries as those pioneered by Dr. Benjamin Carson, Sr., of Johns Hopkins, which are precise and undertaken to heal desperately ill children of all ethnic groups. See O. J. Andy, M.D., "The Neurosurgical Treatment of Abnormal Behavior," *The American Journal of the Medical Sciences,* no. 252 (August 1966): 232–238.

39. Ibid.

40. Ibid.

41. B. J. Mason, "Brain Surgery to Control Behavior: Controversial Options Are Coming Back as Violence Curbs," *Ebony,* February 1973, p. 68.

42. Mark Vernon and Frank Erwin, *Violence and the Brain* (New York: Harper & Row, 1970), pp. 39–51.

43. Glenn Frankel, "Today's Psychosurgeons Defend Techniques: New Generation of Psychosurgeons Defends Techniques Series: The Lobotomy Era; Last of a Series," *Washington Post,* April 8, 1980.

44. Ross, Friedman, and Walsh, "Minority Children in Pediatric Research."

45. Gould, *The Mismeasure of Man,* p. 145.

46. Ross, Friedman, and Walsh, "Minority Children in Pediatric Research," p. 319; Walsh and Ross, "Are Minority Children Under- or Overrepresented in Pediatric Research?" pp. 890–895.

47. Some research protocols require such assent by the child in addition to the informed consent of the parent.

48. Glantz, "Research with Children"; see also Robert J. Katerberg, "Institutional Re-

view Boards, Research on Children, and Informed Consent of Parents: Walking the Tightrope Between Encouraging Vital Experimentation and Protecting Subjects' Rights," *Journal of College and University Law* 24, no. 545, p. 562. A passage states: "In respect to nontherapeutic research using minors, it has been noted that 'Consent to research has been virtually unanalyzed by courts and legislatures.' Our research reveals this statement remains as accurate now as it was in 1977."

49. Glantz, "Research with Children," p. 238.

50. "Study: Better Communication Needed for Parents of Kids in Research," *Cancer Weekly*, February 17, 2004, p. 49.

51. Glantz, "Research with Children," pp. 218–219; 222–223.

52. Nia Lewis, "Baltimore Lead Case Echoes Tuskegee Experiment" (2001), NNPA News Service; at www.nnpa.org. See also *Los Angeles Times*, August 28, 1977.

53. Jocelyn Kaiser, "Lead Paint Trial Castigated," *Science Now*, August 28, 2001, p. 4.

54. *Ericka Grimes v. Kennedy Krieger Institute, Inc.* 128 (2000); *Myron Higgins, a Minor, et al. v. Kennedy Krieger Institute, Inc.* 129 (2000).

55. National Report Series, Juvenile Justice Bulletin, "Minorities in the Juvenile Justice System—Disproportionate Minority Confinement Often Stems from Disparity at Early Stages of Processing" (1999), pp. 1–4

56. Mark Roscoe and Reggie Morton, "Disproportionate Minority Confinement Fact Sheet #11" (1994).

57. National Report Series, "Minorities in the Juvenile Justice System—Disproportionate Minority Confinement Often Stems From Disparity at Early Stages of Processing."

58. *Bonner v. Moran,* 126 F2d 121 (D.C. Cir 1941); cited in Katz, *Experimentation with Human Beings,* p. 972.

59. Glantz, "Research with Children"; see also Katz, *Experimentation with Human Beings,* p. 973.

60. M. Robert Hines, "The Spinal Fluid in the New-Born," *Journal of the American Medical Association* 85 (1925): 500–501.

61. Hilda F. Wiese et. al., "Essential Fatty Acids in Infant Nutrition," *Journal of Nutrition* 66 (1958): 345–360; Arild Hansen, "Role of Linoleaic Acid in Infant Nutrition," *Pediatrics* 55, suppl. 1, part 2 (1963): 170–192.

62. Cory Servaas, "Netty Mayersohn and Her Baby AIDS Bill," *Saturday Evening Post,* January–February 1998.

63. Michael Moss, "Heart Troubles: A U.S. Experiment on Young Children Ignites Painful Debate," *Wall Street Journal,* June 12, 1996, p. A1.

64. Undated report, Washington Office on Haiti and the National Vaccine Information, "More Than 2,000 Children in the Port-au-Prince Slum Cité Soleil Were Inoculated with High Doses of Edmonton-Zagreb (EZ)."

65. "U.S. Tests Drug on Haitian Kids," *Weekly News Update on the Americas,* Haiti Information, July 29, 1996.

66. Amy Goldstein, "Infant Death Study Halts Amid Feuding; NIH Cancels $58 Million Project with GU Focusing on D.C. Babies," *Washington Post,* February 2, 1996, p. A.1.

CHAPTER 12: GENETIC PERDITION

1. DNA fingerprinting is simply a method of comparing the DNA of two or more individuals, which varies by only 0.1 percent—that's one difference in a thousand. It was 1984, appropriately enough, when the discoveries of British geneticist Alec Jeffreys enabled the identification and comparison of unique DNA loci, using them as genetic markers. In RFLP (DNA fingerprinting, the technique used in Calvin Johnson's case), the laboratory must first obtain a tissue sample that contains DNA such as blood, semen, or a buccal swab (a painless scraping from the DNA-packed interior of the cheek). Then technicians extract the DNA, "slice" it into short pieces or fragments, and infuse the pieces with radioactivity. The pieces will expose X-ray film held near them, revealing a complex striped pattern that resembles a bar code and that, although not unique, is usually characteristic enough to help identify a person.

2. Adam K. Liptak, "Study Suspects Thousands of False Convictions," *New York Times,* April 19, 2004, p. 15.

3. Bloodsworth, unlike most of the other exonerated men, is white.

4. In December 2000, six Virginia courts rejected the innocence claims of Leroy Washington, a mentally retarded African American man. The courts ruled that the genetic evidence that excluded him from biological candidacy was inconclusive. Neither was definitively exculpatory evidence from a DNA test enough to free Edward Lee Elmore, a South Carolina man who has been on death row for twenty-four years.

5. Dr. Richard Saferstein, former technical director of the New Jersey state police crime lab, said, "For whatever reasons, whether carelessness, negligence, incompetence, ignorance or fraud . . . [Fish] incorrectly reported her laboratory findings."

6. Liptak, "Study Suspects Thousands of False Convictions."

7. "In a country in which some slip-and-fall claims win millions of dollars, it is startling to realize that decades wrongly spent in maximum-security prisons are typically worth nothing," Amanda Ripley noted in her article "After the Exoneration," *Time,* December 11, 2000, p. 96.

8. Kristen Philipkoski, "A Crime Sniffing Network" *Wired News,* August 11, 1998; at www.wired.com/news/technology/0,282,14231,00.html (accessed July 11, 2002).

9. According to a September 2004 study by the Police Professionalism Initiative at the University of Nebraska at Omaha, there have been at least eighteen investigations nationwide in which police did DNA "sweeps" to identify suspects. Only one case ended with an arrest, according to records kept by Smith Alling Lane, a Tacoma, Washington, law firm that represents DNA equipment makers. Theo Emery, "ACLU Asks Cape Cod Police, District Attorney to Halt DNA Collections, Associated Press, January 10, 2005. See also "DNA Dragnets," *The New Atlantis,* no. 8 (Spring 2005), pp. 104–106.

10. "New England Town Abuzz over DNA Dragnet," *Cape Cod Times* (Truro, MA), January 7, 2005: "Men who submitted a swabbed saliva sample also had to provide their name, date of birth and race."

11. Jeffrey S. Grand, "The Blooding of America: Privacy and the DNA Dragnet," *Cardozo Law Review* 23 (2002): 2277.

12. "Technologies: Real-Time PCR [polymerase chain reaction]"; at http://www.nanogen.com.

13. Ron Walters, "New Law Enables Racist DNA Studies," *Washington Informer* 39, no. 17 (2002): 15.

14. Rebecca Sasser Peterson, "DNA Databases: When Fear Goes Too Far," *American Criminal Law Review* 37 (2000): 1219.

15. In fact, presence of a sickle-cell gene, or allele, has come to code for race. When it is found in the occasional white person, this has been presumed tantamount to discovery of an occult black biological heritage.

16. We now know that sickle-cell disease is also endemic among all racial groups in Italy, northern Greece, southern Turkey, Saudi Arabia, India, and North and equatorial Africa—almost anywhere malaria is found. In fact, the first African identified with sickle-cell disease was not black, but Arab.

17. James Bowman, M.D., and Robert F. Murray, Jr., M.D., M.S., *Genetic Variation and Disorders in People of African Origin* (Baltimore: Johns Hopkins University Press, 1990). Author's interviews with James Bowman, M.D., March 13, 2000, and December 2, 2005.

18. Here is a simplified probability model for the incidence of sickle-cell anemia in the mating of two carriers: S = the gene for normal hemoglobin; s = the gene for sickle-cell anemia.

SS = normal, not a carrier
Ss = carrier for sickle cell
ss = person with sickle cell anemia

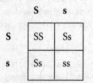

	S	**s**
S	SS	Ss
s	Ss	ss

Boldface type indicates the parents and regular type denotes the offspring. The mating of two carriers will produce one in four (25 percent) offspring who has the normal SS genetic complement; one in four (25 percent) who has sickle-cell anemia with two recessive ss genes; and two in four (50 percent) who will have an Ss complement: they will be healthy carriers.

19. Daniel Kevles, *In the Name of Eugenics* (Cambridge, MA: Harvard University Press, 1995), p. 278.

20. Raymond R. Coletta, *Biotechnology and the Law: Biotechnology and the Creation of Ethics,* 32 *McGeorge Law Review* 89, no. 97 (2000).

21. Kevles, *In the Name of Eugenics.*

22. Ibid.

23. Ibid., pp. 278, 256.

24. Michael Aidoo et al., "Protective Effects of the Sickle Cell Gene Against Malaria Morbidity and Mortality," *The Lancet* 359 (April 13, 2002): 1311–1312.

25. These diseases were caused by two recessive genes or a single dominant gene.

26. Kevles, *In the Name of Eugenics,* p. 255.

27. Ibid., pp. 257–258.

28. Ibid., pp. 277–279; see also Coletta, *Biotechnology and the Law*.

29. Not one of the tested employees had the gene.

30. "Resistance to Chemotherapy Is Found to Vary by Ethnicity, According to New Study," *Sentinel* (Los Angeles), March 29, 2001.

31. Walter A. Kukull and George M. Marti, "APOE Polymorphisms and Late-Onset Alzheimer Disease: The Importance of Ethnicity," *Journal of the American Medical Association* 279, no. 10 (March 11, 1998), 788–789.

32. This condition is marked by a divergent metabolism of the enzyme glucose-6 phosphate dehydrogenase.

33. Today treatment for sickle-cell disease remains symptomatic. Hydroxyurea banishes symptoms without serious side effects in most users, but it is effective for only 15 percent of people with the disease.

34. Untitled article, *Health,* April 1994; see also Harriet A. Washington, "Piece of the Genetic Puzzle Is Left Out," *Emerge,* October 1996.

35. "News and Views: Except as Laboratory Technicians, Blacks Had No Role in the Sequencing of the Human Genome," *Journal of Blacks in Higher Education* 33 (2001): 16.

36. Ibid.: "A JBHE [*Journal of Blacks in Higher Education*] survey of the biology departments of the nation's 25 highest-ranked universities conducted last year found that only 10, or 1.1 percent, of the 932 biology faculty at these universities are black. Our survey also found that there have been 561 African Americans who have earned a Ph.D. in biology over the 1993–1998 period. Not one of these black biologists holds a teaching position at any one of the nation's 25 highest-ranked universities."

37. "New PhRMA Survey Finds 249 Medicines in the Pipeline for African Americans,"; at www.biospace.com/news_story.cfm?StoryID=9961220&full=1 (accessed May 8, 2004).

38. "BiDil for Treatment of Heart Failure in African Americans"; at www.NitroMed. com/BiDil.shtml (accessed January 18, 2004).

39. Jonathan Kahn, J.D., Ph.D., "How a Drug Becomes 'Ethnic': Law, Commerce, and the Production of Racial Categories in Medicine," *Yale Journal of Health Policy, Law, and Ethics* 4, no. 1 (2004); also see Kahn, "Getting the Numbers Right: Statistical Mischief and Racial Profiling in Heart Failure Research," *Perspectives in Biology and Medicine* 46, no. 4 (Autumn 2003): 473–483.

40. "Trials for 'Ethnic' Drug," *Science* 291 (2001): 2547; V. S. Elliot, "FDA May Approve New Heart Drug for Blacks," *American Medical News*.com (March 26, 2001), at http://www.ama-assn.org/sci-pubs/amnews/pick_01/hlsc0326.htm (accessed December 12, 2002); E. Marshall, "Trial for 'Ethnic' Therapy," *Science Now,* March 26, 2001; at http://sciencenow.sciencemag.org/cgi/content/full/2001/326/2 (accessed December 12, 2002).

41. Centers for Disease Control (CDC), "Changes in Mortality from Heart Failure—United States, 1980–1995," *Morbidity and Mortality Weekly Report* 47, no. 30 (1998); at http://www.cdc.gov/mmwr/preview/mmwrhtml/00054249.htm.

42. National Heart, Lung, and Blood Institute (NHLBI), "Data Fact Sheet—Congestive Heart Failure in the United States: A New Epidemic"; at http://www. nhlbi.nih.gov/health/public/heart/other/CHF.htm (accessed December 3, 2002).

See also National Heart, Lung, and Blood Institute (NHLBI), "Morbidity and Mortality: 2002 Chart Book on Cardiovascular, Lung, and Blood Diseases," p. 39 (accessed December 3, 2002).

43. W. W. Dressler, "Social Class, Skin Color, and Arterial Blood Pressure in Two Societies," *Ethnicity and Disease* 1, no. 1 (1991): 60–77; see also W. W. Dressler, "Hypertension in the African American Community: Social, Cultural, and Psychological Factors," *Seminars in Nephrology* 16, no. 2 (1996): 71–82.

44. Press release from NitroMed, Inc., "NitroMed Receives FDA Letter on BiDil®, A Treatment for Heart Failure in Black Patients" (March 8, 2001); at http://www.NitroMed.com/newsindex.html. See also "This Heart Drug Is Designed for African Americans," *Business Week,* March 26, 2001, p. 71.

45. "Noteworthy News: Heart Failure in Blacks May Signal 'Different Disease,' " *Black Issues in Higher Education,* June 20, 2002, p. 26; "Slight Genetic Differences Justify Innovative Medical Treatment," *Chicago Defender,* May 1, 2001; "BiDil for Treatment of Heart Failure in African Americans." BiDil's Web page (www.NitroMed.com/BiDil.shtml) lists the Association of Black Cardiologists (ABC), the National Medical Association (NMA), and the members of the Congressional Black Caucus as part of the A-HeFT coalition.

CHAPTER 13: INFECTION AND INEQUITY

1. Mireya Navarro, "Gauging the Threat of Recalcitrant Patients," *New York Times,* April 14, 1992, p. 1A.

2. Ibid.

3. Michael Winerip, "Rikers Fights an Epidemic Cell by Cell," *New York Times,* May 24, 1992, p. 35.

4. Reluctance to use the vaccine may have been intensified by the tragic consequences of a case in Germany. In 1929–1930, Dr. Georg Deycke, director of Lübeck General Hospital in northern Germany, contaminated an experimental batch with a virulent strain of disease-causing tubercule bacilli. The tainted vaccine caused the deaths of sixty-eight infants in Lübeck. See Julius Moses, *Der Totentanz von Lübeck* (Dresden: Madaus, 1930).

5. This tragic milestone was announced in December 2003. The Web site of Doctors Without Borders adds: "AIDS is caused by the human immunodeficiency virus (HIV). Worldwide, 40 million people have been infected since the AIDS epidemic began, and 28 million of these live in sub-Saharan Africa." MSF (Médecins Sans Frontières), "The Campaign/Target Diseases: HIV/AIDS" (2004).

6. It covers the period between 1999 and 2002.

7. Based upon diagnoses in the thirty-two states with confidential name-based HIV reporting.

8. Nature Publishing Group, news@nature.com; at http://news.nature.com//news/2004/041229/nm0105-5b.html (accessed May 8, 2004).

9. Antony Barnett, "Special Investigation: UK Firm Tried HIV Drug on Orphans: GlaxoSmithKline Embroiled in Scandal in Which Children Were Allegedly Used as 'Laboratory Animals,' " *Observer News* (London), April 4, 2004, p. 2.

10. Liam Scheff, "The House That AIDS Built," *New York Press,* January 28, 2004.

11. Ibid.

12. Jamie Doran, "Guinea Pig Kids," BBC: *This World,* November 30, 2004; transcript at http://news.bbc.co.uk/1/shared/spl/hi/programmes/this_world (accessed April 2006).

13. Sixty-three percent of infected white patients, but only 48 percent of black patients, were offered the antiretroviral drugs. Malcolm Gladwell, "Many Maryland AIDS Patients Not Getting Helpful Drug," *Washington Post,* May 16, 1991, p. A21; see also Richard D. Moore et al., "Racial Differences in the Use of Drug Therapy for HIV Disease in an Urban Community," *The New England Journal of Medicine* 330, no. 11 (1994): 763–768.

14. S. B. Thomas and S. C. Quinn, "The Tuskegee Syphilis Study, 1932 to 1972: Implications for HIV Education and AIDS Risk Education Programs in the Black Community," *American Journal of Public Health* 81, no. 11 (1991): 1498–1505.

15. Ibid.

16. Hanna Rosin, "The Homecoming," *The New Republic,* June 5, 1995.

17. David Perlman, "New Study on How AZT Affects Minorities," *San Francisco Chronicle,* April 17, 1991, p. A13: "The four-year VA study involved 338 people infected with the AIDS virus who did not yet have any symptoms. It showed that early treatment with AZT could effectively delay the onset of the disease in all the participants, but when the VA researchers divided their findings into two population groups—one white and the other all the minorities lumped together—they reported that AZT seemed significantly less effective for the minorities."

18. Linda Villarosa, "Despite Need for H.I.V. Vaccines, Fear Mutes Call for Volunteers," *New York Times,* May 27, 2003, p. 5.

19. There are precedents for investing in vaccines that have been shown to work only in discrete groups. For example, trials revealed that a recent experimental herpes vaccine protects women well, but not men.

20. The p-value is <0.02. See Patricia Kahn, "VaxGen: Are There Hints of Race-Based Effects?" *IAVI Report* 7, no. 1 (February–April 2003).

21. Lawrence K. Altman, "Official Hopes to Explain AIDS Vaccine Disparities," *New York Times,* February 25, 2003, p. 1A.

22. Lawrence K. Altman and Andrew Pollack, "Large Trial Finds AIDS Vaccine Fails to Stop Infection," *New York Times,* February 23, 2003, p. A24: ". . . 5.8 percent of those who received the placebo became infected over the course of the trial, compared with 5.7 percent of those who received the vaccine. The difference was not statistically significant."

23. Villarosa, "Despite Need for H.I.V. Vaccines, Fear Mutes Call for Volunteers."

CHAPTER 14: THE MACHINE AGE

1. The heart had been modified from an earlier version with which celebrated patient volunteer Robert Tools had been implanted.

2. Sheryl Gay Stolberg, "On Medicine's Frontier: The Last Journey of James Quinn," *New York Times,* October 8, 2002, p. D1.

3. Ibid.

4. "Artificial Heart Recipient's Widow Settles," Associated Press, June 14, 2003.

5. Paul D. Simmons, "The Artificial Heart: How Close Are We, and Do We Want

to Get There?" *Journal of Law, Medicine and Ethics* 29, no. 3–4 (Fall–Winter, 2001): 401–406.

6. Kevin A. Schulman, M.D., et al., "The Effect of Race and Sex on Physicians' Recommendations for Cardiac Catheterization," *The New England Journal of Medicine* 340, no. 8 (1999): 618–626.

7. "Death Linked to Heart Device Probed," *Newsday,* September 29, 2004, p. 33.

8. "Cor Artificial-Heart Patient Dies; Trial Nearly Complete" [describes the death of the fourteenth AbioCor artificial-heart subject], *American City Business Journals, Inc.,* 2004.

9. Lindsey Tanner, "Artificial Blood Tested Without Consent," Loyola University Medical Center (Chicago), February 20, 2004; at www.luhs.org (accessed March 8, 2004).

10. Hemoglobin is the oxygen-carrying protein that enables blood to disseminate oxygen throughout the body.

11. W. Osler Abbott, M.D., "The Problem of the Professional Guinea Pig," *Proceedings of the Charaka Club* 10 (1941): 249–260, 253. See also Abbott, *Technique Book for Small Intestinal Studies, 1935–1941.*

12. T. Grier Miller and W. Osler Abbott, "Intestinal Intubation: A Practical Technique," *American Journal of Medical Science* 187 (1934): 595–599; see also Abbott, "The Problem of the Professional Guinea Pig," pp. 250–251.

13. Hans Zinsser, *As I Remember Him: The Biography of R.S.* (Boston: Little, Brown, 1944), pp. 310–311.

14. John O'Neill and Robert Haupt, "Harry Bailey: A Sadist Dressed Up as a Doctor, Or Just Insane?" *Sydney Morning Herald,* August 6, 1988, p. 8.; see also Deborah Cameron and Philip Shenon, "The CIA Link to Deep-Sleep Research," *New York Times/Sydney Morning Herald,* October 8, 1988. And see Brian Stagoll, "One Flew over the Cuckoo's Nest," *Australian and New Zealand Journal of Psychiatry* 37, no. 1 (February 2003): 118.

15. M. H. Pappworth, *Human Guinea Pigs: Experimentation on Man* (Boston: Beacon Press, 1967), pp. 24–25. Maurice H. Pappworth was an English physician whose tome *Human Guinea Pigs* detailed human medical experimentation in greater detail than did the celebrated but more circumspect Boston whistleblower Dr. Henry K. Beecher. Beecher had written a similar exposé of medical research abuse for *The New England Journal of Medicine* in 1966. However, unlike Beecher, Pappworth names names, indicating which physicians performed suspicious experiments, which journals published them, and which groups—students, blacks, children, etc.—were victimized.

CHAPTER 15: ABERRANT WARS

1. Surveys consistently rank George Washington Carver above other American-born scientists in recognition and popularity, and second internationally only to Albert Einstein. In a *People* magazine survey, Carver even outscored such international giants as Louis Pasteur.

2. *Final Report of the Senate Select Committee to Study Governmental Operations with Respect to Intelligence Activities,* book 1, p. 360, April 26, 1976, pp. 522–523.

3. Ibid.

4. Ibid.

5. News accounts often confused not only the Carver Village sites discussed above but also the Florida towns of Carver Village in Broward County and Carver in northern Sumter County. Despite claims in some news accounts, no original evidence has ever been offered for mosquito releases in the latter, northernmost Carver.

6. The *Atlanta Journal* and *Constitution* have since been consolidated into the *Atlanta Journal and Constitution*.

7. Kathy Trocheck, "Savannah Residents Angered by Army's '56 Mosquito Test," *Atlanta Journal*, November 10, 1980.

8. Stephen Lyon Endicott and Edward Hagerman, *The United States and Biological Warfare: Secrets from the Early Cold War and Korea* (Bloomington: Indiana University Press, 1998), p. 142: "The September 1975 Congressional hearings into the activities of the CIA held in the wake of the Watergate scandal that disgraced President Richard Nixon did something to lift the veil of secrecy. The Washington hearings revealed that the CIA had stockpiled substances that cause tuberculosis, anthrax, encephalitis, Rift Valley fever, salmonella, botulism, and smallpox. CIA director William E. Colby told the Congressional hearing that the agency had records of its biological warfare activities going back to 1952, but that now 'the records are very incomplete,' because some documents were destroyed in 1972–73. In response to further questioning, he hedged, stating that he was 'very unsure' of the total destroyed, 'since the agency did not keep an inventory of it.' "

9. Untitled brief, *New York Times*, October 8, 1979, p. 4; see also Bill Richards, "Report Suggests CIA Involvement in Fla. Illness," *Washington Post*, December 17, 1979: "American Citizens for Honesty in Government, a branch of Church of Scientology, reveals Army Chemical Corps used contaminated homing pigeons and turkey feathers in biological warfare tests on oat crops in Watertown, NY, area and in Virgin Islands in '50. Reports that at least 1 test caused the oat crops to be infected with cereal rust, a destructive grain disease. Experiments and effects described. Army silent on reports."

10. *Washington Post*, December 17, 1979, p. A18; Bill Richards, "Report Suggests CIA Involvement in Fla. Illness."

11. Eugene Meyer, "Md. Forest Sprayed in 1969 Tests; Eastern Shore Was Sprayed in Army Tests; Eastern Shore Area Was Used 115 Times to Measure Fallout," *Washington Post*, October 14, 1980, p. C1.

12. Jonathan B. Tucker and Amy Sands, "An Unlikely Threat," *Bulletin of the Atomic Scientists* 55, no. 4 (1999): 46–52.

13. Endicott and Hagerman, *The United States and Biological Warfare*, p. 119.

14. Gavin Cameron, Jason Pate, and Kathleen M. Vogel, "Planting Fear: How Real Is the Threat of Agricultural Terrorism?" *Bulletin of the Atomic Scientists* 57, no. 5 (2001): 38–44.

15. American Citizens for Honesty in Government, "Third Research Report on Chemical and Biological Warfare Testing Involving Human Subjects: Open Air Testing of Biological Agents by the CIA—1955" (1979).

16. Despite this declaration, the United States used napalm in the 1960s and 1970s, ostensibly as a defoliant, but in effect as a lethal biological agent against Vietnamese civilians.

17. Robert Parks, "The Development of Segregation in US Army Hospitals," *Military Affairs* 37, no. 4 (1973): 145–150.

18. Cameron, Pate, and Vogel, "Planting Fear."

19. Tucker and Sands, "An Unlikely Threat," pp. 46–52; see also Jose Vegar, "Terrorism's New Breed: Are Today's Terrorists More Likely to Use Chemical and Biological Weapons?" *Bulletin of the Atomic Scientists* 54, no. 2 (1998): 50–55.

20. Ibid.

21. Tucker and Sands, "An Unlikely Threat."

22. Ibid.

23. In ibid., Tucker and Sands note that "in 1997, however, the FBI opened 74 investigations involving CBW and nuclear materials, and in 1998 it launched 181 investigations. Nevertheless, about 80 percent of these cases turned out to be hoaxes and the remainder were threats, small-scale attacks, and failed attempts at delivery." This, of course, means that 20 percent, or one in five cases investigated, were not hoaxes but actual plans or attempts to mount attacks using biological and chemical agents. The attempts failed because, like the Covenant attack discussed above, they were intercepted by law enforcement action, not through any change of heart on the part of the terrorists.

24. Dan Rosenheck, "WMDs: The Biggest Lie of All; Chemical and Biological Weapons Are a Red Herring. They Are Banned Because They Provide Low-Cost Defence to Poor Nations. Cluster Bombs Are Just as Lethal," *New Statesman,* August, 2003.

25. Jeffrey W. Almond, "Understanding the Molecular Basis of Infectious Disease: Implications for Biological Weapons Development," in *The Devil's Brew I: Chemical and Biological Weapons and Their Delivery Systems,* edited by R. Ranger (Lancaster, UK: Bailrigg Publications, 1996), pp. 39–42.

26. These were followed by more recent efforts to bomb New York's Lincoln Tunnel and a plot—foiled in July 2002—for a rush-hour bombing of a Brooklyn subway station.

27. Marilyn W. Thompson, "Survivor, Brentwood; Leroy Richmond Was Hit with a Biological Weapon in the Line of Duty. His Experience Just Might Be Instructive," *Washington Post Magazine,* March 30, 2003, p. W18. See also Shankar Vedantam and Mary Pat Flaherty, "CDC Rushed Paperwork for Anthrax Vaccinations; 48 Congressional Aides Received Inoculations," *Washington Post,* December 22, 2001, p. 10.

28. Alan Hughes, "Cures for the Privileged? (Newspoints/Washington Report)," *Black Enterprise,* January, 2002, p. 19.

29. Ibid.

30. Bob Woodward and Dan Eggen, "US, FBI and CIA Suspect Domestic Extremists: Officials Doubt Any Links to Bin Laden," *Washington Post,* October 27, 2001, p. A1.

31. Vegar, "Terrorism's New Breed."

32. Ibid.: "The most recent use of chemical weapons was in the 1980s, when the Iraqi army devastated Kurdish villages with chemical attacks."

33. Stephen F. Burgess, Ph.D., and Helen E. Purkitt, Ph.D., "The Rollback of South Africa's Chemical and Biological Warfare Program," Report No. A797704, Air University, Maxwell Air Force Base, AFB AL Center for Aerospace Doctrine Research and Education, April 1, 2001.

34. Ibid.

35. William Finnegan, "The Poison Keeper: Biowarrior, Brilliant Cardiologist, War

Criminal, Spy—Can a Landmark Trial in South Africa Reveal Who Wouter Basson Really Was?" *The New Yorker,* January 15, 2001, p. 58.

36. "Cop Tells of Plan to Poison Chikane's Clothes," *Independent* (Johannesburg), October 21, 2000.

37. Raymond Whitaker, "SA Planned Chemical War on Blacks," *The Independent* (London), June 13, 1998, p. 12: "Hogan Goosen said that during the 1980s Basson often discussed ways to kill then-prisoner Nelson Mandela and Joe Slovo, then leader of the South African Communist Party."

38. Such cosmetic medications already exist, such as those employed in the late 1950s by John Howard Griffin, the white author of *Black Like Me* (Boston: Houghton Mifflin, 1961). Griffin injected himself with chemicals to darken his skin and posed as a black man in order to investigate the racism of the segregated South.

39. Eric Lipton and Kirk Johnson, "A Nation Challenged: The Anthrax Trail; Tracking Bioterror's Tangled Course," *Washington Post,* December 24, 2001, p. A1.

40. Or until 1994; documents do not agree.

41. Max Du Preez, "White Poison: The US Cracks Down on Iraq and Libya over Biological and Chemical Warfare, but Did Not Utter a Word When the Apartheid Regime Did the Same," *The Guardian* (Manchester), August 11, 1998, p. 12; see also Suzanne Daley, "In Support of Apartheid: Poison Whisky and Sterilization," *New York Times,* June 11, 1998, p. A3.

42. See Finnegan, "The Poison Keeper."

43. Marlene Burger and Peta Thornycroft, "Larry the Chemical Charlatan and the Teabags of Death," *Independent* (Johannesburg), March 17, 2000.

44. The military-run Roodeplaat Research Laboratory was part of South Africa's chemical weapons program.

45. Burger and Thornycroft, "Larry and the Teabags of Death."

46. Carl A. Larson, "Ethnic Weapons," *Military Review,* vol. 50, no. 11 (November 1970): 3.

47. Department of Defense, Senate Select Committee on Health and Scientific Research, "Biological Testing Involving Human Testing." The report characterized the United States not as an architect of genocidal bioterrorism but as complicit, claims that are supported by some U.S. scientists' own admissions.

48. See Chandré Gould, "Unwrapping Project Coast: Lessons to Be Learnt from the Exposure of South Africa's Chemical and Biological Programme" (an extract from M. Burger and C. Gould, *Secrets and Lies: Wouter Basson and South Africa's Chemical and Biological Warfare Programme,* Zebra, Cape Town, 2002, Chapter 1), presented to the FOIP (Freedom of Information Programme) Conference: Unlocking South Africa's Nuclear Past, 31 July 2002, at www.wits.ac.za/saha/publications_01.htm.

49. Although the BMA report, "Biotechnology, Weapons and Humanity," made no direct charge, it concluded: "Weapons could theoretically be developed which affect particular versions of genes clustered in specific ethnic or family groups."

50. Antony Barnett, "Police Sniff Out the Mother of All Stink Bombs," *The Observer* (London), February 24, 2002, p. 7.

51. As explained earlier, this gene confers susceptibility to the *P. vivax* strain of malaria.

52. Vegar, "Terrorism's New Breed"; see also Mark Wheelis and Malcolm Dando, "Back to Bioweapons?" *Bulletin of the Atomic Scientists* 59, no. 1 (2003): 40–46.

53. Dean E. Murphy, "U.S. Had Role in S. African Biological Warfare, Witness Alleges," *Los Angeles Times,* August 1, 1998; see also De Wet Potgieter, "Apartheid's Poison Legacy: South Africa's Chemical and Biological Warfare Program" (2001), and Pat Sidley, "South Africa's Doctors Apologise for Apartheid Years," *British Medical Journal* 311, no. 6998 (1995): 148.

54. Interview with Daan Goosen, WGBH/*Frontline* (c. 1998).

55. Whitaker, "SA Planned Chemical War on Blacks."

56. After the U.S. anthrax attacks, at the urging of American friends, Daan Goosen approached the U.S. Department of Defense with an offer of "open cooperation" in sharing Project Coast's extensive research in anthrax vaccines and novel antidotes known as antisera.

57. Joby Warrick and John Mintz, "Lethal Legacy: Bioweapons for Sale: U.S. Declined South African Scientist's Offer on Man-Made Pathogens," *Washington Post,* April 20, 2003, p. A1.

58. Pat Sidley, "South African Doctors Demand Action on 'Unethical' Colleagues," *British Medical Journal* (News), September, 1999.

59. Pat Sidley, untitled article, *British Medical Journal,* September 4, 1999.

60. Zelda Venter, "South Africa's 'Dr. Death' Cleared of Murder by Apartheid Era Judge," *The Independent* (London), April 12, 2002, p. 14.

61. Chris McGreal, "Real Lives: Whiter Than White: This Man Is Charged with Murdering 46 Black People by Using Them as Guinea Pigs for South Africa's Secret Chemical and Biological Warfare Project. The Court Is Due to Deliver Its Verdict Today but He Will Probably Go Free," *The Guardian* (London), April 11, 2002, p. 6.

62. Burgess and Purkitt, "The Rollback of South Africa's Chemical and Biological Warfare Program," p. 1181; Venter, "South Africa's 'Dr. Death' Cleared of Murder by Apartheid Era Judge."

63. "Human Rights and Freedoms: Bringing About Reform Through Investigations of Corruption and Violations of Personal Freedoms," *Church of Scientology International,* March 5, 1980.

64. Author's interview with Dorothy Pelote (2003); author's interview with Dorothy Pelote (2005).

65. U.S. Senate, Ninety-fifth Congress, Hearings before the Subcommittee on Health and Scientific Research of the Committee on Human Resources, Biological Testing Involving Human Subjects by the Department of Defense, 1977; released as *U.S. Army Activities in the U.S. Biological Warfare Programs,* February 24, 1977. These hearings confirmed that between 1949 and 1969, the government released biological agents on nearly 240 residential areas, including neighborhoods in San Francisco, Washington, D.C., Minneapolis, and St. Louis.

EPILOGUE: MEDICAL RESEARCH WITH BLACKS TODAY

1. Lars Noah, "Informed Consent and the Elusive Dichotomy Between Standard and Experimental Therapy," *American Journal of Law and Medicine,* Winter, 2002.

2. Jan-Bart Gewald, *Herero Heroes: A Socio-Political History of the Herero of Namibia, 1890–1923* (Columbus: Ohio University Press, 1999).

3. For a revelatory discussion of white U.S. researchers' attitudes toward and treatment of subjects in Puerto Rico, see Susan E. Lederer, "Porto Ricochet: Joking About Germs, Cancer and Race Extermination in the 1930s," *American Literary History* 4, no. 4 (Winter 2002): 720–746.

4. "Bushmen May Hold Weight Loss Secrets," *CBS Evening News with John Roberts* (2002).

5. Jay Katz, *Experimentation with Human Beings: The Authority of the Investigator, Subject Professions, and State in the Human Experimental Process.* (New York: Russell Sage Foundation, 1972), pp. 663–664.

6. "Vaniqa," Medline; at http://www.nlm.nih.gov/medlineplus/druginfo/uspdi/500227.html (accessed January 2, 2006); see also Don McNeil, Jr., "Profits on Cosmetic Save a Cure for Sleeping Sickness," *New York Times,* February 9, 2001, p. A1.

7. Thalidomide references: "The Return of Thalidomide" (editorial), *New York Times,* September 24, 1997; March of Dimes Birth Defects Foundation Thalidomide, at www.marchofdimes.com/pnhec/159_529.asp, (accessed May 21, 2005); see also "TVAC Position Regarding the Return of Thalidomide," The Thalidomide Victims Association of Canada Web site, at www.thalidomide.ca.

8. IPS-Inter Press Service/Global Information Network, "Nigeria: Lawsuit Revived Against U.S. Company over Testing," October 14, 2003; Muyiwa Adeyemi, "Niger Suspends Boycott," *Guardian,* February 28, 2004; see also George J. Annas, "Faith (Healing), Hope and Charity at the FDA: The Politics of AIDS Drug Trials," 34 VILE. L. REV. (1989), pp. 771, 772, see also 21 CFR [section] 312.34(c) and 21 USC [section] 360bbb (2000).

9. Organisation for Economic Co-operation and Development, "Addressing Africa's Health Workforce Crisis: An Avenue for Action; and Health Workforce Challenges: Lessons from Country Experiences"; see also Clare Nullis-Kapp, "Health Worker Shortage Could Derail Development Goals (News)," *Bulletin of the World Health Organization* 83, no. 1 (January 2005): 5–7.

10. John Murphy, "Polio: A Scourge of the Mid-20th Century Eludes Global Eradication and Begins to Spread as Fearful Nigerians Shun Vaccination," *Baltimore Sun,* January 4, 2004, p. 1A.

11. Sana Loue and David Okello, "Research Bioethics in the Ugandan Context II: Procedural and Substantive Reform," *American Society of Law, Medicine and Ethics* 28, no. 165 (2000).

12. Francis Moore, "Letter to Jay Katz, September 2 1964," reprinted in Katz, *Experimentation with Human Beings,* p. 663.

13. Gina Kolata, "FDA Expands Medical Experimentation; Patients' Consent Not Required," *New York Times,* November 5, 1996. See also section 46.101(i), a waiver of the applicability of the 45 CFR Part 46; Norman Fost, "Waived Consent for Emergency Research," *American Journal of Law and Medicine* 24, no. 163 (Summer–Fall, 1998).

14. Rick Weiss, "Volunteers at Risk in Medical Studies; Complex Research Projects Strain System of Safeguards," *Washington Post* (series: Science on the Ethical Frontier), August 1, 1998, p. 41.

15. Fost, "Waived Consent for Emergency Research"; Michelle H. Biros et al., "Informed Consent in Emergency Research: Consensus Statement from the Coalition Conference of Acute Resuscitation and Critical Care Researchers," *Journal of the American Medical Association* 273 (1995): 1283, 1286; Charles Marwick, "Re-

search in Emergency Circumstances," *Journal of the American Medical Association* 273 (1995): 687–688.

16. Annas, "Protecting Soldiers."

17. Eliot Marshal, "Research Ethics: NIH Examines Standards for Consent," *Science*, June 12, 1998, p. 1688; see also "Protection of Human Subjects; Informed Consent," 60 *Federal Register* 49,086 (September 21, 1995).

BIBLIOGRAPHY

BOOKS

Ackerknecht, Erwin H. *Medicine at the Paris Hospital*. Baltimore: Johns Hopkins University Press, 1967.

Anderson, John Q., and Henry Clay Lewis. *Louisiana Swamp Doctor*. Baton Rouge: Louisiana State University Press, 1962.

Annas, George J. *The Rights of Patients* 3rd ed. Carbondale: Southern Illinois University Press, 2004.

———and Michael A. Grodin. *The Nazi Doctors and The Nuremberg Code: Human Rights in Human Experimentation*. New York: Oxford University Press, 1992.

Altman, L. K. *Who Goes First? The Story of Self-Experimentation in Medicine*. New York: Random House, 1987.

Barnes, J. *The Darkey Phrenologist: A Nigger Absurdity in One Act*. New York: Dick & Fitzgerald, 1826.

Baugh, John. *Out of the Mouths of Slaves: African American Language and Educational Malpractice*. Austin: University of Texas Press, 1999.

Beauchamp, Tom L., and James F. Childress. *Principles of Biomedical Ethics*. 5th ed. Oxford, England: Oxford University Press, 2001.

Beaumont, William. *Experiments and Observations on the Gastric Juice and the Physiology of Digestion*. New York: Dover, 1833.

Benton, Joel. *Life of Hon. Phineas T. Barnum, Comprising His Boyhood Youth, Vicissitudes of Early Life . . . His Genius, Wit, Generosity, Elegance, Christianity, &c., &c., . . . as Told by Joel Benton, Esq.* Philadelphia: Edgewood, 1891.

Bergman, J. P. *Ota Benga: The Man Who Was Put on Display in the Zoo!* 2000. At www.onehumanrace.com/docs/ota_benga.asp (accessed September 18, 2001).

Bernard, C. *An Introduction to the Study of Experimental Medicine*. New York: Dover, 1957.

Blakeley, R. L., and Judith M. Harrington. *Bones in the Basement: Postmortem Racism in Nineteenth-Century Medical Training*. Washington, D.C., and London: Smithsonian Institution Press, 1997.

Bogdan, R. *Freak Show: Presenting Human Oddities for Amusement and Profit*. Chicago and London: University of Chicago Press, 1988.

Borgaonkar, Digamber S. *Chromosomal Variation in Man: A Catalog of Chromosomal Variants and Anomalies.* New York: Liss, 1994.

Bowman, J., M.D., and Robert F. Murray, Jr., M.D., M.S. *Genetic Variation and Disorders in People of African Origin.* Baltimore: Johns Hopkins University Press, 1990.

Bradford, Phillip Verner, and Harvey Blume. *Ota Benga: The Pygmy in the Zoo.* New York: St. Martin's Press, 1992.

Braithwaite, Ronald L., and Sandra E. Taylor. *Health Issues in the Black Community.* San Francisco: Jossey-Bass, 1992.

Brandt, Allan M. *No Magic Bullet? A Social History of Venereal Disease in the United States Since 1880.* New York: Oxford University Press, 1985.

Brown, Henry Box. *Narrative of the Life of Henry Box Brown, Written by Himself.* New York: Oxford University Press, 2002.

Browne, Martha Griffith. *Autobiography of a Female Slave.* New York: Redfield, 1857.

Buckingham, James Silk. *America: Historical and Descriptive.* Vol. 1. London: Fisher, Son & Co., 1841.

Clay, H. L. *Odd Leaves from the Life of a Louisiana Swamp Doctor.* Baton Rouge: Louisiana State University Press, 1997.

Cramer, Clayton E. *Black Demographic Data, 1790–1860: A Sourcebook.* Westport, CT: Greenwood Press, 2003. At http://www.ggnra.org/cramer (accessed May 8, 2001).

Curtin, Philip D. *The Atlantic Slave Trade: A Census.* Madison: University of Wisconsin Press, 1969.

Dain, B. *A Hideous Monster of the Mind: American Race Theory in the Early Republic.* Cambridge, MA: Harvard University Press, 2002.

Darwin, C. *On the Origin of Species by Means of Natural Selection, or the Preservation of Favoured Races in the Struggle for Life.* London: John Murray, 1859.

DeBow, J. D. B. *Statistical View of the United States.* Washington, D.C.: J.D.B. DeBow, 1854.

Douglass, Frederick, J. W. Blassingame, J. R. McKivigan, P. P. Hinks, and G. Fulkerson. *Narrative of the Life of Frederick Douglass, an American Slave.* New Haven: Yale University Press, 2001.

Estes, Mathew. *A Defence of Negro Slavery, as It Exists in the United States.* Montgomery: Press of the University of Alabama Journal, 1846.

Falconbridge, A. *Black Voyage—Eyewitness Accounts of the Atlantic Slave Trade.* Boston: Little, Brown, 1788.

Fauci, Anthony, ed. *Harrison's Principles of Internal Medicine.* New York: McGraw-Hill, 1998.

Foucault, M. *The Birth of the Clinic: An Archaeology of Medical Perception.* New York: Vintage, 1973.

Fry, Gladys-Marie. *Night Riders in Black Folk History.* Chapel Hill and London: University of North Carolina Press, 2001.

Gardiner, Frederick, M.D., *A Mormon Rebel: The Life and Travels of Frederick Gardiner.* Family History Records, Family Ancestral File No. 477D–4H, Pedigree Chart. Historical Department, Church of Jesus Christ of Latter-day Saints, Salt Lake City.

Gilman, S. L. *Difference and Pathology: Stereotypes of Sexuality, Race and Madness.* Ithaca, NY: Cornell University Press, 1985.

Gordon, L. *Woman's Body, Woman's Right: A Social History of Birth Control in America.* New York: Penguin, 1990.

Gordon, M. B. B. *Aesculapius Comes to the Colonies.* Ventnor, NJ: Ventnor, 1949.

Gosney, E. S., and Paul Popenoe. *Sterilization for Human Betterment.* New York: Macmillan, 1930.

Gould, S. J. *The Flamingo's Smile: Reflections in Natural History.* New York and London: W. W. Norton & Company, 1985.

———. *The Mismeasure of Man.* New York and London: W. W. Norton & Company, 1992.

Greer, Germaine. *Sex and Destiny: The Politics of Human Fertility.* New York: Harper & Row, 1984.

Guthrie, Robert V. *Even the Rat Was White: A Historical View of Psychology.* 2nd ed. Boston: Allyn and Bacon, 1998.

Haeckel, E. *The History of Creation.* London: Trübner, 1906.

Harris, Seale, M.D. *Women's Surgeon: The Life Story of J. Marion Sims.* New York: Macmillan, 1950.

Hartmann, B. *Reproductive Rights and Wrongs: The Global Politics of Population Control.* Boston: South End Press, 1995.

Hödl, Klaus. *Gesunde Juden—Kranke Schwarze: Körperbilder im Medizinischen Diskurs.* Berlin: Studien Verlag, 2002.

Hornblum, A. M. *Acres of Skin: Human Experiments at Holmesburg Prison.* New York: Routledge, 1998.

Jacobs, H. A. *Incidents in the Life of a Slave Girl Written by Herself* (Enlarged edition). Cambridge, MA, and London: President and Fellows of Harvard College, 1987.

Jefferson, Thomas. *Notes on the State of Virginia.* Paris: privately published, 1783.

Jones, J. H., and Tuskegee Institute. *Bad Blood: The Tuskegee Syphilis Experiment.* New York and London: Free Press, 1981.

Kalish, Richard A., and David K. Reynolds. *Death and Ethnicity: A Psychocultural Study.* Los Angeles: University of Southern California Press, 1976.

Katz, J., M.D. *Experimentation with Human Beings: The Authority of the Investigator, Subject Professions, and State in the Human Experimentation Process.* New York: Russell Sage Foundation, 1972.

Kevles, Daniel. *In the Name of Eugenics.* Cambridge, MA: Harvard University Press, 1995.

Kiple, K. F., and Virginia H. King. *Another Dimension to the Black Diaspora: Diet, Disease and Racism.* Cambridge, England: Cambridge University Press, 1981.

Knox, Robert. *The Races of Man: A Fragment.* London: Henry Renshaw, 1850.

Lederer, Susan E. *Subjected to Science: Human Experimentation in America Before the Second World War.* Baltimore: Johns Hopkins University Press, 1995.

Leopold, Nathan Freudenthal. *Life Plus 99 Years.* Garden City, NY: Doubleday, 1958.

Lewis, H. C., with Felix Octavius Carr Darley, illustrator. *The Swamp Doctor's Adventures in the South-West. Containing the Whole of the Louisiana Swamp Doctor; Streaks of Squatter Life; and Far-Western Scenes; in a Series of Forty-Two Humorous Southern and Western Sketches, Descriptive of Incidents and Character.* Chapel Hill: Academic Affairs Library, University of North Carolina, 1998, reprinted 2004.

Lewis, Julian Herman, *The Biology of the Negro.* Chicago: University of Chicago Press, 1942.

Lewis, Sinclair. *Arrowsmith.* New York: Harcourt, Brace, 1945.

Linnaeus, C. *Systemae Naturae per Regna Tria Naturae, Secundum Classes, Ordines, Genera, Species, cum Characteribus, Differentiis, Synonymis, Locis.* Stockholm: Laurentii Salvii, 1735.

Lusane, C. *Hitler's Black Victims: The Historical Experience of Afro-Germans, European Blacks, Africans and African Americans in the Nazi Era.* New York: Routledge, 2000.

Martin, C. D. *The White African American Body: A Cultural and Literary Exploration.* New Brunswick, NJ: Rutgers University Press, 2002.

Martineau, Harriet. *Retrospect of Western Travel.* Armonk, NY: M. E. Sharpe, 2000.

McGregor, D. K. *From Midwives to Medicine: The Birth of American Gynecology.* New Brunswick, NJ: Rutgers University Press, 1998.

McKitrick, E. L. *Slavery Defended: The Views of the Old South.* Englewood Cliffs, NJ: Prentice-Hall, 1963.

Miller, Judith, et al. *Germs: Biological Weapons and America's Secret War.* New York: Touchstone, 2002.

Mills, Kay. *This Little Light of Mine: The Life of Fannie Lou Hamer.* New York: Plume, 1994.

Mitford, Jessica. *Kind and Usual Punishment: The Prison Business.* New York: Alfred A. Knopf, 1972.

Morais, H. M. *The History of the Afro-American in Medicine.* Cornwell Heights, PA: The Publishers Agency, Inc., 1979.

Numbers, R. L., and Todd L. Savitt. *Science and Medicine in the Old South.* Baton Rouge and London: Louisiana State University Press, 1989.

Pappworth, M. H. *Human Guinea Pigs: Experimentation on Man.* Boston: Beacon Press, 1967.

Parran, T. *Shadow on the Land: Syphilis.* New York: Reynal & Hitchcock, 1937.

Pernick, M. S. *The Black Stork: Eugenics and the Death of 'Defective' Babies in American Medicine and Motion Pictures Since 1915.* New York: Oxford University Press, 1996.

Peterson, Merrill D., ed. *Visitors to Monticello.* Charlottesville: University Press of Virginia, 1989.

Rawick, George P., ed. *The American Slave: A Composite Autobiography.* Westport, CT: Greenwood Press 1972.

Regis, Edward. *The Biology of Doom: The History of America's Secret Germ Warfare Project.* New York: Henry Holt, 1999.

Reverby, S. M. *Tuskegee's Truths: Rethinking the Tuskegee Syphilis Study.* Chapel Hill: University of North Carolina Press, 2000.

Roberts, D. *Killing the Black Body; Race, Reproduction, and the Meaning of Liberty.* New York: Vintage, 1997.

Sanger, Margaret. *The Pivot of Civilization.* Project Gutenberg Presents, 1999 (originally published 1922). At http://digital.library.upenn.edu/webbin/gutbook/lookup?num=1689 (accessed June 2, 2005).

Sappol, M. *A Traffic of Dead Bodies: Anatomy and Embodied Social Identity in Nineteenth-Century America.* Princeton, NJ: Princeton University Press, 2001.

Satel, Sally, P.C., M.D. *How Political Correctness Is Crippling Medicine.* New York: Basic Books, 2000.

Savitt, T. L. *Medicine and Slavery: The Diseases and Health Care of Blacks in Ante-bellum Virginia*. Urbana: University of Illinois Press, 1978, reprinted 1992, 2002.

———, ed. *Disease and Distinctiveness in the American South*. Knoxville: University of Tennessee Press, 1988.

Shaw, George Bernard. *The Doctor's Dilemma* (play). New York: Penguin, 1908.

Shryock, R. H. *The Development of Modern Medicine: An Interpretation of the Social and Scientific Factors Involved*. New York: Alfred A. Knopf, 1947.

Sims, J. Marion. *Story of My Life*. New York: D. Appleton, 1884.

Stephens, M. *The Treatment: The Story of Those Who Died in the Cincinnati Radiation Tests*. Durham, NC: Duke University Press, 2002.

Twain, M. *Adventures of Huckleberry Finn*. New York: Random House, 1996.

Veney, B. *The Narrative of Bethany Veney, A Slave Woman, with Introduction by Rev. Bishop Mallalieu and Commendatory Notices from Rev. V. A. Cooper, Superintendent of Home for Little Wanderers, Boston, Mass., and Rev. Erastus Spaulding, Millbury, Mass.* Worcester, MA: George H. Ellis, 1889.

Washington, H. A. *Living Healthy with Hepatitis C*. New York: Ballantine, 2000.

Weld, Theodore D. *American Slavery as It Is: Testimony of a Thousand Witnesses*. New York: Arno Press, 1839, reprinted 1968.

Welsome, Eileen. *The Plutonium Files*. New York: The Dial Press, 1999.

Weyers, Wolfgang. *The Abuse of Man: An Illustrated History of Dubious Medical Experimentation*. New York: Ardor Scribendi, 2003.

Wright, Richard. *American Hunger*. New York: Perennial, 1993.

Yerkes, R., ed. *Psychological Examining in the United States Army*. Washington, D.C.: National Academy of Sciences, 1921.

Zinsser, Hans. *As I Remember Him: The Story of R.S.* Boston: Little, Brown, 1940.

BOOK SECTIONS

Almond, Jeffrey W. "Understanding the Molecular Basis of Infectious Disease: Implications for Biological Weapons Development." In *The Devil's Brew I: Chemical and Biological Weapons and Their Delivery Systems*. Washington, D.C.: Center for Defense and International Studies, 1996.

Borgaonkar, Digamber S. "Cytogenic Screening of Community-Dwelling Males." In *Genetic Issues in Public Health and Medicine*. Edited by Abraham M. Lilienfeld, Bernice H. Cohen, and Pien-Chien Huang. Springfield, Ill: Thomas Publishing, 1978.

———, and Saleem A. Shah. "The XYY Chromosome Male—or Syndrome?" In *Progress in Medical Genetics*, vol. 10 (1974): 135–222. Edited by A. G. Steinberg and A. G. Bearn. New York: Grune, 1974.

Breeden, James O. "Disease as a Factor in Southern Distinctiveness." In *Disease and Distinctiveness in the American South*. Edited by Todd Savitt and James Henry Young. Knoxville: University of Tennessee Press, 1988.

Calhoun, John C. "Disquistion on Government"; "Speech on the Reception of Abolition Petitions"; and "Speech on the Importance of Domestic Slavery." In *Slavery Defended: The Views of the Old South*. Edited by Eric L. McKitrick. Englewood Cliffs, NJ: Prentice-Hall, 1963.

Carrigan, Jo Ann. "Yellow Fever: Scourge of the South." In *Disease and Distinctiveness in the American South.* Edited by Todd Savitt and James Henry Young. Knoxville: University of Tennessee Press, 1988.

Cartwright, Samuel. "The Prognathous Species of Mankind." In *Slavery Defended: The Views of the Old South.* Edited by Eric L. McKitrick. Englewood Cliffs, NJ: Prentice-Hall, 1963.

Combahee River Collective. "A Black Feminist Statement." In *This Bridge Called My Back: Writings by Radical Women of Color.* Edited by Cherrie Moraga and Gloria Anzaldua. Watertown, MA: Persephone Press, 1981.

Cooter, Roger. "The Society for the Social History of Medicine and British Paediatric Association." In *The Name of the Child: Health and Welfare, 1880–1940.* London and New York: Routledge, 1992.

Douglass, Frederick. "The Claims of the Negro, Ethnologically Considered." In *Negro Social and Political Thought, 1850–1920: Representative Texts.* Edited by H. Brotz. New York: Basic Books, 1966.

Griggs, S. "On the Dissection Board." In *Imperium in Imperio,* 139–160. Miami: Mnemosyne Publishers, 1969.

Humphreys, Margaret, "Whose Body? Which Disease? Studying Malaria While Treating Neurosyphilis," in *Useful Bodies: Humans in the Service of Medical Science in the Twentieth Century.* Edited by Jordan Goodman, Anthony McElligott, and Lara Marks. Baltimore: Johns Hopkins University Press, 2003.

Jefferson, Thomas. "Thomas Jefferson to James C. Cabell, May 16." In *Early History of the University of Virginia as Contained in the Letters of Thomas Jefferson and Joseph C. Cabell Hitherto Unpublished.* Edited by Nathaniel F. Cabell. Richmond, VA: J. W. Randolph, 1856.

Mather, Cotton. "The Angel of Bethesda. An Essay upon the Common Maladies of Mankind." In George Lyman Kittredge, *Cotton Mather's Scientific Communications to the Royal Society.* Reprinted from The Proceedings of the American Antiquarian Society. Worcester, MA, 1916.

McGregor, D. K. "Sexual Surgery and the Origins of Gynecology: J. Marion Sims and His Patients." In *Garland Studies in Historical Democracy.* New York: Garland, 1989.

Pernick, M. " 'They Don't Feel It Like We Do': Social Politics and the Perception of Pain." In *A Calculus of Suffering: Pain, Professionalism, and Anesthesia in Nineteenth-Century America,* 148–167. New York: Columbia University Press, 1975.

Semmes, Clovis. "Reconstruction and Freedom's Ironies." In *Racism, Health, and Post-Industrialism: A Theory of African-American Health.* Westport, CT: Praeger, 1996.

Smith, James McCune. "Facts Concerning Free Negroes." In *A Documentary History of the Negro People in the United States.* Edited by Herbert Aptheker. New York: Citadel Press, 1844.

Stevenson, Robert Louis. "The Body Snatcher." In *The Black Man and Other Tales.* New York: Scribner, 1881.

Warner, John Harley. "The Idea of Southern Medical Distinctiveness: Medical Knowledge and Practice in the Old South." In *Sickness and Health in America: Readings in the History of Medicine and Public Health.* Edited by Judith Walzer Leavitt and Ronald L. Numbers. Madison: University of Wisconsin Press, 1985.

Washington, Harriet. "Interview with K. Anthony Appiah." In *The Bell Curve Debate:*

History, Documents, Opinions. Edited by R. Jacoby and N. Glauberman. New York: Random House, 1995.

————. "Stereotyping the Karyotype: A Case History in the Genetics of Aggression." In *Twentieth Century Ethics of Human Subjects Research: Historical Perspectives on Values, Practices and Regulations.* Edited by Volker Roelcke and Giovanni Maio. Stuttgart: Franz Steiner Verlag, 2004.

REPORTS AND LEGAL DOCUMENTS

Advisory Committee on Human Radiation Experiments (ACHRE). Pacific Northwest Research Foundation. "Proposal for Atomic Energy Commission Division of Medicine and Biology." 1963.

————. "DOE Openness: Human Radiation Experiments." Especially chapter 9: History of Prison Research Regulation. 1995.

————. Memorandum to Members of the Advisory Committee on Human Radiation Experiments. 1994.

Ahmann, Rosemary. "National Symposium on Children in Jail." United States Office of Juvenile Justice and Delinquency Prevention, National Coalition for Jail Reform, and University of Illinois at Urbana-Champaign Community Research Forum, 1981.

American Citizens for Honesty in Government. "Third Research Report on Chemical and Biological Warfare Testing Involving Human Subjects: Open Air Testing of Biological Agents by the CIA—1955." 1979.

American Medical Association. "Requirements or Incentives by Government for the User of Long-Acting Contraceptives." Board of Trustees Report. *Journal of the American Medical Association* 267, no. 13 (1992): 1818 (4).

Atomic Energy Commission. "Atomic Energy Commission Document 07075001." 1947.

Bowman, James E. "Genetic Screening Programs and Public Policy." W. E. B. Du Bois Conference on the Health of Black Populations, 1976.

Branson, Herman R. "Producing More Black Doctors: Psychometric Barriers, from a Talk Prepared for the Education Research Center Colloquium." Cambridge, MA: Massachusetts Institute of Technology Education Research Center, 1968.

Burgess. Stephen F., Ph.D., and Helen E. Purkitt, Ph.D. "The Rollback of South Africa's Biological Warfare Program," Montgomery, AL: Air University, Maxwell Air Force Base Center for Aerospace Doctrine Research and Education, 2001.

Burger, Marlene, and Chandré Gould. 2001. "Trial Report: Forty-One; the Chemical and Biological Warfare Research Project." Rondebosch, South Africa: Centre for Conflict Resolution, 2001. At http://ccrweb.ccr.uct.ac.za/archive/cbw/41.html (accessed February 4, 2006).

Centers for Disease Control, NHANES III (National Health and Nutrition Examination Survey). "Viral Hepatitis." 2001.

"Characteristics of Prisoners in State and Federal Correctional Institutions, 1997 [by Sex, Race, Age, Marital Status, Educational Attainment, and Citizenship]." *Sourcebook of Criminal Justice Statistics, 1999.*

Contraceptive Use in the United States, 1982–90. National Center for Health Statistics Advance Data, no. 26045. CFR Subtitle A, Sections 46.103 and 46.107.

Department of Health, Education and Welfare. *Final Report of the Tuskegee Syphilis Study Ad Hoc Advisory Panel.* 1974.

Ericka Grimes v. Kennedy Krieger Institute, Inc. 128 (2000).

National Commission for the Protection of Human Subjects of Biomedical and Behavioral Research. "Report and Recommendations: Research Involving Children." 1977.

National Report Series, Juvenile Justice Bulletin. "Minorities in the Juvenile Justice System—Disproportionate Minority Confinement Often Stems from Disparity at Early Stages of Processing." 1999.

"Proceedings of the National Symposium on Children in Jail." Washington, D.C.: U.S. Department of Justice Office of Juvenile Justice and Delinquency Prevention, 1980.

Reynolds, P. Preston. "The Nuremberg Code, 1946–1949." In *Trials of War Criminals Before the Nürnberg Military Tribunals Under Control Council No. 10.* Washington D.C.: Government Printing Office, 1949–1953.

Senate Select Committee to Study Governmental Operations with Respect to Intelligence Activities. "Final Report," 522–523. 1976.

Smith, Brenda V., and Cynthia Dailard. "Black Women's Health in Custody." In *National Black Women's Health Project Symposium Report.* Washington, D.C., 2003.

Smith, James McCune, M.D. "The Memorial of 1844 to the U.S. Senate." Reproduced in *New York Tribune,* May 5, 1844, and in *The Liberator,* May 31, 1844.

U.S. Department of Energy, Human Radiation Experiments. "Human Radiation Studies: Remembering the Early Years [An Oral History of Health Physicist Karl Z. Morgan, Ph.D.]." 1995.

U.S. Statistical Department. "Compilation of the Enumeration of the Inhabitants and Statistics of the United States, as Obtained at the Department of State, from the Returns of the Sixth Census." 1841.

Washington Office on Haiti and the National Vaccine Information Center. "More Than 2,000 Children in the Port-au-Prince Slum Cité Soleil Were Inoculated with High Doses of Edmonston-Zagreb (EZ)," April 1999.

JOURNAL ARTICLES

Ackerman, Terrence F., Ph.D., and Rebecca P. Winsett, Ph.D. "Ethics and Regulation in Organ Procurement Research." *Progress in Transplantation* 12, no. 4 (2002): 257–265.

Alexander, Caleb, and Ashwini R. Sehgal. "Barriers to Cadaveric Renal Transplantation Among Blacks, Women and the Poor." *Journal of the American Medical Association* 280 (1998): 1148–1152.

Allen, Garland E. "The Eugenics Record Office at Cold Spring Harbor, 1910–1940: An Essay in Institutional History." *Osiris* 2 (2nd series, 1986): 225–264.

Allen, L. C. "The Negro Health Problem." *American Journal of Public Health* 5 (1915): 194–203.

Allen, Lane. "Grandison Harris, Sr., Slave, Resurrectionist and Judge." *Bulletin of the Georgia Academy of Science* 34 (April 1976): 192–199.

Anderson, Warwick. "Immunities of Empire: Race, Disease, and the New Tropical Medicine, 1900–1920." *Bulletin of the History of Medicine* 70, no. 1 (Race and Acclimatization in Colonial Medicine, 1996): 94–118.

Andy, O.J., M.D. "The Treatment of Abnormal Behavior." *American Journal of the Medical Sciences* 252 (August 1966): 232–238.

Annas, George J. "Protecting Soldiers from Friendly Fire: The Consent Requirement for Using Investigational Drugs and Vaccines in Combat." *American Journal of Law and Medicine* (Summer–Fall, 1998).

Baer, Hans A. "Toward a Systematic Typology of Black Folk Healers." *Phylon* 43, no. 4 (1982): 327–343.

Bain, R. P., R. S. Greenberg, and J. P. Whitaker. "Racial Differences in Survival of Women with Breast Cancer." *Journal of Chronic Diseases* 39, no. 8 (1996): 631–642.

Balaban, E., J. S. Alper, and Y. L. Kasamon. "Mean Genes and the Biology of Aggression: A Critical Review of Recent Animal and Human Research." *Journal of Neurogenetics* 11, nos. 1, 2 (1996): 1–43.

Bazelon, E. "Grave Offense." *Legal Affairs* (July–August 2002). At http://www.legal affairs.org/issues/July-August-2002/story_bazelon_julaug2002.html (accessed August 17, 2005).

Begley, Sharon. "Polio Vaccines Given Decades Ago Carried Carcinogenic Virus Sv40," *New York Times Science Journal,* July 19, 2002.

Belzer, Edwin G., Jr., et al. "A Method to Increase Informed Consent in School Health Research." *Journal of School Health* 63, no. 7 (1993): 316(2).

"Birth Control or Race Control? Sanger and the Negro Project." *The Margaret Sanger Papers Project Newsletter,* Fall 2001, at http://www.nyu.edu/projects/sanger/bc_or_race_control.htm.

Bishop, Christopher. "Reviled Zimbabwe Doc Sent to Jail." *British Medical Journal* (1999).

———. "Doctor in Zimbabwe Race Row Out on Bail." *British Medical Journal* (February 11, 1995): 310–350.

Boney, F. N. "Doctor Thomas Hamilton: Two View of a Gentleman of the Old South." *Phylon* 28, no. 3 (1967): 288–292.

Bowser, Rene. "The Degenerate Black Patient, Excerpted from *Racial Bias in Medical Treatment.*" *Dickinson Law Review* (Spring 2001): 365–383.

Boyd, Mark F., and S. F. Kitchen. "Observations on Induced Falciparum." *American Journal of Tropical Medicine* 17 (1937): 213–235.

Brandt, Allan M. "Racism and Research: The Case of the Tuskegee Syphilis Experiment." *Hastings Center Report* 8 (1978): 21–29.

Breeden, J. O. "States-Rights Medicine in the Old South." *Bulletin of the New York Academy of Medicine* 52 (March–April 1976): 348–472.

Brody, Janet L., John P. Gluck, and Alfredo S. Aragon. "Participants' Understanding of the Practice of Psychological Research: Informed Consent." *Ethics and Behavior* 10 (2000): 13–15.

Brown, A. M., M.D. Editorial. *Journal of the National Medical Association* (January 1909): 50–56.

Brown, Anthony J., M.D. "Sexual Intercourse Questioned as Source of Most HIV Infections in Africa." *International Journal for the Study of STDs and AIDS* 14 (2003): 144–173.

Cameron, Gavin, Jason Pate, and Kathleen M. Vogel. "Planting Fear: How Real Is the Threat of Agricultural Terrorism?" *Bulletin of the Atomic Scientists* 57, no. 5 (2001): 38–44.

Campion, Edward W., M.D. "Why Unconventional Medicine?" *The New England Journal of Medicine* 328, no. 4 (1993): 282–283.

"Cardiac Care and Catheterization." *The New England Journal of Medicine* 340 (February 24, 1999): 618–626.

Caron, Simone M. "Birth Control and the Black Community in the 1960s: Genocide or Power Politics?" *Journal of Social History* 31, no. 3 (1998): 25.

Carrigan, Jo Ann. "Yellow Fever in New Orleans, 1853: Abstractions and Realities." *The Journal of Southern History* 25, no. 3 (1959): 339–355.

Cartwright, S. "Report on the Diseases and Physical Peculiarities of the Negro Race." *De Bow's Review Southern and Western States* 7, no. 11 (1851): 692–696.

"The Carver Village Controversy." *Tequesta: The Journal of the Historical Association of Southern Florida* 50 (1990): 39–51.

Charles, McDonald, M.D. "The Contribution of the Tuskegee Study to Medical Knowledge." *Journal of the National Medical Association* 66 (1974): 1–7.

Chasnoff, I. J., H. J. Landress, and M. E. Barrett. "The Prevalence of Illicit-Drug or Alcohol Use During Pregnancy and Discrepancies on Mandatory Reporting in Pinellas County, Florida." *The New England Journal of Medicine* 322 (1990): 1202–1206.

Cherek, D. R. and S. D. Lane. "Effects of D,L-Fenfluramine on Aggressive and Impulsive Responding in Adult Males with a History of Conduct Disorder." *Psychopharmacology* 146 (1999): 473–481.

Clery, Daniel. "Elite Science in a Poor Country." *Science* 268, no. 5215 (1995): 1281.

"Clinical Trial Tales Raise Hackles of HHS, Government Panel." *Medical Industry Today,* June 12, 1998.

Cobb, W. Montague, M.D. "Surgery and the Negro Physician: Some Parallels in Background." *Journal of the National Medical Association* 43, no. 3 (1951): 145–151.

———. "Human Material in American Institutions Available for Anthropological Study." *American Journal of Physical Anthropologists* 17 (suppl., 1933): 1–45.

———. "Municipal History from Anatomical Records." *Scientific Monthly* 40, no. 2 (1935): 157–162.

———. "The Negro as a Biological Element in the American Population." *Journal of Negro Education* 8, no. 3 (1939): 336–348.

———. "Education: Priority Number One." *Phylon* 4, no. 4 (1943): 305–310.

———. "Not to the Swift: Progress and Prospects of the Negro in Science and the Professions." *Journal of Negro Education* 27, no. 1 (1958): 120–126.

"Contraceptive Use in the United States, 1982–90." National Center for Health Statistics Advance Data No. 260 (1995).

Darrity, William A., and Castellano B. Turner. "Fears of Genocide Among Black Americans as Related to Age, Sex, and Region." *American Journal of Public Health* 63 (1973).

———. "Family Planning, Race Consciousness and the Fear of Race Genocide." *American Journal of Public Health* 62 (1972).

Davidson, Stuart N. "The Perilous Pathway from Laboratory to Patient." *The Healthcare Forum Journal* 39, no. 4 (1996): 16.

Deibert, A. V., and M. C. Bruyere. "Untreated Syphilis in the Male Negro. III. Evidence of Cardiovascular Abnormalities and Other Forms of Morbidity." *Journal of Venereal Disease Information* 27 (1936): 301–314.

Deutsch, Albert. "The First U. S. Census of the Insane (1840) and Its Use as Pro-Slavery Propaganda." *Bulletin of the History of Medicine* 15 (1944): 469–482.

Dexter, Aaron, and John Warren. "Memorial & Petition for the Removal of Med. Lect. to Boston," February 20, 1810. John C. Warren papers, Massachusetts Historical Society.

Dingell, John D. "Misconduct in Medical Research." *The New England Journal of Medicine* 328, no. 22 (1993): 1610–1615.

"Do the Dead Tell Tales After All? Colonial-Era Burial Project Provides Clues to Africans' Struggle for Human Rights." *NLM Newsline* 56, no. 1 (January–June 2000), at http://www.nlm.nih.gov/pubs/nlmnews/janjun01/jj01_dead.html (accessed July 10, 2001).

"Dr. Louis T. Wright and the NAACP: Pioneers in Hospital Racial Integration." *American Journal of Public Health* 90, no. 6 (2000): 883–892.

Drake, Daniel. "Diseases of the Negro Population—In a Letter to Rev. Mr. Pinney." *Southern Medical and Surgical Journal,* n. s., 1 (1845): 342.

Drucker, Ernest. "Children of War: The Criminalization of Motherhood." *The International Journal on Drug Policy* 1, no. 4 (1990): 11.

Dublin, L. "The Problem of Negro Health as Revealed by Vital Statistics." *Journal of Negro Education* 6 (1937): 268–275.

Du Bois, W. E. B. "Black Folk and Birth Control." *Birth Control Review* 12, no. 8 (the "Negro Number," 1938): 90.

Duffy, John. "Eighteenth Century Health Conditions." *The Journal of Southern History* 18, no. 3 (1952): 289–302.

———. "Sectional Conflict and Medical Education in Louisiana." *The Journal of Southern History* 23, no. 3 (1957): 289–306.

———. "A Note on Ante-Bellum Southern Nationalism and Medical Practice." *The Journal of Southern History* 34, no. 2 (1968): 266–276.

———. "Medical Practice in the Ante Bellum South." *The Journal of Southern History* 25, no. 1 (1959): 53–72.

Eblen, Jack E. "Growth of the Black Population in Ante Bellum America, 1820–1860." *Population Studies* 26 (1972): 273–289.

Editorial. *Journal of the National Medical Association* 2, no. 2 (1910).

English, W. T. "The Negro Problem from the Physician's Point of View." *Atlanta Journal-Record of Medicine* 5 (October 1903): 461.

Eve, Paul F. "An Essay Read Before the Medical Society of Augusta, January 10, 1839." *Southern Medical and Surgical Journal* 3 (March 1839): 329.

"Eighteenth Century Slaves as Advertised by Their Masters." *Journal of Negro History* 1, no. 2 (1916): 163–216.

Farber, I. E. and Jolydon West, "Brainwashing, Conditioning and DDD." *Sociometry* 20, no. 4 (1957): 271–295.

Farrell, Walter C., and J. Oliver, "Genocide Fears in a Rural Black Population: An Empirical Examination." *Journal of Black Studies* 14, no. 1 (1983): 49–67.

Fenner, E. D. "Dirt-Eating Among Negroes." *Southern Medical Reports* 1, no. 194 (1849): 436.

Ferguson, G. O. "The Intelligence of Negroes at Camp Lee, Virginia." *School and Society* 11, no. 233 (1919): 721–726.

Fisher, Walter. "Physicians and Slavery in the Antebellum Southern Medical Journal." *Journal of the History of Medicine and Allied Sciences* 23 (1968): 145–152.

"Follow-Up of Deaths Among U.S. Postal Service Workers Potentially Exposed to Bacillus Anthracis—District of Columbia, 2001–2002." *MMWR Weekly* 52, no. 39 (October 3, 2002): 937–938.

Fortson, Leigh. "Biomedical Research Warfare." *Black Issues in Higher Education* 16, no. 2 (1999): 24.

Fost, Norman. "Waived Consent for Emergency Research (Law, Medicine and Socially Responsible Research)." *American Journal of Law and Medicine* 24, nos. 2 and 3 (1998): 163–168.

Foster, G. "The Limitations of Federal Health Care for Freedmen, 1860–1868." *The Journal of Southern History* 48 (1982): 349–372.

Fuentes, Annette. "Quick Fix; Pushing a Medical Cure for Youth Violence." *Institute for Public Affairs* 22, no. 15 (1998): 14.

Furr, L. Allen. "Perceptions of Genetics Research as Harmful to Society: Differences Among Samples of African-Americans and European-Americans." *Genetic Testing* 6, no. 1 (2002): 25–31.

Genovese, Eugene D. "The Medical and Insurance Costs of Slaveholding in the Cotton Belt." *Journal of Negro History* 45, no. 3 (1960): 141–155.

Glantz, Leonard H. "Research with Children." *American Journal of Law and Medicine* 24, no. 213 (1998): 238.

Gordon, Robert. "The Venal Hottentot Venus and the Great Chain of Being." *African Studies* 51, no. 2 (1992): 191.

Grand, Jeffrey S. "The Blooding of America: Privacy and the DNA Dragnet." *Cardozo Law Review* 23, no. 6 (2002): 2277–2323.

Graves, Marvin L. "The Negro a Menace to the Health of the White Race." *Southern Medical Journal* 9 (1916): 407–413.

Greenberg, Daniel S. "When Institutional Review Boards Fail the System (News)." Statistical data included. *The Lancet* (May 22, 1999).

Greene, John C. "The American Debate on the Negro's Place in Nature, 1780–1815." *Journal of the History of Ideas* 15, no. 3 (1954): 384–396.

Grill, Johnpeter Horst, and Robert L. Jenkins. "The Nazis and the American South in the 1930s: A Mirror Image?" *The Journal of Southern History* 58, no. 4 (1992): 667–694.

Gurri Glass, Gregory E. "Emerging Infectious Diseases." *MMWR Weekly* 6, no. 3 (March–April 2000).

———, et al. "Using Remotely Sensed Data to Identify Areas at Risk for Hantavirus Pulmonary Syndrome." *MMWR Weekly* 6, no. 3 (March–April 2000).

Haller, J. S. "The Negro and the Southern Physician: A Study of Medical and Racial Attitudes, 1800–1860." *Medical History* 16, no. 3 (July 1972): 238–253.

Haller, John S., Jr. "The Species Problem: Nineteenth-Century Concepts of Racial Inferiority in the Origin of Man Controversy." *American Anthropologist* 72, no. 6 (1970): 1319–1329.

Halsey, R. I. "How the President Thomas Jefferson and Dr. Benjamin Waterhouse Established Vaccination as a Public Health Procedure." *Bulletin of the New York Academy of Medicine* (1936): 58.

Hansen, Arild. "Role of Linoleaic Acid in Infant Nutrition." *Pediatrics* 55, suppl. 1 (part 2, 1963): 170–192.

Harden John M. B., M.D. "Some Experiments to Determine the Relative Areas of the Trunks and Branches of Arteries." *Southern Medical and Surgical Journal, n.s.,* 2 (June 1846): 330–333.

Harris, Juriah. "What Constitutes Unsoundness in the Negro?" *Savannah Journal of Medicine* 1 (1858): 145–152.

Harris, R. P. "The Operation of Gastro-Hysterotomy (True Caesarian Section)." *American Journal of the Medical Sciences, n.s.,* 75 (April 1878): 336–339.

Harris, S. N. "Report on the Treatment of Some Cases of Cholera Occurring on the Savannah River." *Charleston Medical Journal and Review* 4 (1849): 581–585.

Harris, W. T., Jr. (undated memo). "Flash Burn Studies in Volunteers": 1–2.

Heller, J. R., Jr., and P. T. Bruyere. "Untreated Syphilis in the Male Negro: Mortality During 12 Years of Observation." *Journal of Venereal Disease Information* 27 (1946): 34–38.

Herrick, J. B. "Peculiar Elongated and Sickle-Shaped Red Blood Corpuscles in a Case of Severe Anemia." *Archives of Internal Medicine* 6 (1910): 517–521.

Herzig, R. "Removing Roots: North America Hiroshima Maidens and the X-ray." *Technology and Culture* 40, no. 4 (1999): 723–745.

Herzig, Rebecca. "In the Name of Science: Suffering, Sacrifice, and the Formation of American Roentgenology." *American Quarterly* 53, no. 4 (2001): 563–589.

Hornaday, William T. "Suicide of Ota Benga, the African Pygmy." *Zoological Society Bulletin* 19, no. 3 (1916): 1356.

Hornblum, A. M. "They Were Cheap and Available: Prisoners as Research Subjects in Twentieth Century America." *British Medical Journal* 315 (1997): 1435–1441.

Hughes, John S. "Labeling and Treating Black Mental Illness in Alabama, 1861–1910." *The Journal of Southern History* 58, no. 3 (1992): 435–460.

Humphrey, David C. "Dissection and Discrimination: The Social Origin of Cadavers in America, 1760–1915." *Bulletin of the New York Academy of Medicine* 49, no. 9 (1973): 819–827.

Humphreys, Margaret, M.D., Ph.D. "Whose Body? Which Disease? Studying Malaria While Treating Neurosyphilis," lecture delivered Tuesday, December 11, 2001, at the New York Academy of Medicine.

Hunt, James. "On Ethno-Climatology; Or the Acclimatization of Man." *Transactions of the Ethnological Society of London* 2 (1863): 74–75.

"Interview with Daan Goosen, 1998," WGBH/*Frontline*, PBS Online. At www.pbs .org/wgbh/pages/frontline/shows/plague/sa/ (accessed February 6, 2005).

Jarvik, L. F., et al. "Human Aggression and the Extra Y Chromosome: Fact or Fantasy?" *American Psychologist* 28 (1973): 674–682.

Jarvis, E., M. D. "Insanity Among the Coloured Population of the Free States." *American Journal of the Medical Sciences, 1844,* 7 (1843): 74–75.

———. "Preliminary Report." *Boston Medical and Surgical Journal* 27 (1843): 126–132, 281–282.

Johns Hopkins Hospital. "Consent Form for Chromosome Study of Institutionalized Juvenile Delinquents." 1970.

Jones, W. F. "On the Utility of the Applications of Hot Water to the Spine in the Treatment of Typhoid Pneumonia." *Virginia Medical and Surgical Journal* 3 (1854): 108–110.

Kahn, Jonathan, J.D., Ph.D. "How a Drug Becomes 'Ethnic': Law, Commerce, and the Production of Racial Categories in Medicine." *Yale Journal of Health Policy, Law, and Ethics* 4, no. 1 (2004): 1–46.

Kiple, Virginia, and Kenneth Kiple. "The African Connection: Slavery, Disease and Racism." *Phylon* 41, no. 3 (1980): 211–222.

Landenheim, J. C. "The Doctor's Mob of 1877." *Journal of the History of Medicine* 5 (1950): 23–36.

Lederer, Susan E. "Porto Ricochet: Joking About Germs, Cancer, and Race Extermination in the 1930s." *American Literary History* 14, no. 4 (Winter 2002): 720–746.

LeDuc, J. W., J. E. Childs, and G. E. Glass. "The Hantaviruses, Etiologic Agents of Hemorrhagic Fever with Renal Syndrome: A Possible Cause of Hypertension and Chronic Renal Disease in the United States." *Annual Review of Public Health* 13 (1992): 79–98.

Lewis, J. H. "Contribution of an Unknown Negro to Anesthesia." *Journal of the National Medical Association* 23 (1931) 23–24.

Macintosh, J. A. "The Etiology of Granuloma Inguinale." *Journal of the American Medical Association* 87 (1926): 996–1002.

Mall, F. P. "Anatomical Material—Its Collection and Preservation at the Johns Hopkins Anatomical Laboratory." *Bulletin of Johns Hopkins Hospital* 16 (1905): 38–39.

Matas, R. "The Surgical Peculiarity of the Negro: A Statistical Inquiry Based upon the Records of the Charity Hospital of New Orleans (Decennium 1884–1894)." *Transactions of the American Surgical Association* 14 (1894): 485–609.

Mathias, R. "Developmental Effects of Prenatal Drug Exposure May Be Overcome by Postnatal Environment." *NIDA Notes* 14, no. 1 (1992): 14–17.

Mayes, L. C. T. "The Problem of Prenatal Cocaine Exposure: A Rush to Judgment." *Journal of the American Medical Association* 267 (1992): 406.

McGee, W. J. "Anthropology at the Louisiana Purchase Exposition." *Science* 22, no. 573 (Dec. 22, 1905): 811–826.

Mettauer, J. P. "On Vesico-vaginal Fistula." *Boston Medical Journal* 22 (1840): 154–155.

Miller, D. J. F. "The Effects of Emancipation upon the Mental and Physical Qualifications of the Negro in the South." *North Carolina Medical Journal* 38 (1896): 286.

Nott, J. "The Mulatto a Hybrid—Probable Extermination of the Two Races if the Whites and Blacks Are Allowed to Intermarry." *American Journal of the Medical Sciences* 6 (1843): 256.

Reiss, B. "PT Barnum, Joice Heth and the Antebellum Spectacles of Race." *American Quarterly* 51, no. 1 (1999): 78–107.

Rivers, E., et. al. "Twenty Years of Follow Up Experience in a Long Range Medical Study." *Public Health Reports* 68 (1953): 381–395.

Roberts, D. E. "Punishing Drug Addicts Who Have Babies: Women of Color, Equality and the Right of Privacy." *Harvard Law Review* 104, no. 7 (1991): 1419–1482.

Roy, B. "The Tuskegee Syphilis Experiment: Medical Ethics, Constitutionalism, and Property in the Body." *Harvard Journal of Minority Public Health* 1, no. 1 (1995): 11–15.

Rush, Benjamin. "Observations Tended to Favor a Supposition That the Black Color as It Is Called of the Negroes Is Derived from the Leprosy." *Transactions of the American Philosophical Society* 4, no. 9 (1799): 289–297.

Samples, L. T. "Greenbrier County, West Virginia—160th Anniversary Booklet," part 13. At http://ftp.rootsweb.com/pub/usgenweb/wv/greenbrier/history/160th13.txt (accessed May 8, 2001).

Sanger, Margaret. "Birth Control or Race Control? Sanger and the Negro Project." *Margaret Sanger Papers Project Newsletter* 28 (2001).

Savitt, Todd L. "Slave Life Insurance in Virginia and North Carolina." *The Journal of Southern History* 43, no. 4 (1977): 583–600.

———. "The Use of Blacks for Medical Experimentation and Demonstration in the Old South." *The Journal of Southern History* 48, no. 3 (1982): 331–348.

———, and M. F. Goldberg. "Herrick's 1910 Case Report of Sickle Cell Anemia: The Rest of the Story." *Journal of the American Medical Association* 261 (1989): 266–271.

Shryock, R. H. "Medical Sources and the Social Historian." *American Historical Review* 41 (1936): 465.

Sims, J. M. "On the Treatment of Vesico-Vaginal Fistula." *American Journal of the Medical Sciences* 45 (January 1852): 59–82.

Thomas, S. B., and S. C. Quinn, "The Tuskegee Syphilis Study, 1932 to 1972: Implications for HIV Education and AIDS Risk Education Programs in the Black Community." *American Journal of Public Health* 81, no. 11 (1991): 1498–1505.

Tucker, Jonathan B., and Amy Sands. "An Unlikely Threat." *Bulletin of the Atomic Scientists* 55, no. 4 (1999): 46–52.

Van De Wetering, Maxine. "A Reconsideration of the Inoculation Controversy." *The New England Quarterly* 58, no. 1 (1985): 45–46.

Vetter, R. T., M.D. "Vaccines and the Power of Immunity." *Post Graduate Medicine* 101, no. 6 (1997): 154.

Vonderlehr, R. A., T. Clark, O. C. Wenger, and J. R. Heller, Jr. "Untreated Syphilis in the Male Negro: A Comparative Study of Treated and Untreated Cases." *Venereal Disease Information* 17 (1936): 260–265.

Waite, F. C. "Grave Robbing in New England." *Medical Library Association Bulletin* 33 (July 1945): 272–294.

Walker, L. R. "George Pray and the 'Wild, Rude Set of Med Students.' " *Michigan Today* (Grave Images, Fall 1999). At http://www.umich.edu/~newsinfo/MT/99/Fal99/mt1f99d.html (accessed April 17, 2003).

Wall, L. L. "Fitsari 'Dan Duniya: An African (Hausa) Praise Song About Vesicovaginal Fistulas." *Obstetrics and Gynecology* 100, no. 6 (2002): 1328–1332.

Wallis, Brian. "Black Bodies, White Science: The Slave Daguerreotypes of Louis Agassiz. *Journal of Blacks in Higher Education* 12 (1996): 102–6.

Walsh, Catherine, B.S., and Lainie F. Ross, M.D., Ph.D. "Are Minority Children Under- or Overrepresented in Pediatric Research?" *Pediatrics* 112 (2003): 890–895.

Wheelis, Mark, and Malcolm Dando. "Back to Bioweapons?" *Bulletin of the Atomic Scientists* 59, no. 1 (2003): 40–46.

Windley, L. A. "Runaway Slave Advertisements of George Washington and Thomas Jefferson." *Journal of Negro History* 63, no. 4 (1978): 373–374.

Wright, Louis, M.D., 1910–1925. Diary. Louis T. Wright Papers, Manuscript Collections, Moorland-Springarn Research Center, Washington D.C.

Wright, Peter B. "An Unusual Case of Paget's Disease; Presenting an Extraordinary Degree of Osteoblastic Activity." *American Journal of Bone and Joint Surgery* 33, no. A:1 (1951): 239–244.

Zuckerman, B. " 'Crack Kids': Not Broken." *Pediatrics* 89 (1992): 337.

NEWSPAPER AND MAGAZINE ARTICLES

Adams-Wade, Norma. "Slave Passage Estimates Among History's Debated Numbers." *Dallas Morning News*, September 16, 1997.

Ahuja, Anjana. "Pioneer or Sadist? Suspicions Linger About 'Hero': He Developed the Space Suit and Led Studies on Jet Lag. But Did Hubertus Strughold Also Oversee Terrible Experiments on Jews at Dachau to Help His Research?" *The Times* (London), April 2, 2001.

"AIDS Is SA's New Apartheid, Says Tutu." *Independent-Reuters*, October 7, 2001.

"Alabama Prisons to End Drug Tests: 'Substantial Defects' Found in Private Research." *New York Times*, May 31, 1969, p. 32A.

Altman, Lawrence K. "Official Hopes to Explain AIDS Vaccine Disparities." *New York Times*, February 25, 2003, p. A25.

———., and Andrew Pollack. "Large Trial Finds AIDS Vaccine Fails to Stop Infection." *New York Times*, February 23, 2003, p. A1.

Anderson, David C. "When Should Kids Go to Jail?" *The American Prospect*, May–June 1998, p. 72.

"Attempt to Kill a Whole Family." *Provincial Freeman*, 1856.

"Aventis to Donate Sleeping-Sickness Drugs." Reuters News Service, May 3, 2001.

Barnett, Antony. "Special Investigation: UK Firm Tried HIV Drug on Orphans: GlaxoSmithKline Embroiled in Scandal in Which Children Were Allegedly Used as 'Laboratory Animals.' " *The Observer* (London), April 4, 2004, p. 2.

———. "Police Sniff Out the Mother of All Stink Bombs." *The Observer* (London), February 24, 2002, p. 7.

Barrett, George. "Convicts to Get Cancer Injection; 96 at the Ohio State Prison to Aid Fight on Disease; Convicts to Get Cancer Injection to Help Try to Solve the Disease; Live Cells to Be Injected." *New York Times*, May 23, 1956, p. 1.

Barnum, P. T. "Adventures of an Adventurer, Being Some Passages in the Life of Barnaby Diddleum." *New York Atlas* 1841 (series).

Bauer, Diane. "Maryland Tests for Criminal Potential." *Washington Daily Times*, n.d. [c. 1970], p. 7.

———. "XYY Tests Stop." *Washington Daily News*, n.d. [c. 1970], p. 5.

———. "Criminal-Prone Tests Resumed." *Washington Daily News*, n.d. [c. 1970], p. 1.

"Benefits of Slavery." *The Colored American*, n.d. [c. 1838].

Burling, Stacey, "Life, but at What Cost?" *Philadelphia Inquirer*, September 29, 2002.

Buncombe, A. "Nuclear Site Where Deep South's Old Attitudes Live On." *The Independent* (London), August 13, 2002.

Burger, Marlene, and Peta Thornycroft, "Larry and the Teabags of Death." *Independent Online*, March 11, 2000.

"Burking in Baltimore." *The Baltimore Sun*, December 13, 1886.

"Can Contraception Reduce the Underclass? (editorial)." *Philadelphia Inquirer*, December 12, 1990.

"Canada 'Looting' South African Doctors." *Independent Online*, February 14, 2001.

Caruso, David B.. "Inmates Subjected to Medical Tests Lose Bid to Win Compensation." Associated Press, September 25, 2002.

"Circus and Museum Freaks—Curiosities of Pathology." *Scientific American*, March 28, 1908.

Cobb, C. L. "Students Charge BCH's Obstetrics Unit with Excessive Surgery." *Boston Globe,* Month 10, 1972, p. 1A.

Cockburn, Alexander. "Beat the Devil: Karl Popper and the March of Science." *The Nation* 258, no. 4 (1994): 116.

Connolly, Ceci. "Vaccine Plan Revives Doubts on Anthrax Policy." *Washington Post,* December 24, 2001, p. A1.

Davis, Angela. "Masked Racism: Reflections on the Prison Industrial Complex." *Color Lines Magazine* 1, no. 2 (1998): 11.

"Death Linked to Heart Device Probed." *Newsday,* 2004.

DeMuth, J. "Sick and Tired of Being Sick and Tired." *The Nation* 549 (1964): 549–556.

"Do the Dead Tell Tales After All? Colonial-Era Burial Project Provides Clues to Africans' Struggle for Human Rights." *NLM Newsline* 56 (2001).

Dobnik, Verena. "Aggression Study of Kids Assailed; Critics Say Drug Dose Put Minority Boys at Risk." *American Statesman* (Austin), April 18, 1998, p. A2.

Du Preez, Max. "White Poison: The US Cracks Down on Iraq and Libya over Biological and Chemical Warfare, but Did Not Utter a Word When the Apartheid Regime Did the Same." *The Guardian* (Manchester), August 11, 1998, p. 12.

"Edmund Andrews and the Body Snatchers." *Michigan Today,* March, 1999. At www.umich.edu/~newsinfo/MT/99/Fal99/mtlf99b.html (accessed May 3, 2002).

Egelko, Bob. "Inmates Sue State over Health Care; State Hit with Huge Class Action over Health Care in Prisons." *San Francisco Chronicle,* April 6, 2001, p. 3B; at http://www.sfgate.com.

"The Executions at Charleston, Virginia." *The National Era* (Charleston, VA), December 22, 1859.

Finnegan, William. "The Poison Keeper: Biowarrior, Brilliant Cardiologist, War Criminal, Spy—Can a Landmark Trial in South Africa Reveal Who Wouter Basson Really Was?" *The New Yorker,* January 15, 2001.

Frankel, Glenn. "D.C. Neurosurgeon Pioneered 'Icepick' Lobotomy Method," *Washington Post,* April 7, 1980, p. A1.

Gabriel, M. S., M.D. "Ota Benga Having a Fine Time: A Visitor at the Zoo Finds No Reason for Protests About the Pygmy." *New York Times,* September 13, 1906, p. 6.

García-Barrio, C. "African-Americans Under the Big Top." *American Legacy Magazine* (Fall 1999): 338–348.

Gates, William H. "Humane Research." *Wall Street Journal,* January 27, 2003, p. 16A.

Gatty, Bob. "Bill Seeks to Overturn Medical Patents." *Physician's Management* 35 (1995): 27.

Gillon, J. K. "The Story of Burke and Hare"; at http://members.fortunecity.com/gillonj/burkeandhare/ (accessed February 1, 2006).

Gladwell, Malcolm. "Many Maryland AIDS Patients Not Getting Helpful Drug AZT." *Washington Post,* May 16, 1991, p. A21.

Goldstein, Amy. "Infant Death Study Halts Amid Feuding; NIH Cancels $58 Million Project with GU [Georgetown University] Focusing on D.C. Babies." *Washington Post,* February 2, 1996, p. 1A.

Goodman, Walter. "Doctors Must Experiment on Humans, but What Are the Patient's Rights? Experiments on Humans (Cont.)" *New York Times,* July 2, 1967, p. 125.

Gordon, Neve. "Rape Used as Control in U.S. Prisons." *National Catholic Reporter,* September 14, 2001.

Gurganus, A. "P. T. Barnum and My Great-Great-Granddad's Slaves." *Harper's*, June 2, 2000.

Hartnack, Michael. "Court Jails Anaesthetist." *Business Day* (Harare, Zimbabwe), March 12, 1999, p. 17.

"How the Business Is Managed at Indianapolis: Twelve 'Resurrectionists' Engaged in It." *Indianapolis Herald* (January 1875). At www.hcgs.net/bodysnatch.html (accessed February 7, 2006).

Hughes, Alan. "Cures for the Privileged? Government Officials Receive Anthrax Treatment Prior to Post Office Employees (Washington Report)." *Black Enterprise*, January, 2002, p. 19.

Jelinek, Pauline. "Judge Halts Forced Anthrax Shots for Troops." Associated Press, December, 22, 2003.

Jensen, Brennen. "Blood Money." *City Paper Online* at www.citypaper.com/news/story.asp?id=2541 (March 18, 1998; accessed January 3, 2006).

Johnston, Richard J. H. "Leopold Receives Parole in 1924 'Thrill' Slaying; Vows to 'Justify Faith' in Him—Touhy Gains in Fight for Freedom." *New York Times*, February 21, 1958, p. 1A.

Jones, Solomon. "Under Their Skin: Experiments Performed on Philadelphia Inmates Decades Ago Still Pack Horrific Power." *Philadelphia Weekly*, May 15, 2002.

Kahn, Jeffrey P. "Prison Research: Does Locked Up Mean Locked Out?" September 6, 1999. At http://www.cnn.com/HEALTH/bioethics/9909/prison.research (accessed January 10, 2006).

Kamen, Al. "Hospital Allegedly Let Some Newborns Die; Quality-of-Life Criteria Challenged." *Washington Post*, May 9, 1985, p. A3.

Kealey, Terence. "Don't Blame Eugenics, Blame Politics." *The Spectator* 286, no. 9006, March 17, 2001, pp. 10–11.

Krauthammer, C. Editorial, *Washington Post*, July 30, 1989.

Lardner, George Jr. "Army Report Details Germ War Exercise in N.Y. Subway in '66." *Washington Post*, May 9, 1980.

Lardner, James. "After 4 Months, Body Found at Lab." *Washington Post*, January 5, 1978, p. 1B.

Larson, Carl A. "Ethnic Weapons." *Military Review* 50, no. 11 (November, 1970).

Laurence, William L.. "New Drugs to Combat Malaria Are Tested in Prisons for Army." *New York Times*, March 5, 1945, p. 1A.

Lowinger, Paul. "The Detroit Case: Psychosurgery." *The New Republic*, April 13, 1974.

"Malaria Remedy Tested in Prison," *New York Times*, July 23, 1944. p. 36.

McGreal, Chris. "Whiter than White: This Man Is Charged with Murdering 46 Black People by Using Them as Guinea Pigs for South Africa's Secret Chemical and Biological Warfare Project." *The Guardian* (London), April 11, 2002, p. 6.

Muck, Patti. "Apartheid Killings Recounted; Ex-Officer Says He Dumped Corpses of Prisoners into the Sea." *Houston Chronicle*, April 23, 1993, p. 31.

Muwakkil, Salim. "Biowar and the Apartheid Legacy." *In These Times*, June 6, 2003. At www.alternet.org/story/16095/ (accessed January 2, 2006).

"New Guidelines for Inmate Medical Studies." *New York Times*, October 16, 1999, p. A9.

Newman, Richard J. "A Five-Month U.S. News Investigation Shows That Transfusions Are Riskier than Patients Are Led to Believe." *U.S. News & World Report*, June 27, 1994.

"Orphanage Babies 'Used as Guinea Pigs.' " SAPA (South African Press Association)–AFP (Australian Free Press, Melbourne), November 6, 1997.

"Ota Benga Now a Real Colored Gentleman; Little African Pygmy Being Taught Ways of Civilization at Howard Colored Orphan Asylum." *New York Daily Globe,* September 19, 1906.

"Pigmy Chased by Crowd." *New York Times,* September 22, 1906.

"Plague Wars: A Report on Biological Weapons Threats and How the Soviet Union Secretly Amassed an Arsenal of Bio-Weapons." WGBH/*Frontline,* PBS Online; at www.pbs.org/wgbh/pages/frontline/shows/plague/sa/ (accessed February 6, 2005).

"Prison Official in Illinois Halts Malaria Research with Inmates." *New York Times,* April 28, 1974, p. 50.

"Prisons Boss in the Soup for Saying Blacks Die More Easily." *Independent Newspapers* (London), n.d. [c. 1998].

"Reports New Drug to Fight Malaria." *New York Times,* November 18, 1947.

Rusk, M.D., Howard A. "Prisoners and Medicine." *New York Times,* August 3, 1969, p. 67.

———. "Tests Among Volunteers Demonstrate Need for Penology Research, Too." *New York Times,* n.d. [c. 1962].

———. "Drugs and Prisoners; Tests Among Volunteers Demonstrate Need for Penology Research, Too; Volunteers Won Release Aid to Self-Esteem; 50 Prisoners Used Indeterminate Sentences." *New York Times,* November 11, 1962, p. 74.

"SA Troops Used as Guinea Pigs: Basson." SAPA (South African Press Association), September 7, 2001.

Sarlat, Rick. "Dollars Lured Former Prisoners into Labs: Stories Detail Abuses by Researchers." *Philadelphia Tribune,* October 10, 1998, p. 1A.

———. "Prison Experiments Leave Legacy of Pain." *Philadelphia Tribune,* October 10, 1998, p. 1A.

Schoofs, Mark. "Half-Truths and Consequences: Did Doctors Mislead the Parents of Kids They Experimented On?" April 29, 1998.

"The Science of Apartheid." *Harper's,* September, 1998, p. 297.

Scott, Jeffry. "Daughter Loses Round in Suit over Mom's Body." *Atlanta Journal-Constitution,* December 2, 2003, p. 2B.

———. "Woman Sues over Display of Mom's Skeleton." *Atlanta Journal-Constitution,* March 17, 2003, p. 1A.

Servaas, Cory. "Nettie Mayersohn and Her Baby AIDS Bill." *Saturday Evening Post,* January/February 1998.

Sidley, Pat. "South Africa's Doctors Apologise for Apartheid Years." *British Medical Journal* (News) 148 (July 1995).

———. "South African Doctors Demand Action on 'Unethical' Colleagues." *British Medical Journal* (News), September 1999.

———. "South Africa to Tighten Control on Drug Trials After Five Deaths." *British Medical Journal* (News), April 15, 2000.

———. "Proceedings Start Against Former Chemical Warfare Chief (News)." *British Medical Journal* 320, no. 1426, May 27, 2000.

"South Carolina Hospital Cited for Illegal Drug Tests." *New York Times,* February 24, 1994.

Stolberg, Sheryl Gay. " 'Unchecked' Experiments on People Raise Concern." *New York Times,* May 14, 1997, p. 1A.

"Studies on Boys Given Diet Drug Criticized as Risky, Racist." Associated Press, April 18, 1998.

Sullivan, W. "Scientist Reports Isolating 2 Strains of Hepatitis." *New York Times,* June 29, 1961.

Susman, Ed. "Artificial Blood Gets OK in South Africa." United Press International; at www.AEGIS_UPI.com (April 12, 2001; accessed April 21, 2003).

Talvi, Silja J. A. "The Prison as Laboratory." *In These Times* (2002).

Trafford, Abigail. "Bitter Medicine." *Washington Post,* July 2, 1996, p. Z6.

"Tuberculosis Test Reported Success." *New York Times,* December 11, 1934.

"UDC Official Broadus N. Butler, 75, Dies." *Washington Post,* January 15, 1996. p. B4.

"U.S. Hospital Allowed to Use Artificial Blood In Crisis Situations." Baxter Healthcare's HemAssist, *Independent Newspapers* (South Africa), 1997.

Vedantam, Shankar, and Mary Pat Flaherty. "CDC Rushed Paperwork for Anthrax Vaccinations; 48 Congressional Aides Received Inoculations." *Washington Post,* December 22, 2001, p. 10A.

Venter, Zelda. "Basson Trial Gets Set for Session in U.S." *The Independent* (London), September 2, 2000, p. 14.

———. "South Africa's 'Dr. Death' Cleared of Murder by Apartheid Era Judge." *The Independent* (London), April 12, 2002, p. 14.

Washington, Harriet A. "Tracking the Risks of Birth Control." *Heart and Soul,* February 1996.

———. "Gene Blues?" *Essence,* September 2001, p. 88.

———. "Hospitals Test Medicine's Moral Responsibility." *Emerge,* July 1994.

"We Used Troops as Guinea Pigs—Basson." *Independent Online* (South Africa); at www.io1.co.za (September 7, 2001; accessed February 8, 2006).

Weiss, R. "Volunteers at Risk in Medical Studies; Complex Research Projects Strain System of Safeguards." *Washington Post,* August 1, 1998, p. 1A.

Wharton D. "Prisoners Who Volunteer Blood, Flesh, and Their Lives." *The American Mercury* 79 (1954), p. 53.

Whitaker, Joseph D. "City Told to Pay $53,000 in Case of Unidentified Body." *Washington Post,* November 22, 1979, p. B7.

Whitaker, R. "SA Planned Chemical War on Blacks." *The Independent* London, June 13, 1998.

"Wits Fires Cancer Researcher." SAPA (South African Press Association), March 10, 2000.

Young, Perry Deane. "A Surfeit of Surgery." *Washington Post,* May 30, 1976, B1.

INDEX

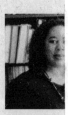

DATE DUE

		MAY 3 1 2017
OCT 1 9 2016	JAN 1 3 2022	
	FEB 14 2022	
	May 14 '22	
DEC 0 5 2016	APR 2 2 2023	
FEB 2 5 2017		
MAR 3 1 2020		
MAR 3 1 2020		
NOV 1 9 2022		
JUN 0 6 2023		

GAYLORD   #3523PI   Printe

has worke
Knight Fel
forums as
of Medicin